ANNUAL EDITIONS

Nutrition 11/12

Twenty-Third Edition

EDITOR

Amy Strickland, MS, RD
University of North Carolina–Greensboro

Amy Strickland is an Academic Professional Instructor, the Director of the Didactic Program in Dietetics, and Undergraduate Director in the Nutrition Department at the University of North Carolina at Greensboro. She currently teaches Nutrition Education, Management Practices in Dietetics, Nutrition Assessment, and Medical Nutrition Therapy. In past semesters she has taught sections of Introductory Nutrition, Advanced Clinical Dietetics, and Food Safety/Sanitation as a certified ServSafe Instructor/Proctor with the National Restaurant Association. Recent emphasis in her work at UNCG includes overseeing service learning projects in which UNCG students create and implement nutrition education programs for elementary-school-aged children, with special emphasis on educating children of low income families.

   Prior to working at UNCG, Amy worked six years as a clinical dietitian, one year as a consultant dietitian, and five years in a biomedical laboratory. She is a member of The American Dietetic Association, American Society for Nutrition, American Society for Parenteral and Enteral Nutrition, North Carolina Dietetic Association, and the Greensboro District Dietetic Association.

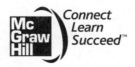

McGraw Hill — Connect Learn Succeed™

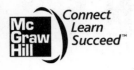

The McGraw·Hill Companies

Connect
Learn
Succeed™

ANNUAL EDITIONS: NUTRITION, TWENTY-THIRD EDITION

Published by McGraw-Hill, a business unit of The McGraw-Hill Companies, Inc., 1221 Avenue of the Americas, New York, NY 10020. Copyright © 2012 by The McGraw-Hill Companies, Inc. All rights reserved. Previous edition(s) 2011, 2010, 2009. No part of this publication may be reproduced or distributed in any form or by any means, or stored in a database or retrieval system, without the prior written consent of The McGraw-Hill Companies, Inc., including, but not limited to, in any network or other electronic storage or transmission, or broadcast for distance learning.

Some ancillaries, including electronic and print components, may not be available to customers outside the United States.

Annual Editions® is a registered trademark of The McGraw-Hill Companies, Inc.
Annual Editions is published by the **Contemporary Learning Series** group within the McGraw-Hill Higher Education division.

1 2 3 4 5 6 7 8 9 0 QDB/QDB 1 0 9 8 7 6 5 4 3 2 1

ISBN 978-0-07-351557-1
MHID 0-07-351557-4
ISSN 1055-6990 (print)
ISSN 2158-4117 (online)

Managing Editor: *Larry Loeppke*
Developmental Editor II: *Debra A. Henricks*
Senior Permissions Coordinator: *Shirley Lanners*
Marketing Specialist: *Alice Link*
Senior Project Manager: *Joyce Watters*
Design Coordinator: *Margarite Reynolds*
Buyer: *Susan K. Culbertson*
Cover Designer: *Kristine Jubeck*

Compositor: Laserwords Private Limited
Cover Images: © BananaStock/PunchStock (inset); Photodisc (background)

Editors/Academic Advisory Board

Members of the Academic Advisory Board are instrumental in the final selection of articles for each edition of ANNUAL EDITIONS. Their review of articles for content, level, and appropriateness provides critical direction to the editors and staff. We think that you will find their careful consideration well reflected in this volume.

ANNUAL EDITIONS: Nutrition 11/12
23rd Edition

EDITOR

Amy Strickland, MS, RD
University of North Carolina–Greensboro

ACADEMIC ADVISORY BOARD MEMBERS

Editors/Academic Advisory Board continued

Preface

In publishing ANNUAL EDITIONS we recognize the enormous role played by the magazines, newspapers, and journals of the public press in providing current, first-rate educational information in a broad spectrum of interest areas. Many of these articles are appropriate for students, researchers, and professionals seeking accurate, current material to help bridge the gap between principles and theories and the real world. These articles, however, become more useful for study when those of lasting value are carefully collected, organized, indexed, and reproduced in a low-cost format, which provides easy and permanent access when the material is needed. That is the role played by ANNUAL EDITIONS.

Many of the articles in *Annual Editions: Nutrition 11/12* are based on the areas of concentration identified in the recently released report for the 2010 U.S. Dietary Guidelines. The Dietary Guidelines are published every five years by the U.S. federal government to address the latest nutrition related research findings and how they apply to the health of U.S. citizens. A summary of the key health and nutrition related concerns and recommendations published in the 2010 Dietary Guidelines report is provided in the unit overview for Unit 1.

Annual Editions: Nutrition 11/12 is composed of seven units that review current knowledge and controversies in the area of nutrition. The first unit describes current trends in the field of nutrition with emphasis on areas of concentration identified in the 2010 U.S. Dietary Guidelines, such as the availability of affordable healthy foods for low-income Americans, improving nutrition literacy, and adopting aspects of the "Mediterranean diet." Nutrition trends other than those topics from the dietary guidelines are also included in this unit. Trends such as the rise in people following a gluten-free diet and changes that are occurring in businesses that have historically provided "junk foods" to the U.S. markets are also included in Unit 1.

Unit 2 includes seven articles on the function and food sources of nutrients and antioxidants. Vitamin D, sodium, fiber, and fats are all emphasized in the 2010 Dietary Guidelines report as nutrients of concern for Americans and are represented in articles in this section. The guidelines devote considerable attention to consuming omega-three fatty acids and monounsaturated fatty acids rather than the conventional omega-six, saturated, and trans fatty acids found in the typical American diet.

Units 3 through 5 include topics that focus on the relationship between nutrition and chronic diseases. Recent research findings on the role nutrients and diet play on diabetes, heart disease, hypertension, and obesity are emphasized.

Unit 6 covers food safety/technology including information on the growing incidence of bacteria and viruses in our food supply as well as what the reader can do to prevent contracting a food borne illness.

Unit 7 focuses on hunger, nutrition, and sustainability of our food and water supply. Articles on the growing amount of nitrogen added to our environment, genetically altered grain crops, the supply of fresh water, and sustainability efforts of the food industry make up this section.

Annual Editions: Nutrition is updated annually with the latest topics and controversies in the field as a way to keep students who study nutrition informed of the latest research findings, changes in policy, and trends in nutrition-related topics. Keeping up with all of the nutrition research and policy changes is a challenging task, but thanks to books like the updated versions of *Annual Editions,* you can easily review the latest nutrition information taken from reputable sources.

Annual Editions: Nutrition 11/12 is to be used as a companion to a standard nutrition text so that it may update, expand, or emphasize certain topics that are covered in the text or present totally new topics not covered in a standard text. We hope that students will develop critical thinking and be empowered to ask questions and to seek answers from credible sources.

Two new learning features have been added to this edition to aid students in their study and expand critical thinking about each article topic. Located at the beginning of each unit, *Learning Outcomes* outline the key concepts that students should focus on as they are reading the material. *Critical Thinking* questions, located at the end of each article, allow students to test their understanding of the key concepts. A *Topic Guide* assists students in finding other articles on a given subject within this edition, while a list of recommended *Internet References* guides them to the best sources of additional information on a topic.

Your input is most valuable to improve this anthology, which we update yearly. We would appreciate your comments.

Amy Strickland
Editor

Contents

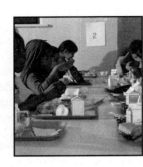

UNIT 1
Nutrition Trends

The concepts in bold italics are developed in the article. For further expansion, please refer to the Topic Guide.

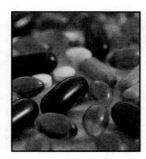

UNIT 2
Nutrients

The concepts in bold italics are developed in the article. For further expansion, please refer to the Topic Guide.

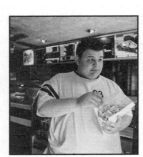

UNIT 3
Diet and Disease

The concepts in bold italics are developed in the article. For further expansion, please refer to the Topic Guide.

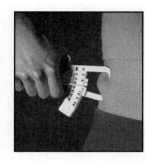

UNIT 4
Obesity and Weight Control

The concepts in bold italics are developed in the article. For further expansion, please refer to the Topic Guide.

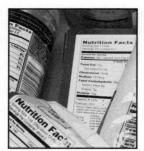

UNIT 5
Health Claims

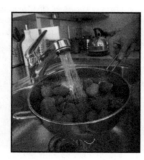

UNIT 6
Food Safety/Technology

The concepts in bold italics are developed in the article. For further expansion, please refer to the Topic Guide.

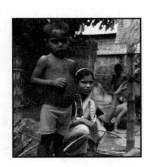

UNIT 7
Hunger, Nutrition, and Sustainability

The concepts in bold italics are developed in the article. For further expansion, please refer to the Topic Guide.

Correlation Guide

The *Annual Editions* series provides students with convenient, inexpensive access to current, carefully selected articles from the public press. **Annual Editions: Nutrition 11/12** is an easy-to-use reader that presents articles on important topics such as *nutrition trends, obesity and weight control, sustainability,* and many more. For more information on *Annual Editions* and other *McGraw-Hill Contemporary Learning Series* titles, visit www.mhhe.com/cls.

This convenient guide matches the units in **Annual Editions: Nutrition 11/12** with the corresponding chapters in two of our best-selling McGraw-Hill Nutrition textbooks by Schiff and Wardlaw/Smith.

Annual Editions: Nutrition 11/12	Nutrition for Healthy Living, 2/e by Schiff	Contemporary Nutrition: A Functional Approach, 2/e by Wardlaw/Smith	Contemporary Nutrition, 8/e by Wardlaw/Smith
Unit 1: Nutrition Trends	**Chapter 1:** The Basics of Nutrition **Chapter 2:** Evaluating Nutrition Information **Chapter 3:** Planning Nutritious Diets	**Chapter 1:** What You Eat and Why **Chapter 2:** Guidelines for Designing a Healthy Diet	**Chapter 1:** What You Eat and Why **Chapter 2:** Guidelines for Designing a Healthy Diet
Unit 2: Nutrients	**Chapter 5:** Carbohydrates **Chapter 6:** Fats and Other Lipids **Chapter 8:** Vitamins	**Chapter 4:** Carbohydrates **Chapter 5:** Lipids **Chapter 9:** Nutrients that Function as Antioxidants **Chapter 10:** Nutrients Involved in Bone Health	**Chapter 4:** Carbohydrates **Chapter 5:** Lipids **Chapter 8:** Vitamins
Unit 3: Diet and Disease	**Chapter 10:** Energy Balance and Weight Control **Chapter 13:** Nutrition for a Lifetime	**Chapter 7:** Energy Balance and Weight Maintenance **Chapter 16:** Pregnancy and Breastfeeding **Chapter 17:** Nutrition from Infancy through Adolescence **Chapter 18:** Nutrition during Adulthood	**Chapter 7:** Energy Balance and Weight Control **Chapter 15:** Nutrition from Infancy through Adolescence **Chapter 16:** Nutrition during Adulthood
Unit 4: Obesity and Weight Control	**Chapter 10:** Energy Balance and Weight Control	**Chapter 7:** Energy Balance and Weight Maintenance	**Chapter 7:** Energy Balance and Weight Control
Unit 5: Health Claims	**Chapter 8:** Vitamins **Chapter 9:** Water and Minerals	**Chapter 9:** Nutrients that Function as Antioxidants **Chapter 10:** Nutrients Involved in Bone Health	**Chapter 8:** Vitamins **Chapter 9:** Water and Minerals
Unit 6: Food Safety/Technology	**Chapter 12:** Food Safety Concerns	**Chapter 15:** Food Safety	**Chapter 13:** Safety of Food and Water
Unit 7: Hunger, Nutrition, and Sustainability	**Chapter 13:** Nutrition for a Lifetime	**Chapter 14:** Undernutrition throughout the World	**Chapter 12:** Undernutrition throughout the World

Topic Guide

This topic guide suggests how the selections in this book relate to the subjects covered in your course. You may want to use the topics listed on these pages to search the Web more easily.

On the following pages a number of websites have been gathered specifically for this book. They are arranged to reflect the units of this Annual Editions reader. You can link to these sites by going to www.mhhe.com/cls

All the articles that relate to each topic are listed below the bold-faced term.

Adolescents
2. Healthy Food Looks Serious: How Children Interpret Packaged Food Products
21. Food for Thought: Exploring the Potential of Mindful Eating
23. Underage, Overweight

Agriculture
38. Fixing the Global Nitrogen Problem
39. Perennial Grains: Food Security for the Future
40. Draining Our Future: The Growing Shortage of Freshwater

Alzheimer's disease
14. Seafood Showdown: Fatty Acids vs. Heavy Metals
18. We Will Be What We Eat
31. Brain Food

Attitudes/knowledge
3. 10 Urban Food Legends: Things Aren't Always as Simple as They Seem
4. Eat Like a Greek
14. Seafood Showdown: Fatty Acids vs. Heavy Metals
15. The Fairest Fats of Them All (and Those to Avoid)
16. Vitamins, Supplements: New Evidence Shows They Can't Compete with Mother Nature
21. Food for Thought: Exploring the Potential of Mindful Eating
24. Engaging Families in the Fight against the Overweight Epidemic among Children
27. In Your Face: How the Food Industry Drives Us to Eat

Cancer
13. Fiber Free-for-All
17. Antioxidants: Fruitful Research and Recommendations
18. We Will Be What We Eat

Carbohydrates
19. Sugar Overload: Curbing America's Sweet Tooth
20. Fructose Sweeteners May Hike Blood Pressure

Children
2. Healthy Food Looks Serious: How Children Interpret Packaged Food Products
19. Sugar Overload: Curbing America's Sweet Tooth
23. Underage, Overweight
24. Engaging Families in the Fight against the Overweight Epidemic among Children
25. Birth Weight Strongly Linked to Obesity
27. In Your Face: How the Food Industry Drives Us to Eat

Communication
29. Influencing Food Choices: Nutrition Labeling, Health Claims, and Front-of-the-Package Labeling
33. Miscommunicating Science

Controversies
1. Can Low-Income Americans Afford a Healthy Diet?
2. Healthy Food Looks Serious: How Children Interpret Packaged Food Products

6. Have a Coke and a Tax: The Economic Case against Soda Taxes
12. Keeping a Lid on Salt: Not So Easy
14. Seafood Showdown: Fatty Acids vs. Heavy Metals
20. Fructose Sweeteners May Hike Blood Pressure
27. In Your Face: How the Food Industry Drives Us to Eat

Coronary heart disease
4. Eat Like a Greek
5. Definition of the Mediterranean Diet Based on Bioactive Compounds
9. A Burger and Fries (Hold the Trans Fats)
12. Keeping a Lid on Salt: Not So Easy
14. Seafood Showdown: Fatty Acids vs. Heavy Metals
15. The Fairest Fats of Them All (and Those to Avoid)
17. Antioxidants: Fruitful Research and Recommendations
18. We Will Be What We Eat
20. Fructose Sweeteners May Hike Blood Pressure
21. Food for Thought: Exploring the Potential of Mindful Eating

Diabetes
4. Eat Like a Greek
18. We Will Be What We Eat
22. The Best Diabetes Diet for Optimal Outcomes
25. Birth Weight Strongly Linked to Obesity

Diet/disease
4. Eat Like a Greek
5. Definition of the Mediterranean Diet Based on Bioactive Compounds
11. Color Me Healthy: Eating for a Rainbow of Benefits
12. Keeping a Lid on Salt: Not So Easy
18. We Will Be What We Eat
19. Sugar Overload: Curbing America's Sweet Tooth
20. Fructose Sweeteners May Hike Blood Pressure
21. Food for Thought: Exploring the Potential of Mindful Eating
22. The Best Diabetes Diet for Optimal Outcomes
23. Underage, Overweight

Food
2. Healthy Food Looks Serious: How Children Interpret Packaged Food Products
3. 10 Urban Food Legends: Things Aren't Always as Simple as They Seem
4. Eat Like a Greek
7. Pepsi Brings in the Health Police
11. Color Me Healthy: Eating for a Rainbow of Benefits
15. The Fairest Fats of Them All (and Those to Avoid)
16. Vitamins, Supplements: New Evidence Shows They Can't Compete with Mother Nature
27. In Your Face: How the Food Industry Drives Us to Eat

Food safety/technology
14. Seafood Showdown: Fatty Acids vs. Heavy Metals
34. H_2 Uh–Oh: Do You Need to Filter Your Water?
35. Produce Safety: Back to Basics for Producers and Consumers
36. Irradiation of Fresh Fruits and Vegetables
37. Is Your Food Contaminated?
39. Perennial Grains: Food Security for the Future

Internet References

The following Internet sites have been selected to support the articles found in this reader. These sites were available at the time of publication. However, because websites often change their structure and content, the information listed may no longer be available. We invite you to visit www.mhhe.com/cls for easy access to these sites.

Annual Editions: Nutrition 11/12

General Sources

American Dietetic Association
www.eatright.org

This consumer link to nutrition and health includes resources, news, marketplace, search for a dietician, government information, and a gateway to related sites. The site includes a tip of the day and special features.

The Blonz Guide to Nutrition
www.blonz.com

The categories in this valuable site report news in the fields of nutrition, food science, foods, fitness, and health. There is also a selection of search engines and links.

CSPI: Center for Science in the Public Interest
www.cspinet.org

CSPI is a nonprofit education and advocacy organization that is committed to improving the safety and nutritional quality of our food supply. CSPI publishes the *Nutrition Action Healthletter,* which has monthly information about food.

Food Guide Pyramid
www.mypyramid.gov

Visit this website and find out your daily needs for kilocalories and for protein intake.

Institute of Food Technologists
www.ift.org

This site of the Society for Food Science and Technology is full of important information and news about every aspect of the food products that come to market.

International Food Information Council Foundation (IFIC)
www.FoodInsight.org

IFIC's purpose is to be the link between science and communications by offering the latest scientific information on food safety, nutrition, and health in a form that is understandable and useful for opinion leaders and consumers to access.

U.S. National Institutes of Health (NIH)
www.nih.gov

Consult this site for links to extensive health information and scientific resources. Comprised of 24 separate institutes, centers, and divisions, the NIH is one of eight health agencies of the Public Health Service, which, in turn, is part of the U.S. Department of Health and Human Services.

UNIT 1: Nutrition Trends

Celiac Disease Foundation
www.celiac.org

The celiac disease foundation website provides comprehensive information on celiac disease, diet and lifestyle, resources, and shopping guides.

Food Science and Human Nutrition Extension
www.fshn.uiuc.edu

This extensive Illinois State University site links to latest news and reports, consumer publications, food safety information, and many other useful nutrition-related sites.

Mediterranean Diet
www.webmd.com/diet/features/the-mediterranean-diet

Web MD reviews the popular diets of the world. This link reviews the principles and foods of the Mediterranean diet and offers medical explanation of the health benefits.

Revolution Foods
www.revfoods.com

Web Revolution Foods caters healthy breakfasts and lunches to schools in eight states, serving over 30,000 students healthy foods. Revolution foods is making strides in changing the food culture for school aged kids.

US Dietary Guidelines Report
www.cnpp.usda.gov/DGAs2010-DGACReport.htm

The 2010 Dietary Guidelines for Americans was recently released. This link is to the entire report from the USDA and HHS Advisory Committee.

UNIT 2: Nutrients

Dietary Supplement Fact Sheet: Vitamin D
http://ods.od.nih.gov/factsheets/vitamind.asp

The Office of Dietary Supplements fact sheet on vitamin D.

Food and Nutrition Information Center
www.nal.usda.gov/fnic

Use this site to find dietary and nutrition information provided by various USDA agencies and to find links to food and nutrition resources on the Internet.

NutritionalSupplements.com
www.nutritionalsupplements.com

This source provides unbiased information about nutritional supplements and prescription drugs, submitted by consumers with no vested interest in the products.

Office of Dietary Supplements: Health Information
http://ods.od.nih.gov/Health_Information/Health_Information.aspx

The Office of Dietary Supplements, a division of the National Institute of Health is the leading source on nutritional and botanical supplements. This website provides comprehensive information on the supplement industry.

U.S. National Library of Medicine
www.nlm.nih.gov

This site permits you to search databases and electronic information sources such as MEDLINE, learn about research projects, and keep up on nutrition-related news.

Internet References

UNIT 3: Diet and Disease

American Cancer Society
www.cancer.org

Open this site and its various links to learn the concerns and lifestyle advice of the American Cancer Society. It provides information on alternative therapies, tobacco, other Web resources, and more.

American Diabetes Association
www.diabetes.org

The American Diabetes Association is the primary resource for type 1, type 2, and gestational diabetes.

American Heart Association (AHA)
www.americanheart.org

The AHA offers this site to provide the most comprehensive information on heart disease and stroke as well as late-breaking news. The site presents facts on warning signs, a reference guide, and explanations of diseases and treatments.

The Center for Mindful Eating
www.tcme.org

The Center for Mindful Eating sets out to help professionals and institutions implement principles of mindful eating.

The Food Allergy and Anaphylaxis Network
www.foodallergy.org

The Food Allergy Network site, which welcomes consumers, health professionals, and reporters, includes product alerts and updates, information about food allergies, daily tips, and links to other sites.

LaLeche League International
www.lalecheleague.org

Important information to mothers who are contemplating breast feeding can be accessed at this website. Links to other sites are also possible.

National Eating Disorders Association
www.nationaleatingdisorders.org

Offers information on the different types of eating disorders, programs, events, research, resources, insurance coverage, and a support line.

UNIT 4: Obesity and Weight Control

American Society of Exercise Physiologists (ASEP)
www.asep.org

The goal of the ASEP is to promote health and physical fitness. This extensive site provides links to publications related to exercise and career opportunities in exercise physiology.

Calorie Control Council
www.caloriecontrol.org

The Calorie Control Council's website offers information on cutting calories, achieving and maintaining healthy weight, and low-calorie, reduced-fat foods and beverages.

Centers for Disease Control and Prevention: Overweight & Obesity
www.cdc.gov/obesity

The Centers for Disease Control and Prevention is a component of the Dept. of Health and Human Services. It monitors and tracks the general health of Americans, conducts research, and implements health prevention strategies.

Shape Up America!
www.shapeup.org

At the Shape Up America! website you will find the latest information about safe weight management, healthy eating, and physical fitness. Links include Support Center, Cyberkitchen, Media Center, Fitness Center, and BMI Center.

UNIT 5: Health Claims

Federal Trade Commission (FTC): Diet, Health & Fitness
www.ftc.gov/bcp/menus/consumer/health.shtm

This site of the FTC on the Web offers consumer education rules and acts that include a wide range of subjects, from buying exercise equipment to virtual health "treatments."

Food and Drug Administration (FDA)
www.fda.gov/default.htm

The FDA presents this site that addresses products they regulate, current news and hot topics, safety alerts, product approvals, reference data, and general information and directions.

National Council against Health Fraud (NCAHF)
www.ncahf.org

The NCAHF does business as the National Council for Reliable Health Information. At its Web page it offers links to other related sites, including Dr. Terry Polevoy's "Healthwatcher Net."

Office of Dietary Supplements: Health Information
http://ods.od.nih.gov/Health_Information/Health_Information.aspx

The Office of Dietary Supplements, a division of the National Institute of Health is the leading source on nutritional and botanical supplements. This website provides comprehensive information on the supplement industry

QuackWatch
www.quackwatch.com

Quackwatch Inc., a nonprofit corporation, provides this guide to examine health fraud. Data for intelligent decision making on health topics are also presented.

UNIT 6: Food Safety/Technology

American Council on Science and Health (ACSH)
www.acsh.org

The ACSH addresses issues that are related to food safety here. In addition, issues on nutrition and fitness, alcohol, diseases, environmental health, medical care, lifestyle, and tobacco may be accessed on this site.

Centers for Disease Control and Prevention (CDC)
www.cdc.gov

The CDC offers this home page, from which you can obtain information about travelers' health, data related to disease control and prevention, and general nutritional and health information, publications, and more.

FDA Center for Food Safety and Applied Nutrition
www.fda.gov/food/foodsafety/default.htm

It is possible to access everything from this website that you might want to know about food safety and what government agencies are doing to ensure it.

Internet References

Food Safety Project (FSP)
www.extension.iastate.edu/foodsafety

This site from the Cooperative Extension Service at Iowa State University has a database designed to promote food safety education via the Internet.

USDA Food Safety and Inspection Service (FSIS)
www.fsis.usda.gov

The FSIS, part of the U.S. Department of Agriculture, is the government agency "responsible for ensuring that the nation's commercial supply of meat, poultry, and egg products is safe, wholesome, and correctly labeled and packaged."

UNIT 7: World Hunger, Nutrition, and Sustainability

Food and Agriculture Organization of the United Nations (FAO)
www.fao.org/economic/ess/food-security-statistics/en

The FAO is the premier site for information on food production, consumption, deprivation, malnutrition, poverty, and food trade of countries around the globe. The FAO hunger map is a tool that is commonly used to demonstrate the areas of the world that suffer from malnutrition and food insecurity.

Population Reference Bureau
www.prb.org

A key source for global population information, this is a good place to pursue data on nutrition problems worldwide.

U.S. Sustainable Agriculture Research and Education Program, University of California-Davis
www.sarep.ucdavis.edu/concept.htm

This UC-Davis sponsored site describes the main concepts of sustainable agriculture principles and practices.

World Health Organization (WHO)
www.who.int/en

This home page of the World Health Organization will provide you with links to a wealth of statistical and analytical information about health and nutrition around the world.

UNIT 1
Nutrition Trends

Unit Selections

Learning Outcomes

After reading this unit, you should be able to

- Define the Thrifty Food Plan (TFP) and evaluate whether the TFP is an effective way to determine the lowest cost for a healthy diet in the United States.
- Explain how a nutrient-profiling tool (such as the Nutrient Rich Foods Index) could be used in conjunction with food price analysis to evaluate the cost of a healthy diet in the United States.
- Judge if marketing non-nutritious foods as fun and entertaining to kids will have long-term consequences on health.
- Describe the history of what researches have defined as the "Mediterranean diet".
- Explain why cutting 3,500 calories may not equate to the loss of one pound of body fat for everyone.
- Identify seven steps to incorporating the Mediterranean lifestyle.
- Differentiate the antioxidant and non-antioxidant bioactive compounds commonly found in the Mediterranean diet.
- Criticize the definition of dietary fiber as non-starch polysaccharides and lignin. Defend why resistant starch should be included in quantification of dietary fiber.
- Discuss the pros and cons of implementing a tax on soda. Determine whether you support or do not support the soda tax.
- Describe how PepsiCo is changing its business model to improve the nutrient density of its food and beverage items.
- Defend the requirement that chain restaurants must post nutrition information on their menus. In your response, consider the perspective of a restaurant owner, a politician, and a nutritionist.
- Explain how restaurants have eliminated trans fats from their menus.
- Explain why trans fats are considered "bad fats" as well as how you can best avoid them in your diet.
- Describe the benefits of establishing a farm-to-college program at your college/university.

Student Website

www.mhhe.com/cls

Internet References

Celiac Disease Foundation
www.celiac.org

Food Science and Human Nutrition Extension
www.fshn.uiuc.edu

Mediterranean Diet
www.webmd.com/diet/features/the-mediterranean-diet

Revolution Foods
www.revfoods.com

US Dietary Guidelines Report
www.cnpp.usda.gov/DGAs2010-DGACReport.htm

The hottest trends in nutrition policy today revolve around reducing the incidence of obesity in the United States, especially among children, ensuring that healthy foods are available to low-income populations, and holding the food industry and restaurants accountable for providing healthy foods to Americans. These trends are central themes found in the report of the 2010 Dietary Guidelines for Americans. The Dietary Guidelines for Americans are published every five years by the United States Department of Agriculture (USDA) and the Department of Health and Human Services (HHS) to address latest nutrition-related research findings and how they apply to the health of the United States. In the 2010 report, the USDA and HHS offer overall key recommendations to improve the most significant concerns plaguing the health status of Americans as well as recommendations to change the U.S.'s food environment to promote healthful lifestyle patterns.

Key recommendations identified by the USDA and HHS from review of recent research:

- Reduce the incidence and prevalence of overweight and obesity of the U.S. population by reducing calorie intake and increasing physical activity.
- Shift food patterns to a more plant-based diet and increase intake of seafood and low-fat dairy, with only moderate amounts of lean meats, poultry, and eggs (similar to the Mediterranean diet).
- Reduce the intake of foods containing added sugars and solid fats.
- Meet the 2008 Physical Activity Guidelines for Americans.

Recommendations to change the U.S. food environment to promote healthful lifestyle patterns:

- Improve nutrition literacy and cooking skills with emphasis on families with children preparing healthy foods at home.
- Increase health, nutrition, and physical education programs in U.S. schools and preschools, including food preparation, food safety, and cooking skills.
- Create financial incentives to purchase, prepare, and consume a healthy diet.
- Improve the availability of affordable fresh produce.
- Increase environmentally sustainable production of vegetables, fruits, and fiber-rich whole grains.
- Improve and expand aquaculture practices to increase the availability of seafood to all segments of the population.
- Improve the distribution of information to ensure that consumers make informed choices in seafood selection.
- Improve access to adequate amounts of foods that are nutritious and safe to eat.
- Encourage restaurants and the food industry to offer health-promoting foods that are low in sodium, added sugars, refined grains, and solid fats.

The Dietary Guidelines for Americans define the nutrition trends of the United States and influence the direction of health policies, changes in funding for food and agriculture programs, the creation of food and nutrition programs, public health education, childhood health and nutrition initiatives, school lunch

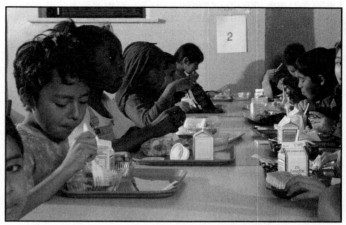

© Photodisc

programs, and to some extent, how the food industry operates. Unit 1 addresses current trends in the field of nutrition with emphasis on areas of concentration identified in the 2010 U.S. Dietary Guidelines, such as the availability of affordable healthy foods for low-income Americans, improving nutrition literacy, and adopting aspects of the "Mediterranean diet."

Considering the economic instability of the past years, more Americans are living at or below the poverty level. The changes in our economy and employment rates lead many Americans in general to spend less money on food for themselves and their families. It is possible to consume fresh and nutritious foods on a tight budget, but it is challenging in our current food culture. "Can Low-Income Americans Afford a Healthy Diet?" explains some of the challenges that low-income populations face in obtaining nutritious foods and what can be done to improve the accessibility of nutritious foods for those that struggle to feed their families.

The Mediterranean diet is widely accepted as a healthy way of eating. This acceptance by the medical community and popular press are encouraging Americans to adopt principles and foods of the Mediterranean lifestyle. "Eat Like a Greek" from *Consumer Reports on Health* leads the reader through practical steps of how to incorporate the Mediterranean lifestyle into daily life. "Definition of the Mediterranean Diet Based on Bioactive Compounds" evaluates the Mediterranean diet and suggests a new definition of the diet based on the dietary fat profile, phytochemical, and fiber content of the diet. The 2010 Dietary Guidelines report makes many references to the health benefits of the Mediterranean diet and strongly recommends Americans adopt the Mediterranean diet and lifestyle.

The most common foods known to Americans from the Mediterranean region is Italian food. However, the Mediterranean diet is not pizza, lasagna, and other cheese, meat, refined pasta dishes. None of the meals commonly served in Italian restaurants in the US are consistent with how scientists define the Mediterranean diet. The Mediterranean diet is composed of fruits, non-starchy vegetables, nuts, whole grains, legumes, and fish. The fat source in the diet is preliminary olive oil, which is a great source of the heart health monounsaturated fatty acids

(MUFA's). The history of the creation of the "Mediterranean diet" is covered in the 10 Urban Food Legends article published in the Nutrition Action Newsletter.

The problem of childhood obesity and unhealthy "kid friendly" foods marketed to kids in the United States is in the forefront of many nutrition professionals and policymakers. Think of the foods that are commonly eaten by children in the United States: chicken nuggets, fries, pizza, hamburgers, sweetened cereals, sweetened snacks, and the occasional carrot stick with ranch dressing will come to mind. "Healthy Food Looks Serious: How Children Interpret Packaged Food Products" by Charlene Elliott will show a different perspective on the marketing techniques of "fun foods" to kids. Our food environment for childhood nutrition is in the process of change, albeit slow change.

An example of trends within the food industry to provide more healthy foods can be seen in the changes that are occurring at PepsiCo. PepsiCo, the parent company of soft drinks and snack foods, is working to improve its image and ensure that it is positioned to meet the demand for healthier snack foods and beverages. Indra Nooyi, the CEO of PepsiCo, is leading the company that traditionally has provided foods laden with added sugar, salt, and fats to a company that is leading the industry on research and development of healthier versions of snack foods and beverages.

Other recent trends that encourage healthier food choices include recent action by city and state municipalities to ban trans fats in restaurants in some cities and require restaurants to post calorie and saturated fat contents of their foods either on the menu or by the register. Thankfully, the current trends are moving away from non-nutritious convenience foods to foods with higher nutrient density and quality.

The premise of eating locally grown, in-season foods, commonly referred to as the "locavore" movement, is expanding into higher education through such initiatives as farm-to-college programs. College and University students across the United States are advocating for the purchase of foods that are in season and grown by local farmers. This locavore movement can be seen in increased use of local farmers markets as well as initiatives such as farm to school programs.

Can Low-Income Americans Afford a Healthy Diet?

Many nutritional professionals believe that all Americans, regardless of income, have access to a nutritious diet of whole grains, lean meats, and fresh vegetables and fruits. In reality, food prices pose a significant barrier for many consumers who are trying to balance good nutrition with affordability. The Thrifty Food Plan, commonly cited as a model of a healthy, low-cost diet, achieves cost goals by relaxing some nutrition constraints and by disregarding the usual eating habits of the American population. Diet optimization techniques, when sensitive to cost and social norms, can help identify affordable, good-tasting, nutrient-rich foods that are part of the mainstream American diet. *Nutr Today.* 2009;44(6):246–249.

ADAM DREWNOWSKI, PHD AND PETRA EICHELSDOERFER, ND, MS, RPH

When incomes drop and family budgets shrink, food choices shift toward cheaper but more energy-dense foods. The first items dropped are usually healthier foods—high-quality proteins, whole grains, vegetables, and fruits. Low-cost, energy-rich starches, added sugars, and vegetable fats represent the cheapest way to fill hungry stomachs.[1,2]

Lower diet quality separates lower-income from the more affluent Americans.[3] Higher-income households are more likely to buy whole grains, seafood, lean meats, low-fat milk, and fresh vegetables and fruits. Lower-income households purchase more cereals, pasta, potatoes, legumes, and fatty meats. Their vegetables and fruits are often limited to iceberg lettuce, potatoes, canned corn, bananas, and frozen orange juice.

Many nutritionists insist that all Americans have equal access to healthy fresh foods; if only they made the effort.[4] In reality, energy-dense sweets and fats are tasty, cheap, readily available, and convenient. Where kitchen facilities, cooking skills, money, or time is limited or absent, they offer satisfying, but nutrient-poor, options. They also help reduce waste, spoilage, and cooking costs. Not surprisingly, they are often chosen in preference to fresh produce and other more nutrient-rich foods by lower-income groups.[5]

Nutritious Diets at Low Cost

The US Department of Agriculture food plans are cited to support arguments that healthy diets can be inexpensive.[6] The computer-generated Thrifty, Low-Cost, Moderate-Cost, and Liberal Food Plans were designed to illustrate how nutritious diets can be obtained at different income levels.

In June 2008, the lowest-cost Thrifty Food Plan (TFP) was estimated at $588.30 per month, or around $20 per day, for a reference family of 4. Cost estimations of nutritious diets are significant because the TFP cost is used to set maximal benefits available from the Supplemental Nutrition Assistance Program (SNAP, previously called "food stamps").[7]

One way that the TFP achieves its cost objectives is by using inexpensive foods. In the 1999 TFP, most of the energy came from oil, shortening and mayonnaise, white bread, sugar, potatoes, and beans. The only fresh fruit choices were low-cost oranges, apples, bananas, and grapes. Although vegetable servings technically met the guidelines, the amounts of fresh tomatoes or lettuce in the TFP were very small.

Another way that the TFP achieves its low-cost objectives is by ignoring the current eating habits of the American population. In its 2006 revision, the TFP was dramatically different from the observed patterns of consumption. The goals of the TFP could be achieved only by pushing the consumption of rarely eaten foods (eg, legumes or whole-grain pasta) to unacceptable amounts, sometimes exceeding current amounts by a factor of 20 or more. By contrast, the consumption of other food groups (eg, citrus juices and whole milk) would need to drop to zero. There is nothing in the food marketing or nutrition education literature to indicate that such massive shifts from existing eating habits are even feasible. Keeping the TFP closer to the actual eating habits of the population would, of course, entail higher costs.

Time poverty presents an additional problem. Decades ago, many American households included at least one person with sufficient time to shop for and prepare meals "from scratch."

The 2006 TFP recognized that workforce demographic shifts necessitated more convenience foods, yet after modifications, the estimated time required to purchase, prepare, and cook the TFP foods is still higher than the American norm.

In other words, low-cost nutritious diets can be created, in principle, by the TFP framework. However, such diets may be low in palatability and variety, require dramatic shifts in eating habits, and be time intensive to prepare. Working mothers can follow TFP guidelines and prepare low-cost nutritious foods or can have a paying job outside the home but may find it difficult to do both.

The benefits of SNAP are intended to provide low-income families with sufficient food purchasing power to obtain a nutritious diet. However, good nutrition does go beyond mere survival and should include taste, convenience, and variety and be consistent with societal norms. Some suggestions on how low-income families can improve their diets have lost track of these basic facts. Low-income families face a bad situation, which is worsening in the present economic climate.[8]

The "Dinner Plate of Healthy Foods"

A November 2008 article in the Economic Research Service/US Department of Agriculture publication[4] asserted that SNAP provided low-income households with ample purchasing power to afford healthy diets. A prominent photograph, composed mostly of steamed and fresh vegetables, was entitled "a dinner plate of healthy foods." The suggestion was that low-income food assistance recipients move them to the "center of their plates and budgets."

We purchased the pictured foods from a local chain supermarket in the smallest quantities necessary (see Table 1). Purchased were 3 brussels sprouts, 12 green beans, 3 olives, 1 mushroom, 1 red pepper, and 1 head of romaine lettuce, exactly as pictured by the Economic Research Service. Purchases of grated carrots, pasta, and grapes were limited by the smallest purchasable size. Produce preparation included washing, trimming, coring, slicing, boiling, and draining while the noodles were boiled. Estimated preparation time totaled 40 minutes. Reported consumption frequencies were obtained from the 1999–2002 National Health and Nutrition Examination Survey (NHANES) database. Nutrient composition analysis was performed using the Food Processor for Windows program (version 8.5.0; ESHA Research, Salem, Oregon).

The minimum purchase price for one person was $9.28. Because some foods had to be purchased in minimum quantities, the per-person cost of the pictured dinner dropped to $4.17 per person for a reference family of four. That amount exceeded 80% of that family's maximal SNAP benefits for one day, with the foods selected falling far short of a full day's total nutrient needs.

The healthy dinner weighed 458 g (1 lb) yet supplied just 335 kcal, mostly from carbohydrates. Protein content

Table 1 USDA/ERS "Dinner Plate of Healthy Food": Ingredients, Weights, Preparation Time, Prices, and Frequency of Consumption

Food	Net Purchase Weight, g	Purchase Price, $	Total Preparation Time, min	Portion Shown, g	Kcal per Portion Shown	Cost per Portion Shown, $	Total Price/4 Servings, $	Cost/100 kcal, $	Frequency of Consumption[a]
Romaine lettuce	440	1.79	4	33	6	0.13	1.79	2.39	312
Brussels sprouts	78	0.54	8	76	27	0.51	2.16	1.87	5
Green beans, whole	77	0.50	8	70	25	0.47	2.00	1.91	71
Mushroom, crimini	28	0.36	2	9	2	0.12	0.72	5.84	100
Carrots, shredded	233	1.79	1	30	12	0.23	1.79	1.87	1265
Whole-wheat thin spaghetti, boxed	371	1.50	8	132	164	0.18	1.50	0.11	2
Red pepper	200	1.50	6	48	12	0.36	3.00	2.88	69
Grapes, green seedless[b]	120	1.03	2	74	51	0.65	2.65	1.27	823
Olives	13	0.27	1	13	37	0.27	1.08	0.74	138
Total		9.28	40	485	335	2.92	16.69		

Abbreviations: ERS, Economic Research Service; NHANES, National Health and Nutrition Examination Survey; USDA, US Department of Agriculture.

[a]Reported frequency of consumption, listed in NHANES, as purchased and consumed, without added salt or fat.

[b]Grapes from Metropolitan Market, where they could be purchased in small quantities.

was inadequate (13 g), whereas percentage energy from fat was 13% (5 g). Overall energy density was 0.7 kcal/g, less than half that of the typical American diet without beverages (1.6 kcal/g). The pictured low-income "dinner" was nutritionally unbalanced and based on expensive and rarely eaten foods. Of the foods shown, only shredded carrots, grapes, and romaine lettuce were consumed with any regularity by NHANES study adults. Reported consumption of whole-wheat pasta or brussels sprouts in NHANES was close to zero.

What Are the Affordable Nutrient-Rich Foods?

More realistic dietary guidelines would do well to emphasize nutrient-rich foods that are affordable, appealing, and part of the mainstream American diet. This may require 2 novel research tools. First, nutrient profiling techniques can help calculate nutrients per calorie and nutrients per unit cost for individual foods or food groups.[9] Second, diet optimization techniques, similar to the TFP framework, but more sensitive to consumption constraints, can help translate dietary guidelines into more concrete food plans for consumers at every income level.[10]

Nutrient profiling involves systematically ranking or classifying foods on the basis of nutrient content, through calculation of key nutrient content, relative to dietary energy. Nutrient-rich foods provide relatively more nutrients than calories. For example, the Nutrient-Rich Foods index (NRF) is based on 9 nutrients that should be encouraged: protein; fiber; vitamins A, C, and E; calcium; iron; potassium; and magnesium, and on 3 nutrients that should be limited: saturated fat, added sugar, and sodium, with all amounts calculated per 100 kcal of food or per serving size.

Combining nutrient profiling with food price analyses allows researchers to directly evaluate nutrients per calorie and nutrients per unit cost, allowing "energy cost" comparisons across foods and food groups. Preliminary data already suggest that milk, yogurt, eggs, beans, potatoes, carrots, cabbage, citrus juices, and fortified cereals offer high nutrient density at low cost, as do many canned and frozen foods. Dietary guidelines ought to combine sound nutritional advice with analysis of cost.

Diet optimization models can be used to translate dietary recommendations into food plans at different levels of nutritional quality and cost. Such models should minimize the difference between the observed and the recommended diets by setting consumption limits based on the eating habits of the referent population. To prevent the food plan from including excessive amounts of any one food group, lower and upper bounds for consumption are included in the model. Food plans based on dietary guidelines can then be designed for different population subgroups. For those with good dietary habits, the recommended dietary changes may be small and achievable. On the other hand, those with poor baseline diets may find it difficult to achieve the recommended goals. The

development of dietary guidelines ought to be accompanied by a feasibility analysis.

Toward 2010 Dietary Guidelines for All Americans

Reducing food expenditures below a certain amount virtually ensures an energy-dense diet with low nutrient content. With affordable good nutrition the theme of the day, identifying affordable nutrient-rich foods becomes a matter of prime concern to dietary guidelines.

Affordable good nutrition requires reconciling nutrient density, nutrient cost, and current consumption patterns or social norms. These diverse factors must be considered to develop dietary guidelines truly applicable to all segments of American society. The current economic situation demands that the 2010 Dietary Guidelines Advisory Committee take food prices and the food choices made by real people into account.

References

1. Darmon N, Briend A, Drewnowski A. Energy-dense diets are associated with lower diet costs: a community study of French adults. *Public Health Nutr.* 2004;7:21–27.
2. Andrieu E, Darmon N, Drewnowski A. Low cost diets: more energy, fewer nutrients. *Eur J Clin Nutr.* 2006;60:434–436.
3. Drewnowski A, Specter SE. Poverty and obesity: the role of energy density and energy costs. *Am J Clin Nutr.* 2004;79:6–16.
4. Golan E, Stewart H, Kuchler F, Dong D. Can low-income Americans afford a healthy diet? *Amber Waves.* 2008;5:26–33.
5. Drewnowski A, Darmon N. The economics of obesity: dietary energy density and energy cost. *Am J Clin Nutr.* 2005;82(suppl):265S–273S.
6. Carlson A, Lino M, Juan W-Y, Hanson K, Basiotis PP. Thrifty Food Plan, 2006. US Department of Agriculture, Center for Nutrition Policy and Promotion, CNPP-19. 2007. www.cnpp.usda.gov/Publications/FoodPlans/MiscPubs/TFP2006Report.pdf. Accessed December 8, 2008.
7. Hanson K, Andrews M. Rising food prices take a bite out of food stamp benefits. US Department of Agriculture, Economic Research Service, EIB–41. December 2008. www.ers.usda.gov/Publications/EIB41/. Accessed December 23, 2008.
8. Tillotson J. Why does my food suddenly cost so much? *Nutr Today.* 2009;44:31–37.
9. Drewnowski A, Fulgoni V III. Nutrient profiling of foods: creating the nutrient rich foods index. *Nutr Rev.* 2008; 66(I):23–39.
10. Masset G, Monsivais P, Maillot M, Darmon N, Drewnowski A. Diet optimization methods can help translate dietary guidelines into a cancer prevention food plan [published online ahead of print June 17, 2009]. *J Nutr.*

Critical Thinking

1. According to the Thrifty Food Plan, what is the lowest cost required to feed a healthy diet to a family of four in the United States?
2. Explain how time poverty affects the dietary intake of lower-income U.S. households.

3. How does the Thrifty Food Plan affect U.S food assistance programs such as SNAP?

4. What is nutrient profiling?

ADAM DREWNOWSKI, PhD, is director of the Nutritional Sciences Program, the Center for Public Health Nutrition, and the University of Washington Center for Obesity Research. He is a professor of epidemiology and medicine and a joint member of the Fred Hutchinson Cancer Research Center. **PETRA EICHELSDOERFET,** ND, MS, RPh, is a postdoctoral research fellow funded through the National Centers for Complementary and Alternative Medicine. A naturopathic physician, certified nutritionist, and pharmacist, she is affiliated with the Bastyr University Research Institute. Her research interests include public health, obesity, and the gut microbiota. **ADAM DREWNOWSKI,** PhD, was supported by the US Department of Agriculture grant CSREES 2004-35215-14441 on "Poverty and Obesity: The Role of Energy Density and Cost of Diets" and by The Nutrient Rich Food Coalition. Petra Eichelsdoerfer, ND, MS, RPh, was supported by National Centers for Complementary and Alternative Medicine grant 2 T32AT000815. Corresponding author: Adam Drewnowski, PhD, University of Washington, 305 Raitt Hall, Box 353410, Seattle, WA 98195 (adamdrew@u.washington.edu).

From *Nutrition Today,* 44:6, November/December 2009, pp. 246–249. Copyright © 2009 by Lippincott, Williams & Wilkins/Wolters Kluwer Health. Reprinted by permission via Rightslink.

Healthy Food Looks Serious: How Children Interpret Packaged Food Products

CHARLENE D. ELLIOTT

"The fun starts here." Such was the promise—and the slogan—of Kraft Foods' 1999 campaign to promote its sweetened Post cereals to children. The campaign included, among other things, television and Internet advertising, coupon promotions, retail displays, redesigned packaging with greater "shelf impact," and cartoon stickers included in Post cereal boxes. Post's marketing push sought to capitalize on the 8.5% growth seen in its cereals from the previous year while the company affirmed its "commitment to innovation with its kid-targeted cereal brands" (Thompson, 1999b, p. 19).

This "commitment to innovation" in child-oriented food products was not unique to Kraft. The trend, which formally began in the 1950s with the sugar-laden cereals targeted at children (McNeal, 1992, p. 8), had significantly advanced by the 1999 campaign. Indeed, the fun *had* started by 1999, for in that year alone: Quaker Oats allocated U.S.$15 million just to market Cap'n Crunch Cereal (Thompson, 1999a, p. 8); Yoplait launched its enormously successful[1] GoGurt kids' yogurt tubes (Thompson, 2000, p. 30); Kellogg announced it was "bringing fun" into the cereal aisle by putting Sesame Street mini bean-bag toys into specially marked cereal boxes (Kellogg Company, 1999); and marketer James McNeal devoted an entire chapter of *The Kids Market* to careful instructions on how to "kidize" packaging. Specifically, McNeal (1999) explained how marketers could shift from the "A to K" (adult to kid) in package design, so as to better serve the "end user" (that is, the child) (p. 88).

The "fun start" promised by Post's campaign threads throughout contemporary children's food marketing. In 2001, Kraft Foods extended its "fun cereal" motif to the snack food category, with the U.S.$25 million launch of Lunchables Fun Snacks. "Some snacks have all the fun" was the slogan for these cookie or brownie snacks, which children could frost and decorate with sprinkles (Thompson, 2001, p. 45). Innovation, joined with theme of fun, is now standard in contemporary child-targeted foods. Kidized packaging is commonplace, and *fun* represents an entire category of food products. In today's supermarket, *fun foods* can be found in every food category. They populate the dry goods, dairy, meat, and refrigerated and frozen foods sections (Elliott, 2008b), and equally target every major meal. Such children's foods are not junk or confectionary products; instead, they are regular foods whose packaging and contents specifically and unambiguously target children.

In the supermarket, children's foods are cued by their unusual product names and unconventional flavours or colours, by their cartoon images and (child-related) merchandizing tie-ins, and by their direct reference or allusion to fun/play on the package. Fun foods rest on the key themes that food is fun and eating is entertainment—these products emphasize foods' play factor, interactivity, artificiality, and general distance from ordinary or "adult" food (Elliott, 2008a; Elliott, 2008b). Yet no data has been collected on how this U.S.$15 billion industry (Gates, 2006, p. 38)[2] is influencing children's food preferences and dietary habits, or, more specifically, how children interpret the packaged food messages that are directly targeted at them. Although the childhood obesity epidemic has prompted sustained, critical scrutiny of food marketing to children (Federal Trade Commission, 2008; Harris, Pomeranz, Lobstein, & Brownell, 2009; Hastings, Stead, McDermott, Forsyth, MacKintosh, Rayner, Godfrey, Caraher, & Angus, 2003; Hawkes, 2004; Horgan, Choate, & Brownell, 2001; IOM, 2006) the focus has been predominantly on television advertising to children.[3] Even though recent studies have expanded in scope to probe online food marketing to children, such as advergaming (Alvy & Calvert, 2008; Moore, 2006) or product placement (Moore, 2004; Auty & Lewis, 2004; Tiwsakul, Hackley, & Szmigin, 2005), the powerful communicator of *food packaging* is routinely overlooked. Indeed, it appears that the only people dealing seriously and primarily with children's food packaging are the marketers themselves.[4]

Along with the tendency to overlook children's food packaging (and the types of supermarket products targeted at children), a clear gap also exists when it comes to asking children what this kid friendly food communicates to them. This reality is underscored by a recent Canadian policy consensus conference examining "Obesity and the impact of marketing on children." Hosted by the Chronic Disease Prevention Alliance of Canada (CDPAC) in March 2008, the conference assembled leading national and international experts to present the most current sociocultural, legal, and scientific evidence on the problem of marketing and childhood obesity. The panel of assessors, in developing their consensus statement, observed that:

> Advertising is but one component of marketing. Today's marketing is much more. We were not presented with any thorough research on the many dimensions of marketing in today's world, including but not limited to: pricing . . . labelling; branding, packaging; in-store displays . . . character creation and celebrity endorsements; and many other platforms that marketing now employs. (CDPAC, 2008)

The panel further remarked, "The health of Canadian children and the reduction of childhood obesity are at the centre of this discussion. In our view, the voices of children and youth themselves are missing in this process and they must be heard" (CDPAC, 2008).

It is within this context that the current research project was designed. The goal of this study extends beyond simply observing that food is marketed to children using child-friendly appeals (Elliott, 2008b; Linn & Novosat, 2008; Page, Montgomery & Ponder, 2008; Schor & Ford, 2007). Instead, it investigates how children interpret food packaging and, heeding the panel's call at CDPAC, seeks to bring children's voices into the discussion. Specifically, this project explores:

1. how children understand and respond to child-oriented foods—both in terms of packaging and the foods themselves;
2. how this understanding and response varies by age and/or gender; and
3. how children determine and classify what is healthy (both in general, and in relation to packaged goods).

Drawing from a series of focus groups of children from grades 1 to 6, separated according to age and gender, the project aims to provide some introductory probes into an overlooked topic. The question was *not* about whether fun foods contribute to childhood obesity (which is a complex, multi-factorial problem), but rather to probe the meaning and appeal of these packaged foods to children. To this end, the article first contextualizes the research on children and marketing and then outlines the research design and methodology. The research findings, along with the concluding section titled "Making sense of fun food," suggest some of the substantial implications of this type of symbolic marketing. Fun in food absolutely matters to these children, who fully appreciate the aesthetic, gustatory, tactile, and/or interactive features that these foodstuffs offer. However, although the children reveal extensive knowledge about the packaging cues they deem relevant to them, there is a remarkably limited literacy when it comes to health or nutrition. One unintended consequence of symbolically framing kids food as fun is that healthy food is seen as plain—and drab.

Contextualizing Research on Children and Food Marketing

The childhood obesity epidemic has fueled much of the recent scholarly and policy interest in food marketing to children. With 26 percent of children being over-weight or obese, Canada has one of the highest rates of childhood obesity in the developed world (Standing Committee, 2007). This problem of childhood obesity has pulled the food industry and its marketing practices into the spotlight. Food marketing is critiqued for establishing an "obesogenic" (Swinburn, Egger, & Raza, 1999) or "toxic environment" (Brownell & Horgen, 2004)—one where food is symbolically overvalued and always available (Ulijaszek, 2007). Referring specifically to childhood obesity, Schwartz and Brownell argue that the food industry makes "relentless efforts to market their brands to children" in a food environment that "promotes over-consumption of calorie-dense, nutrient-poor foods" (Schwartz & Brownell, 2007). Their critique is warranted: the Federal Trade Commission's (July 2008) report summarizing industry expenditures on marketing food to children revealed that 44 food and beverage companies spent over $1.6 billion in 2006 advertising foodstuffs directly to youth using the "full spectrum of promotional techniques and formats" (FTC, 2008). Most of these expenditures were used to promote precisely the types of poorly nutritious products that contribute to childhood obesity, including carbonated beverages, fast foods, and sugar-laden cereals.

Obesity aside, other interesting issues pertain to the relationship between food and children's perspectives, although (as previously noted) children's voices receive significantly less airtime. Even though academic research about children's culture and consumer practices/preferences has "grown at what seems to be an exponential rate" over the past two decades (Cook, 2008b, p. 220), critical studies on children's perspectives on food—especially supermarket foods—are rare. Marketing literature, however, provides some insight. Charles Atkin provided one approach in his 1978 study conducted in the supermarket, which observed parent-child "decision-making in the selection of breakfast cereals" (1978, p. 41). His study design called for unobtrusive observations of the parent-child negotiation over cereals, where a researcher (impersonating a store clerk carrying a clipboard) recorded "a verbatim description of the sequence of parent-child exchanges on a standardized form" (Atkin, 1978, p. 42). Basically, the children's voices were recorded, even though their opinions were not asked. Marketer James McNeal (1992) attempted to assess children's perspectives through a different method, using drawing exercises. McNeal asked a sample of 1,330 children (aged 4 to 12) to draw "what comes to your mind when you think about going shopping" (p. 60). A good percentage of the children (40.2%) thought of the supermarket first and crayoned supermarket carts filled with packaged goods and some produce. More recent studies (Cooke & Wardle, 2005; Wardle, Sanderson, Gibson, & Rapoport, 2001) have used food preference questionnaires to determine what foods children like—although these studies tend to focus on single foods (e.g., apples), mixed foods (e.g., lasagna), and condiments (e.g., jam) instead of packaged foods (see Cooke & Wardle, 2005).

In short, children's thoughts on supermarket packaged foods are not the subject of academic inquiry. Even Martin Lindstrom's BRANDchild, promoted as "the world's most extensive study of tween attitudes and brand relationships" (Lindstrom, 2004, p. 311),[5] does not address branded/packaged foods (with the exception of a cursory nod to branded colas). In Canada, some insight into the topic of children's preference was provided by Health Canada's Nutrition Programs Unit, which, in 1995, published the results of a national study on children's broad perceptions of healthy eating concepts (Nutrition Programs Unit, 1995). The report documented children's views about their own eating behaviours and the factors influencing their food choices. While this study proves helpful in detailing children's observations about healthy eating in general, it is now extremely dated and provides no guidance with regard to the category of packaged foods or children's interpretation of the foods (and food labels) targeted specifically at them.

Research Design and Methods

Assessing children's perspectives on packaged foods is perfectly suited to qualitative research methodology and principles. Qualitative research methods are an excellent choice when:

1. a concept or phenomenon is immature because of a lack of previous research in the area (Kitzinger, 1995);
2. the research problem fits well with the insistence in qualitative research that interpretations include the perspectives and voices of the people being studied (Lunt & Livingstone, 1996); and
3. when the nature of the concept (because of its seminal connection to the context in which it occurs) is not well suited to quantitative measures (Lunt & Livingstone, 1996).

All of these criteria apply to a study on child-responses to fun food.

In light of this, a series of focus groups were conducted with children from grades 1 to 6. Focus group research is designed to help understand what people think and why; as such, it provides an ideal research method for exploratory work on children's responses to fun food (Deacon, Pickering, Golding, & Murdock, 1999; Heary & Hennessy, 2002; Morgan, Gibbs, Maxwell, & Britten, 2002). Using a blend of random sampling and convenience sampling, a total of 36 children were recruited for 6 separate focus groups held in Ottawa in February 2007.[6] The groups were divided so that three separate focus groups were held for girls (grades 1/2, 3/4, and 5/6), and three separate focus groups were held for boys (with the same grade segmentation). This allowed the researchers to note differences in perspective according to both gender and age. (Participants were not screened specifically for family income or ethnic background.) The study was conducted in facilities where researchers could view and listen in on the groups via a two-way mirror and closed-circuit audio in an adjacent room. Heeding recommendations regarding the optimal size and length of children's focus groups (Deacon et al., 1999; Levine & Zimmerman, 1996; Morgan et al., 2002) the research design aimed for 4-6 children per group, with each session lasting approximately 60 minutes.

The focus groups were led using a customized moderator's guide that asked participants to select from and discuss various child-oriented foods and food packages. Questions probed children's food preferences, how they categorize different types of food (i.e., what they like and what they feel is healthy), and how they make sense of nutrition information/claims on fun food packaging. Specifically, children were asked to: draw their favourite dinner, conduct mock shopping trips (where they selected from an array of packages and discussed packaging appeals), sample and discuss their preferred selections of fun foods, and explain their thoughts on nutrition and nutrition information. Responses were audio-taped and subsequently transcribed (with pseudonyms used for all participants); field notes were also recorded by the researchers during and after each session. A provisional list of codes was created from the conceptual framework and the overarching research questions outlined in the project objectives (described above), and inductive coding techniques (see Strauss & Corbin, 1998) were used to create a content analysis of particular topics. Salient themes were identified and coded following a grounded theory approach. For the purposes of this article, the goal is less to quantify the focus group findings than to provide a more nuanced exposition of children's perceptions and perspectives.

Please note that in the following discussion on the focus groups findings, for ease of readability, the term "children" refers *specifically* and solely to the children interviewed in the focus groups. As a small, exploratory study, it does not presume to speak for the preferences of all children.

What Would You Pick as Your Favourite Dinner?

At the outset of each focus group, the children were given a sheet of paper containing the image of an empty dinner plate. They were invited to draw their favourite meal and to explain why they chose the foods they did. Regardless of age or gender, children consistently drew a similar selection of foods. Pizza, fries, and "junk food" were top choices, with 84 percent of the participants selecting one (or more) of these items as constituting a favourite meal. Specific fruits and vegetables were infrequently mentioned—only 25 percent of children identified a fruit or vegetable as part of their meal. Likely this is unremarkable, since favourite meals may not contain the types of foodstuffs that children think they *ought* to eat. Yet the reasons children gave to explain *why* these foods were their favourite are worth noting. Several participants revealed that they love foods precisely because they are not "healthy" foods. In children's classification of foods, it appears junk food is enticing because it is junk (and perhaps in opposition to adult foods).

John (Grade 1) (G1): I like fries because it's junk food.

This same theme is elaborated on in the Moderator's (M) discussion with Kim (G2):

M: Can you tell us what you put on your dinner plate?
Kim (G2): Chips and treats.
M: And, why did you pick those for dinner?
Kim (G2): I like treats.
M: You like treats. What do you like the most about treats?
Kim (G2): Because they're junky.

Notions of junk were underscored by the general sense of imbalance characterizing some of the children's meals. Children were asked to draw their favourite meal, but the moderator was clear that the meal was dinner.[7] Several of the responses revealed complete indifference to balance in this meal:

M: Okay, do you want to tell us what you put for your dinner?
Shannon (G1): Pizza . . . and chicken nuggets. And, I was going to put fries. And, a spring roll.
James (G1): Donuts, fries, and chocolate. . . . I like the donut because it tastes like chocolate, and the fries are so good.
Olivia (G3): I made a pizza with a chocolate crust, caramel as a sauce, and then . . . no, wait. With chocolate sauce and caramel for the cheese.

Yet, as previously noted, the majority of children identified some variant of the "pizza/fries and something sweet/junky" (often ice cream) combination. Branded foods were notably absent from this dinnertime discussion, with the exception of four mentions (Coke [twice], Caramilk chocolate, and Rice Krispies Squares). Children in this study clearly did not associate their favourite meals with either branded food or fast foods.

Selecting from Child-Oriented Packaged Foods

At this point in the focus group, participants were asked to go on pretend shopping trips and to select the package they found most appealing. Two shopping stations were set up, displaying various fun and regular food packages of products in the same food category. To ensure participants were not influenced by the selections of others in the group, children went to each station one-by-one with a clipboard and recorded their choices in secret. They then returned to the table and explained the reasons for their selections.

Shopping Station 1 contained the same options for all of the focus groups, three boxes of chicken nuggets: a box of President's Choice® (PC) Mini Chefs™ Jungle Buddies™ breaded chicken nuggets, a box of Janes Kids© Disney© Pixar Buzz Lightyear "fun-shaped breaded" chicken nuggets, and a box of President's Choice® breaded chicken nuggets.

Shopping Station 2 contained a selection of either six children's breakfast cereals or nine fruit snacks. Breakfast cereal or fruit snack packages were rotated between groups, so as to provide a broader scope of perspectives.

It was in this pretend shopping that differences in perspectives according to age started to emerge. The youngest children (G1/2) unanimously selected the fun shaped nuggets—either PC® Mini Chefs Jungle Buddies™ or Janes Kids© Disney© Pixar Buzz Lightyear. Their focus was on the shape of the nuggets (50 percent of participants noted this) and the merchandizing tie-in with Buzz Lightyear (33%). Some children (17%) observed that the fun nuggets looked like they would taste better. The older children (G3/4 and G5/6) were less likely to indicate that they selected a package because of its fun shapes (11 percent and 13 percent, respectively), and none of them mentioned the merchandizing tie-in as a reason for their choice. For grades 3/4, all of the boys and half of the girls selected the regular chicken nuggets as their top choice—which was also the choice for all of the girls and 4 out of 6 boys in grades 5/6. The reasons provided were considerably more focused on the aesthetics of the package and/or a focus on taste: almost 56 percent of grade 3/4 participants and 67 percent of grade 5/6 participants made some direct reference to package aesthetics or the product "looking tastier" as the reason for their selection. The girls were more attuned to the package attractiveness, colour, and overall design:

Kristen (G5): I picked number 3 [the regular nuggets] because it looks pretty and, I don't know, I just like it.
M: You find the food looks pretty?
Kristen (G5): The whole box looks pretty.
Susan (G5): I liked number 3 as well; I think it looks a bit more perfect to me. It also just, looking at the way it is displayed, it looks more appetizing. The other ones just don't look as good tasting.

Kristen (G5): I also notice that it looks like it is from a restaurant because it's in a small basket with the cloth and the little vegetables in the background. That makes it look prettier.

At first blush, it appears that these children's preferences matured from a focus on fun and shapes (G1/2) to an appreciation of aesthetics and taste (G3/4 & 5/6). However, the older children's responses were deeply informed by a concern about how their selections might appear to the rest of their peer group. When it came to the chicken nuggets, the older children were resistant to selecting packages that were "too young for them."

Carly (G5): I like number 3 because I look at number 1 [Jungle Buddies] and I saw it was in animal shapes and I had that when I was four. And with the little persons [Buzz Lightyear package], I thought it looked like for little kids . . .
Hailey (G6): I had the same one as Carly. I think it is maybe because sometimes, depending on what age you are, you don't necessarily like certain shapes that maybe younger kids would like. . . . If you were to have younger kids in the group, they would have probably gone for those [the other selections].
Susan (G5): [PC nuggets] It's just more appropriate for me.

Again, this appeared to be driven solely by the children's desire to be perceived by their peers as mature. When they were asked which product they thought *their friends* might like, half of the older children selected the fun shaped nuggets instead of the plain ones, and provided rather enthusiastic explanations as to why.[8]

Children's Cereals and Fruit Snacks

Shopping Station 2 provided a greater array of packaged products, yet the children's selections (and their explanations) generally mirrored the trends observed in their first shopping venture. Grade 1/2 children were more likely to cite cross-merchandizing as a reason for choosing a product (although it was not a dominant reason), whereas older children were more likely—far more likely—to specifically comment on the packaging or package aesthetics. None of the children in grades 1 to 4 referred to packaging to explain why they selected particular cereals or fruit snacks, whereas 50 percent of the girls and 43 percent of the boys in grades 5/6 made mention of it.

Mavis (G5): [Explaining why she liked one package over the other choices] It's yeah, the colour. It makes it stand out. I think if you go to a store and you were to walk by, you wouldn't see C since the colours, well they don't pop out to you as much as the other ones do. If you have a better package for it, then someone may look at it more than people usually would.
Kristen (G5): I agree. If you had like highlighters, you would say "oh it's highlighters" . . . your eyes are attracted to it. And with the colours, why I chose B is because of the colours . . . the green and the yellow, and that's why . . .

Aesthetic reasons were also provided for why a product was not chosen:

Simon (G5): I hate the box, the box is ugly. . . . The other ones probably taste better and have a little bit more flavour.

Daniel (G5): It doesn't really stand out as much, and it [the cereal] is small, and people don't want to pick small things. It's not that interesting because there's just this bowl standing still with a bunch of cereal.

Daniel's comment reveals the degree to which fun matters to children, irrespective of the older children's desire to distance themselves from little kids' food. In fact, concerns over selecting packages that were too young were largely absent in the children's discussion of cereals and fruit snacks. It is important to emphasize that older children do *not* associate fun with little kids. (They have no problem with the concept of fun!) Moreover, all of the children showed considerable interest in the unique product claims or play aspects the packages trumpeted, as well as their surface appearance.

Shawn (G3): [Discussing Betty Crocker Tongue Talk Tattoo fruit snacks] You can get a tattoo from it and you can roll it up into a ball and suck on it. I like to put it around my finger.

James (G1): [Discussing Sun-Ripe Squiggles fruit snacks] It's junk food and I love it. It's very long and they squiggle like a worm.

Lindsay (G2): The Polly Pockets [fruit snacks] look fun because they have sparkles and everything.

Tyler (G2): [Discussing General Mills Chocolate Lucky Charms] The marshmallows are magical and each one has a power. And I like the colours on the box.

Simon (G5): [Discussing Chocolate Lucky Charms] It looks delicious.

M: What makes it look tastier than the other ones?

Simon (G5): Because of the rainbow things. And, it's in a pot of gold.

Jake (G6): It looks kinda cool. The box looks cool with streaks of colour coming out.

The Appeal of Fun Foods

Interest in surface appearance and play extended, not surprisingly, to the foods themselves. Children were asked to select their top choice from a tray containing samples of nine child-oriented cereals or fruit snacks. Selections were rotated in each session so that the children who examined cereal packages during their shopping trip sampled fruit snacks, and vice versa. (Children were able to taste/eat the snacks they selected.) Then all of the children had the opportunity to choose from an array of child-oriented yogurts or pudding snacks (and taste their choice). No packages or identifying material accompanied the samples; children selected them based on the look of the foodstuff alone. (An exception is the yogurts/puddings, which were individually packaged in tubes or cups.)

Again, the theme of play factored strongly; children were intrigued by the foods' unusual colours and shapes and often indicated that they selected a sample because of these unique characteristics. The more unusual the colour or unique the feature, the better. Ryan (G5) selected pudding because "the [blue] colour stood out, and it looked good"; Jake (G6) picked pink pudding for the same reason ("the pink stood out"). Some participants were drawn to Yogo's fruit snacks because of their "neat" multi-colours, but also because "you can throw them up in the air" (Kim, G2) or because "they look like you can roll them" (Brendan, G2). In short,

a general feeling expressed in all the focus groups is that fun or play remains an important variable.

Interactivity versus Aesthetics

Differences in gender emerged in the discussion of why certain products were chosen over others. Interest in a food's interactivity was substantially more pronounced for boys, whereas girls (particularly the older ones [G5/6]) generally focused on the aesthetic qualities of food. In the case of the yogurt/pudding samples, all children were invited to select from nine products. This included yogurt in brightly coloured portable tubes (Babang and Kaboum flavours), as well as Squeeze N Go pudding (also in a tube). A number of portable pudding snacks (in clear plastic) were offered, including bubblegum and cotton candy flavours (coloured bright pink and robin blue, respectively), Chocolate Splat! pudding (brown), and layered parfait-style puddings (one chocolate and vanilla, and the other, Oreo cookie layered puddings). Gendered differences to these options were remarkable. All of the boys (except two) chose the yogurt or pudding *tubes*— packages that allowed kids to squirt its contents into their mouths (often holding the tubes far up in the air with head tilted back to catch it), or squeeze the product onto their lips, or suck it up all in at once, as if through as straw. Although the boys did not usually articulate that the tube motivated their choice, they were absolutely drawn to this form of packaging.[9]

In contrast, all of the girls selected the parfait-style puddings. Unlike Eric's (G4) observation that "when things look fancier, they taste worse," the girls appreciated the "pretty" components of the product, and the fact that (unlike the squirtable tubes) they could be savoured:

Gwen (G4): [Discussing the chocolate/vanilla parfait pudding] I can enjoy it more and I can save it for later, but with the tubes, it finishes very fast.

Isabella (G6): I thought it was a pretty package.

M: So, you like the colour? Why did you pick it over the tube things?

Isabella (G6): I like the stripes.

Mavis (G5): I thought it was interesting how it had stripes. . . . . It looked the most appetizing.

The girls also were more likely to discuss the associational values evoked by the food/package, noting it reminded them of something (be it a movie, family outing, feeling, et cetera). This did not happen with the boys, who provided more concrete explanations or focused on what they could do with the product (i.e., squeeze it, stretch it, twist it, play with it).

Vivienne (G1): [Discussing Oreo striped parfait pudding] I picked it because me and my friend went to a farm of cows, and it reminded me of the cow. Sometimes they are black and white.

Kristen (G5): [Discussing Jungle Buddies chicken nuggets] It looks funner because I like animals. And because, well actually, for the other box [of Buzz Lightyear shaped nuggets] in class we are doing space and it makes me think of homework.

Melissa (G2): [Discussing Froot Loops cereal] At school we made a necklace with Froot Loops, and at the end we got to eat it.

Classifying Healthy: In General, and for Packaged Foods

Classifying healthy is another important question when it comes to probing children's interpretations of packaged food—and food in general. Cereals, fruit snacks, yogurts, cheeses, canned pasta, frozen meals, packaged lunches—all offer fun food for sale. Yet no published research assesses how children classify what is healthy and not healthy in this vast array of consumables. Given this, the focus groups also probed what children consider to be healthy food and how they make sense of the healthfulness of packaged goods.

Without question, Canadians are concerned about food's health qualities. The latest *Tracking Nutrition Trends* surveyed over 2,000 Canadians (18 years and older) and reported that 91% of those polled deemed a food's "healthfulness" either "somewhat important" or "very important" when choosing what to eat (CCFN, 2008, p. 3). But healthfulness is a nebulous concept, both for adults (see CCFN, 2008, p. 2) and for children. Indeed, the children in this study showed a limited understanding of the health qualities of food. When asked to name a healthy food and explain why it was healthy, 67% of the children named a fruit or a vegetable, 17% named bread or pasta, and 7% named yogurt or cheese. Fifteen percent of children said "they didn't know"—comments made more interesting given that the focus group setting allows children to echo another child's response, should they desire.[10]

With 67% of participants naming a fruit or vegetable as a healthy food, it perhaps seems odd to argue that they have limited understanding of the health qualities of food. Yet this logic becomes clear when one considers the range of foods identified: specific fruits and vegetables were mentioned, but dairy, whole grains, lean meats, and fish were rarely given as examples of healthy foods. Consider, too, children's explanations of *why* the food is healthy.

Stuart (G3): Carrots, because it's a vegetable.
Melissa (G2): Apples. . . because, fruits are good for you.
Ryan (G5): I would say fruits and vegetables, because everybody says they're healthier for you.
Mavis (G5): Broccoli. It's a green vegetable, and I heard they are healthy.
Simon (G5): Pasta, because it's good for you . . . I think.

While a number of children (starting from grades 3 up) observed that fruits or vegetables are healthy because they have "vitamins" (and two children identified calcium as the reason cheese/yogurt is healthy), 70% of the children either did not know why the item they selected was healthy or provided a self-evident answer (i.e., oranges because they're fruit). This lack of knowledge over healthy extended to children's evaluation of packages and nutritional claims as well.

"The Box Looks Serious": Children Discuss How to Tell If a Packaged Product Is Good for You

When asked what they looked for on packaging to help them determine whether the food is healthy or not, children pointed to a number of important clues. They mentioned the ingredient list (22%) or the presence of a "smart check" or symbol (17%). Some children conflated the absence of (allergy-inducing) ingredients with product healthfulness, with 14% saying that "a peanut with a circle and a line" on a package is a clue that a food is healthy.

Zack (G5): One of the rules that I always was taught is if there's big words, like really big words that you can't pronounce, it's probably another way to say sugar.

Awareness of the nutrition facts table was remarkably low: only 8% of children (all from grades 5/6) named the nutrition facts table as means of evaluating whether a product is "good for you." While this suggestion was well received by the other participants in the grades 5/6 focus group (some nodded agreement or verbally called out in affirmation), the children could not actually explain what the nutrition facts table "meant." They simply knew to look for it on packages, because they had learned it at school (and for some, at home).

This said, children provided remarkably sophisticated—although not necessarily accurate—explanations about how to tell if a packaged food is healthy. Some of the answers (from 16% of the children, mostly grades 1/2) were completely wrong headed:

Christine (G1): You can tell [it's healthy] by the front cover. If [the food] is shaped, then it may have been cut with a dirty knife.

Yet most of the statements demonstrated a savvy reasoning, even if the answers were incorrect. Kim (G6) used calories as the sole indicator of health ("it has only 130 calories per serving, which makes it really healthy"), whereas 20% of the children relied on some aspect of the package *image* to determine healthy:

Katie (G3): If the box looks serious [it's a healthy food].
Christine (G1): Green means it's healthy.
Brendan (G2): When there is green on the box, it means it's healthy.
Joshua (G3): [Explaining why Honeycomb cereal was a healthy choice] It has honey on the box.

Several children suggested that they can simply tell by looking.

Susan (G5): Usually I know what's healthy; even if you look at the picture you can tell.
Travis (G3): [The box] *looks* really good and healthy.

This reliance on the visual assessments and associational indicators of health also played out in the children's selection of foods. If a serious package or its colour could indicate healthfulness for some children, then so could look of the foodstuff itself. Jake (G6) picked the Kellogg's Fruit Winders fruit snack to eat because, even though he thought the Froot Loops fruit snack "probably tasted better," the Fruit Winders "*looked better for you.*"[11] Zack (G5) explained that Honeycomb cereal was healthy because it was brown. The flipside also held true. Gwen (G4) explained that Lucky Charms cereal probably was *not* healthy "because they have covered the marshmallows in food colouring."

"It Says Fat Free, So You Won't Get Fat": Children's Understanding of Nutrition Claims

Front-of-package labelling has become ubiquitous in recent years, as food manufacturers strive to position their products to capitalize on consumers' interest in health. Canada's decade-old Health Check program (governed by the Heart and Stroke Foundation) exists to "help consumers make healthy food choices within food categories, at the point of purchase, across all eligible food categories" (Heart and Stroke Foundation, 2008, pp. 3–4). Numerous other front-of-pack "nutrition symbols" or food rating systems also exist, since food manufacturers have each created their own logos, slogans, or symbols—as well as their own criteria—as a strategy to communicate a food's healthfulness to consumers.

While certain scholars have criticized the validity of nutrition claims in general (see Elliott, 2008a; Nestle, 2002; Pollan, 2008; Smith, Stephen, Dombrow, & MacQuarrie, 2002), they are also promoted as a strategy for improving people's diets. Even the Standing Committee on Health, which issued the *Healthy Weights for Healthy Kids* report in 2007, suggests that "Increas[ing] Awareness Through Front of Package Labelling" can help to promote healthy weights in children (Standing Committee on Health, 2007, p. 22) and is something that "must be done" to "tackle the issue of childhood obesity" (p. 18).

But this imperative seems wrong-headed, since children in this study revealed little understanding of the meaning of nutrition claims. First, (as earlier noted) they rarely referred to nutrition symbols in explaining the *clues* to use in evaluating whether a packaged food was healthy (17%). When directly asked about particular symbols found on the packaged foods being examined, children were rarely able to demonstrate a comprehension of what it *means* for food to be fat free, organic, or made with whole grains, etc. Children would literally read the claim ("it says fat free") and then come up with their own, reasonable, explanations. Discussing a round, orange symbol that proclaimed *FAT FREE,* participants observed:

Matthew (G1): It says fat free so you won't get fat.

Abigail (G3): You won't get any fatter if you're already very fat.

Geoff (G4): It means you won't get fat.

Regarding a green *CERTIFIED ORGANIC* logo:

Zack (G5): I've not seen it before, but I can tell that it is a sponsor saying that something about this is true. Like for that it means it is good quality food. That company probably has taste testers.

Daniel (G5): I'm not 100% sure what it is. But it says certified organic. So that means organic food and it was tested and looked at to make sure that it actually is organic and it's not just flavours that make it look organic or taste organic.

Kristen (G5): The label is green so it's not mass produced in some greenhouse.

There was also the tendency to assume the symbols cued other diet or health-related qualities. Jake (G6) interpreted the *FAT FREE*

symbol to mean "low in calories, [so] it's good for you." Vivienne (G1), and many others, equated the symbol with healthy ("it means it is really healthy"). Judging from the discussion in these focus groups, it appears that front-of-package labelling is of little help to children in accurately assessing the health of a product. Most of the children did not notice the claims on their own. It is worth noting, however, that some of the older female participants (G5/6) engaged in a lengthy, critical discussion over the use of several nutrition claims on the front of a particular box of sugared cereal. They dismissed the claims as lacking in credibility.

Susan (G5): No one's going to believe it.

Hailey (G6): I don't believe it since chocolate is unhealthy and marshmallows are unhealthy. The only thing healthy is the milk. It's just to get you to buy it.

Yet this was the *only* group to discuss the credibility of package claims. Remarkably, no such skepticism was voiced regarding any of the other semiotic elements on the package.

Making Sense of Fun Food: Discussion and Implications

Although a small-scale study, these focus groups provide fascinating insight into how children make sense of fun food and its packaging. As the sales figures attest, parents and care-givers are certainly purchasing these supermarket products for their children. Children, in turn, show deep appreciation for the aesthetic, gusta-tory, tactile and/or interactive features that these foodstuffs offer. The focus groups consistently revealed how passionate children can be about food; they spoke enthusiastically and extensively about their favourite edibles and about why they selected particular packages. "Loving" food was articulated repeatedly (e.g., "I *love* chocolate," "I *love* the cheese [on pizza]," "It's junk food, and I *love* it," "They're yummy, and I'm in *love* with them").

These children were equally interested in taste, primarily explaining their selections in light of personal taste preferences (i.e., appreciation for chocolate, marshmallows, sweetness, sourness). The food package's *look* factored strongly in the children's comments about taste, and they were very clear about what *looked* tastier. This said, a discernable evolution was present in terms of the appreciation of the aesthetic qualities of packaging. While younger children were more likely to be attracted to cross-merchandizing techniques (i.e., Buzz Lightyear, Spiderman, or Polly Pocket) and fun shapes, older children contemplated the overall look of the package—its colours, design, and their appreciation (or not!) of its images. The oldest girls in particular demonstrated a fairly sophisticated aesthetic sense, commenting on whether products looked tasty and selecting items based on overall display—be it the "pretty" package or "appetizing" nature of the parfait puddings "with the stripes."

Although a clear progression existed with regard to aesthetic appreciation, this study did not reveal any discernable evolution in terms of actual taste. Children, regardless of age, showed, and said, that they *loved* chocolate, junk food, and sugary cereals/ fruit snacks/puddings. They did not grow out of chocolate Lucky Charms cereal by Grade 6, for example—virtually every child in the study (92%) selected it as their top choice.

Of course, the central interest in this study pivoted on children's interpretation of and responses to fun food—and the focus groups revealed that fun *absolutely* matters to children. Food holds a special position in children's lives, and not for nutritive reasons. As Newton (1992) argues in her discussion of popular culture foodways:

> Playing with food—by learning the 'rules' for eating Oreo cookies or spaghetti or Jell-O—quickly becomes part of a child's repertoire of play behaviour. Although this food play is not approved of in most households, often adults and children have a tacit understanding about Jell-O: Jell-O for dessert is license to play. (p. 253)

Yet as the proliferation of fun food underscores, no longer is a "license to play" reserved for Oreos or Jell-O. Scholars such as Buckingham (2000), Seiter (1993), and others have long emphasized that cultural constructions of childhood are defined in opposition to adulthood. This opposition also unfolds with regard to food, and is reinforced by child-oriented food marketing. As Schor and Ford (2007) observe, the symbolic marketing characterizing children's food persuades children "to eat particular foods, not on the basis of their tastiness, or other benefits, but because of their place in a social matrix of meaning" (p. 16). This "place," I suggest, resides squarely within the theme of fun. Food marketers design and offer up fun food for consumption, and in many ways children are merely acting out the scripts provided for them. But these scripts clearly resonate with children.

Researchers probing the relationship between food advertising and childhood obesity affirm that "today, children opt for their own preferred food and drink rather than acquiescing to parental preferences" (Eagle, Bulmer, de Bruin, & Kitchen, 2004, p. 52), and the focus group participants patently demonstrated that these foods were of utmost appeal. Boys were particularly drawn to the interactivity (and transgressive eating practices) promised by the food products; they also liked foods because of their strange colours and "cool" shapes. Girls were more likely to choose products because of their pretty colours and general aesthetic appeal. The fun resided in the colours, "in the sparkles" and the associational elements the food presented—be it a memory, a personal experience with family/friends/at school, or a link to a movie. As a whole, the children were highly attuned to the range of cues that made food fun, quickly identifying the Polly Pocket or SpongeBob Squarepants fruit snacks, the "gushing" quality of Betty Crocker's Fruit Gushers, or the fun tattoo feature of Betty Crocker's Tongue Talk Tattoo Fruit Roll-Ups. Many could (and would spontaneously) identify the special "power" represented by each marshmallow in Lucky Charms. These responses reveal the degree to which young children are embedded in a world of commercial marketing/media—but the children's interest in the packages and products themselves (e.g., colours, interactivity, aesthetics, et cetera) did not stem solely from cross-merchandising or advertising appeals.

While the children discussed the fun aspects of food at length, their understanding of health was quite limited. Their ideal meals certainly did not reflect Canada's Food Guide recommendations, and their discussion of healthy foods often comprised self-evident claims. But it is their evaluation of *how to determine if a packaged food is healthy* that is the most remarkable because, while the nutrition facts table or ingredient list was given a cursory nod, children favoured their own interpretive accounts. These accounts equally tended to conflate certain markers with "healthy"

(e.g., green = healthy, serious = healthy). Policy recommendations for more front-of-pack labelling (such as those suggested by the Standing Committee on Health, 2007) may influence adult food selections, but such labels certainly did not lead to more informed food choices with the children interviewed in these focus groups. Indeed, children's misunderstanding of nutrition (communicated through symbols/logos) also played out in their discussions of why they might pick certain products over another. For instance, Honeycomb cereal was identified as a healthier choice by several participants because of the honey pictured on the box or because it was coloured brown. Alpha Bits cereal was preferred by one participant *because,* she argued, "I don't really like sugared cereals." These kinds of responses underscore the opportunity for further education for children when it comes to determining healthy foods. As already mentioned, the children were highly literate when it came to deciphering packages—just not in the right arenas.

In fairness, the food industry has complicated the issue by putting front-of-pack nutrition claims on products that children do *not* identify as "good for you." So-called "goodness corners" on boxes of sugary, marshmallow-laden cereals are a case in point, and some older children rightfully observed that the presence of these claims worked to undermine the credibility of the product as a whole. But the bigger issue is that children do not associate fun—or fun food—with nutrition. The more fun the package and product appears to be, the less children correlate it with health or classify it as a healthy selection. This raises some interesting challenges for food manufacturers who have developed "fun *and* healthy" product lines for children, but use the exact same techniques (such as cartoon images, unusual shapes, fun product names, wild colours, et cetera) to cue children's food to children and their parents. To reiterate one of the more interesting claims made in the focus groups, some of the children observed that they could tell if a product was healthy simply by seeing whether the package looked serious or not. Serious packages, for children, are healthy food packages. Fun packages, regardless of the presence of nutrition claims, are not evaluated under the lens of health.

But the biggest issue underpinning this fun food marketing is the question of meaning. What are the implications of promising (as did Post's cereal campaign) that "the fun starts here"? There is certainly something problematic about positioning food mainly as fun. Eating for entertainment (or distraction) is one of the main drivers of the current obesity epidemic, and it leads to a distorted relationship with food. (Like food marketing in general, fun food marketing also does not address any notion of portion control.) The fact that children are being taught, through fun food messages, to value food strictly for its play factor is troubling; children learn taste preferences very early on, and they persist over time. When we teach children that "the fun starts" when they sit down in front of processed and pointedly artificial food—comprised of strange shapes, bizarre colours, or magical qualities—we are leading them down a dangerous path. Healthy food, as one child observed, *does* look serious, and (especially in light of the childhood obesity epidemic) it is critical that *serious* food be given prominence in the social matrix of meaning that defines children's fare.

Notes

1. Described as "kid-targeted slurpable yogurt in a tube," Yoplait's Go-Gurt captured $100 million in retail sales within eight months of its launch, "bolstering General Mills to No. 1 in

refrigerated yogurt ahead of Dannon Co." and "trigger[ing] a new growth phase for the category as a whole" (Thompson, 2000, p. 30).

2. Data are not available on the overall sales of fun foods in Canadian supermarkets. However, the sales of food individual brand lines are equally striking. Fun yogurts targeted at children—such as Yoplait's Go-Gurt and Dannon's D'animals line—had sales of U.S.$99.9 million and $94 million, respectively, for the 52-week period ending in March 2007 (Cultured products shine, 2007, p. 16). In Canada, the Toronto-based NDP group identified fruit snacks/rolls as one of the fastest growing snack foods (Cooper, 2006, p. 6). And Canada's President's Choice Mini Chefs brand—launched nationally in December 2004 and targeted specifically at children—has since tripled the number of products in the line.

3. See, for example, Batada, Seitz, Wootan, & Story, 2008; Botterill & Kline, 2006; Consumers International, 1996; Cook, 2008a; Harris, 2008; Gantz, Schwartz, Angelini, & Rideout, 2007; IOM, 2006; Kotz & Story, 1994; Livingstone, 2005; Powell, Szczypka, Chaloupka, & Braunschweig, 2007. As the U.S.-based Institute of Medicine *Committee on Food Marketing and the Diets of Children and Youth* reported "television advertising remains the dominant form of marketing reaching children . . . that is formally tracked" (IOM, 2006, p. 15).

4. In 2006, Palmer and Carpenter observed that marketers spend "over $3 billion annually to design food product packaging that children and youth will want to purchase" (2006, p. 167)—a figure that has undoubtedly increased, particularly in light of the number of supermarket food brands (or sub-brands) aimed exclusively at children. These include, for example, Loblaw's highly popular President's Choice Mini Chefs brand, Safeway's Eating Right Kids line, Nature's Path EnviroKidz brand and Earth's Best Sesame Street line of children's foods.

5. The BRANDchild study spanned seven countries and interviewed thousands of children.

6. Ethics approval and written parental consent was obtained prior to holding the focus groups. Recruits for the convenience sample comprised 32 of the 36 children and were drawn from acquaintances of the research company (Delta Media Inc.) that hosted and moderated the focus groups. To completely fill the groups, four children were recruited randomly using a standard telephone directory listing for Ottawa.

7. The moderator's instructions included: "So, if you could choose what you would have for dinner, what would it be? . . . Remember, there are no right or wrong answers, just do your best to draw your favourite dinner."

8. This enthusiasm over kids' food (despite what the older children might have said) was demonstrated throughout the focus groups. At points, the children were literally crawling on the table to get their first pick of the cereals.

9. The remaining two boys were drawn to the most unnatural shades of pudding—blue and pink.

10. The percentage breakdown (67% fruit/vegetable; 17% bread/pasta; 7% yogurt/cheese; and 15% "don't know") adds up to more than 100 because some children provided more than one example of a healthy food.

11. Neither product was a healthy choice, owing to the high proportion of calories coming from sugar and the fact that the fruit snack would be better classified as a fruit-flavoured snack.

References

Alvy, Lisa & Calvert, Sandra L. (2008). Food marketing on popular children's websites: A content analysis. *Journal of the American Dietetic Association, 108*(4), 710–713.

Atkin, Charles. (1978). Observation of parent-child interaction in supermarket decision-making. *Journal of Marketing, 42*(4), 41–45.

Auty, Susan & Lewis, Charlie. (2004). Exploring children's choice: The reminder effect of product placement. *Psychology & Marketing, 21*(9), 697–713.

Batada, Ameena, Seitz, M. D., Wootan, Margo, & Story, M. (2008). Nine out of 10 food advertisements shown during Saturday morning children's television programming are for foods high in fat, sodium, or added sugars, or low in nutrients. *Journal of the American Dietetic Association, 108*(4), 673–678.

Botterill, Jacqueline & Kline, Stephen. (2006). *Flow, branding and media saturation: Towards a critical analysis of promotional marketing in children's television.* Paper presented at Child and Teen Consumption, 2006, Copenhagen Business School.

Brownell, Kelly, & Horgen, Katherine Battle. (2004). *Food fight: The inside story of the food industry, America's obesity crisis and what we can do about it.* New York: Contemporary Books.

Buckingham, David. (2000). *After the death of childhood.* Cambridge: Polity Press.

CCFN (Canadian Council of Food and Nutrition). (2008). *Tracking nutrition trends VII.* Woodbridge, ON: CCFN.

CDPAC (Chronic Disease Prevention Alliance of Canada). (2008). *Obesity and the impact of marketing on children: Policy consensus statement.* Ottawa, ON. URL: www.cdpac.ca/media .php?mid=433 [August 2009].

Consumers International. (1996). *A spoonful of sugar: Television food advertising aimed at children—An international comparative study.* London: Consumers International.

Cook, Brian. (2008a). *Overview of television food advertising to children.* Championing Public Health Nutrition Conference, October 22–23, Ottawa, ON. URL: www.cspinet.org/ canada/2008conference/presentation/BCook.pdf [August 2009].

Cook, Daniel. (2008b). The missing child in consumption theory. *Journal of Consumer Culture, 8*(2), 219–243.

Cooke, Lucy & Wardle, Jane. (2005). Age and gender differences in children's food preferences. *British Journal of Nutrition, 93,* 741–746.

Cooper, Carolyn. (2006). Snack attack. *Food in Canada, 66*(1), 7.

Cultured products shine on. (2007). *Dairy Foods, 108*(7), 16.

Deacon, David, Pickering, Michael, Golding, Peter & Murdock, Graham. (1999). *Researching communications: A practical guide to methods in media and cultural analysis.* London: Arnold.

Eagle, Lynne, Bulmer, Sandy, de Bruin, Anne & Kitchen, Philip. (2004). Exploring the link between obesity and advertising in New Zealand. *Journal of Marketing Communications, 10*(1), 49–67.

Elliott, Charlene. (2008a). Assessing fun foods: Nutritional content and analysis of supermarket foods targeted at children. *Obesity Reviews, 9,* 368–377.

Elliott, Charlene. (2008b). Marketing fun food: A profile and analysis of supermarket food messages targeted at children. *Canadian Public Policy, 34*(2), 259–274.

(FTC) Federal Trade Commission. (2008). Marketing food to children and adolescents: A review of industry expenditures, activities, and self-regulation: A Federal Trade Commission Report to Congress. URL: www.ftc.gov/os/2008/07/ P064504foodmktingreport.pdf.

Gantz, Walter, Schwartz, Nancy, Angelini, James & Rideout, Victoria. (2007). *Food for thought: Television food advertising to children in the United States.* Menlo Park, CA: Kaiser Family Foundation. URL: www.kff.org/entmedia/upload /7618.pdf [August 2009].

Gates, Kelly. (2006, October 30). Tempting tummies. *Supermarket News, 54*(44), 39–48.

Harris, Jennifer. (2008). *Children and food advertising effects: When are they old enough to resist?* Championing Public Health Nutrition Conference, October 22–23, Ottawa, ON. URL: www.cspinet.org/ canada/2008conference/presentation /Harris.pdf [August 2009].

Harris, Jennifer L., Pomeranz, Jennifer L., Lobstein, Tim & Brownell, Kelly D. (2009). A crisis in the marketplace: How food marketing contributes to childhood obesity and what can be done. *Annual Review of Public Health, 30,* 211–225.

Hastings, Gerard, Stead, Martine, McDermott, Laura, Forsyth, Alasdair, MacKintosh, Anne Marie, Rayner, Mike, Godfrey, Christine, Caraher, Martin, & Angus, Kathryn. (2003). *Review of Research on the Effects of Food Promotion to Children, Final Report.* [Prepared for the UK Food Standards Authority]. London: UK Food Standards Authority; Glasgow, Scotland: Centre for Social Marketing, University of Strathclyde. URL: www.food.gov.uk/ multimedia/pdfs/foodpromotiontochildren1.pdf [August 2009].

Hawkes, Corinna. (2004). *Marketing foods to children: The global regulatory environment.* Geneva, Switzerland: World Health Organization.

Heart and Stroke Foundation. (2008). *Assessing the impact of the Health Check food information program.* URL: www.hsf.ca/ research/images/PDF/final%20rfp%20sept%2025%2008%20eg .pdf [August 2009].

Heary, Caroline & Hennessy, Eilis. (2002). The use of focus group interviews in pediatric health care research. *Journal of Pediatric Psychology, 27*(1), 47–57.

Horgen, Katherine Battle, Choate, Molly, & Brownell, Kelly. (2001). Television food advertising: Targeting children in a toxic environment. In D.G. Singer & J.L. Singer (Eds.), *Handbook of children and the media.* Thousand Oaks, CA: Sage.

IOM (Institute of Medicine). (2006). *Food marketing to children and youth: Threat or opportunity?* Washington, DC: National Academies Press.

Kellogg Company brings fun back into the cereal aisle with Sesame Street Mini-Beans in-pack premium offer. (1999, December 8). *Business Wire.* URL: http://findarticles.com/p/articles/mi_m0EIN/ is_1999_Dec_8/ai_58079654 [August 2009].

Kitzinger, Jenny. (1995). Qualitative research: Introducing focus groups. *British Medical Journal, 311,* 299–302.

Kotz, Krista & Story, Mary. (1994). Food advertisements during children's Saturday morning television programming: Are they consistent with dietary recommendations? *Journal of the American Dietetic Association, 94,* 1296–1300.

Levine, I. S., & Zimmerman, J. D. (1996). Using qualitative data to inform public policy: Evaluating Choose to De-Fuse. *American Journal of Orthopsychiatry, 66*(3), 363–377.

Lindstrom, Martin. (2004). *BRANDchild.* London: Kogan Page.

Linn, Susan & Novosat, Courtney. (2008). Calories for sale: Food marketing to children in the twenty-first century. *The Annals of the American Academy of Political and Social Science, 615,* 133–155.

Livingstone, Sonia. (2005). Assessing the research base for the policy debate over the effects of food advertising to children. *International Journal of Advertising, 24*(3), 273–296.

Lunt, Peter, & Livingstone, Sonia. (1996). Rethinking the focus group in media and communications research. *Journal of Communication, 46*(2), 79–98.

McNeal, James. (1992). *Kids as customers: A handbook of marketing to children.* New York: Lexington Books.

McNeal, James. (1999). *The kids market: Myths and realities.* Ithaca, NY: Paramount Market Publishing.

Moore, Elizabeth S. (2004). Children and the changing world of advertising. *Journal of Business Ethics, 52*(2), 161–167.

Moore, Elizabeth S. (2006). *It's child's play: Advergaming and the online marketing of foods to children.* Menlo Park, CA: Kaiser Family Foundation. URL: www.kff.org/entmedia/7536.cfm [August 2009].

Morgan, Myfanwy, Gibbs, Sara, Maxwell, Krista & Britten, Nicky. (2002). Hearing children's voices: Methodological issues in conducting focus groups with children aged 7-11 years. *Qualitative Research, 2*(1), 5–20.

Nestle, Marion. (2002). *Food politics: How the food industry influences nutrition and health.* Berkeley: University of California Press.

Newton, Sarah E. (1992). The Jell-O Syndrome: Investigating popular culture/foodways. *Western Folklore, 51*(3/4), 249–267.

Nutrition Programs Unit. (1995). Food for thought: Results of a national study on children and healthy eating. *Report.* Ottawa, ON: Nutrition Programs Unit, Health Canada.

Page, Randy, Montgomery, Katie, Ponder, Andrea & Richard, Amanda. (2008). Targeting children in the cereal aisle: Promotional techniques and content features on ready-to-eat cereal product packaging. *American Journal of Health Education, 39*(5), 272–282.

Palmer, Edward & Carpenter, Courtney. (2006). Food and beverage marketing to children and youth: Trends and issues. *Media Psychology, 8,* 165–190.

Pollan, Michael. (2008). *In defense of food.* New York: Penguin.

Powell, Lisa, Szczypka, Glen, Chaloupka, Frand J., & Braunschweig, Carol L. (2007). Nutritional content of television food advertisements seen by children and adolescents in the United States. *Pediatrics, 120,* 576–583.

Schor, Juliet & Ford, Margaret. (2007). From tastes great to cool: Children's food marketing and the rise of the symbolic. *Journal of Law, Medicine & Ethics, 35*(1), 10–21.

Schwartz, Marlene & Brownell, Kelly. (2007). Actions necessary to prevent childhood obesity: Creating the climate for change. *Journal of Law, Medicine & Ethics, 35*(1), 78–89.

Seiter, Ellen. (1993). Utopia or discrimination? Commercials for kids. In E. Seiter, *Sold separately: Children and parents in consumer culture* (pp.115–144). New Jersey: Rutgers University Press.

Smith, Shannon, Stephen, Alison M., Dombrow, Carol & MacQuarrie, Doug. (2002). Food information program. *Canadian Journal of Dietetic Practice and Research, 63*(2), 55–60.

Standing Committee on Health, House of Commons. (2007, March). Healthy weights for healthy kids. *Report.* Ottawa, ON: Rob Merrifield (Chair). URL: http://cmte.parl.gc.ca/Content/HOC/ committee/391/hesa/reports/rp2795145/hesarp07/hesarp07-e.pdf [August 2009].

Strauss, Anselm & Corbin, Juliet. (1998). *Basics of qualitative research: Techniques and procedures for developing grounded theory* (2nd ed.). Thousand Oaks, CA: Sage.

Swinburn, B. A., Egger, G., & Raza, F. (1999). Dissecting the obesogenic environments: The development and application of a framework for identifying and prioritizing environmental interventions for obesity. *Preventative Medicine, 29,* 563–570.

Thompson, Stephanie. (1999a). Cap'n goes AWOL as sales flatten; Quaker redirects cereal brand's marketing budget to focus on kids. *Advertising Age, 70*(48), 8.

Thompson, Stephanie. (1999b). Kraft-y promo: Post gives coins for 'comb.' *Advertising Age, 70*(41), 19.

Thompson, Stephanie. (2000). Go-Gurt. *Advertising Age, 71*(27), 30.

Thompson, Stephanie. (2001). Kraft launches Lunchables for *snack* attacks. *Advertising Age, 72*(11), 45.

Tiwsakul, Rungpaka, Hackley, Chris, & Szmigin, Isabelle. (2005). Explicit, non-integrated product placement in British television programmes. *International Journal of Advertising, 24*(1), 95–111.

Ulijaszek, Stanley. (2007). Obesity: A disorder of convenience. *Obesity Reviews, 8*(1), 183–187.

Wardle, J., Sanderson, S., Gibson, E. L., & Rapoport, L. (2001). Factor-analytic structure of food preferences in four-year-old children in the UK. *Appetite, 37,* 217–223.

Crirtical Thinking

1. What are "fun foods"?

2. What are some marketing techniques that make foods interactive and concentrate on play rather than nutrition?

3. Why can positioning "food as fun" and "eating as entertainment" to kids have negative consequences to taste perceptions/preferences and long-term outcomes on their health?

CHARLENE D. ELLIOTT is Associate Professor of Communication Studies at the University of Calgary.

Acknowledgments—Funding for this research was generously provided by the Canadian Institutes of Health Research. The author would like to thank Bernie Gauthier for his assistance in coordinating and overseeing the focus groups.

10 Urban Food Legends
Things Aren't Always as Simple as They Seem

BONNIE LIEBMAN

Okay. They're not urban. (Neither are most other urban legends.) Nor are they only about food.

Some come from reliable sources, but are out of date. Others were wrong from the get-go. Some may not surprise you. But we're betting that others will.

Some even surprised *us*.

1. You'll Lose a Pound for Every 3,500 Calories You Cut

"Because 3,500 calories equals about 1 pound (0.45 kilogram) of fat, you need to burn 3,500 calories more than you take in to lose 1 pound," explains the Mayo Clinic Web site. "So if you cut 500 calories from your typical diet each day, you'd lose about 1 pound a week (500 calories × 7 days = 3,500 calories)."

If only it were that simple.

If you burn 500 calories more than you take in every day, you will lose about a pound a week. But once you've lost roughly 10 percent of your body weight, cutting 500 calories a day isn't enough to keep losing a pound a week because your body—afraid of starving—starts to burn fewer calories.[1]

"The body becomes a more efficient engine," explains Rudolph Leibel, co-director of the New York Obesity Research Center at Columbia University. "It's gone from being a Cadillac to a motorcycle. It's getting more miles per gallon, and it's a smaller vehicle."

What can help? Move more to burn more calories. And do strength training to build muscle (which burns more calories than fat).

2. Too Much Sugar Is the Main Cause of Diabetes

Diabetes is defined as too much sugar in the blood, so it's reasonable that people would assume that eating too much sugar is the culprit. And it likely is *a* culprit.

For example, women who drink at least one sugar-sweetened soft drink or fruit punch a day have nearly twice the risk of diabetes over four years as women who drink less than one a month.[2]

But it would be a mistake to think that sugar or soft drinks are the entire ball-game. Among other players:

- **Weight & exercise.** More than 80 percent of people with diabetes are overweight or obese. In a landmark study, weight loss cut the risk of diabetes by more than half in people who had pre-diabetes, and the average weight loss was only 9 pounds after three years.[3] The participants also boosted their exercise to 2½ hours of brisk walking a week, but weight loss mattered more.

- **Carbs.** People who eat more white potatoes have a higher risk of diabetes.[4] And people who eat more whole grains have a lower risk.[5] The fiber, magnesium, or chromium in whole grains may make a difference.

- **Fats.** Women who eat more trans fat have a 30 percent higher risk of diabetes, while those who eat the most polyunsaturated fats have a 25 percent lower risk.[6]

- **Meat & Iron.** People who eat about one serving a day of red meat have a 22 percent higher risk of diabetes than those who eat about one serving a week.[7] The heme iron in red meat may damage the pancreas, which produces insulin.

And nitrites in hot dogs, bacon, and lunch meats could explain why men who eat processed meats at least five times a week have a 46 percent higher risk of diabetes than men who eat them less than once a month.[8]

"Apart from obesity, the greatest risk for diabetes is not just the huge amount of sugar, but the displacement of beneficial whole grains by the large amount of refined starch in the American diet," explains Walter Willett, chair of the department of nutrition at the Harvard School of Public Health in Boston.

3. Sandwiches Are Lighter Fare Than Entrées

"I'm not that hungry," you may think. "I'll just have a sandwich." Watch out. At many sit-down restaurants, the sandwiches have as many calories as the entrées. Take The Cheesecake Factory.

Its Chicken Salad, Grilled Chicken & Avocado Club, Chicken Parmesan, and Crabcake sandwiches each has 1,100 to 1,500 calories without the fries or green salad that comes on the side. That's about as many calories as you'd get from most Cheesecake Factory steaks, chops, or even some chicken dishes.

And sandwiches range from 600 to 1,000 calories at Panera and from 500 to 700 calories at Au Bon Pain.

Sandwiches are no longer a shmear of tuna or egg salad on two thin slices of bread that people used to buy at the local lunch counter. They likely come with supersize rolls (or wraps), cheese, and dressings or spreads. Today's sandwiches typically weigh three-quarters of a pound.

Want something light? Eat half a sandwich . . . and skip the fries.

4. Fruits & Vegetables Prevent Most Cancers

"Eating vegetables doesn't stop cancer," declared the headline in *The New York Times* in April.

That's a bit of an exaggeration, given that the study cited by *The Times*—which tracked 335,000 women and 140,000 men in 10 European countries for nine years—did find that people who ate more vegetables and fruit had a 3 percent lower risk of "all cancers" added together (which doesn't necessarily apply to each individual cancer).[9]

And among those in the study at high risk of cancer due to smoking, cancer risk was 10 percent lower in heavy drinkers who ate the most vegetables. That makes sense, since earlier studies suggested that fruits and vegetables might help prevent cancers of the mouth, throat, larynx, esophagus, lung, and stomach. All are more likely in people who smoke and/or drink.

But researchers don't have good evidence that fruits and vegetables can lower the risk of breast, prostate, colon, and most other cancers.

So, can you dispense with the salads, stir-fries, and fruits-and-vegetables-as snacks? On the contrary, they appear to lower the risk of heart disease and stroke.[10]

What's more, their low calorie density means that they can help keep off unwanted pounds. And that's critical because being overweight or obese *does* raise the risk of cancers of the breast, colon, kidney, uterus, and esophagus.

"The bottom line is to eat plenty of fruits and vegetables because the health benefits are substantial," says Harvard's Walter Willett. "But for cancer prevention, it's much more important to avoid smoking and to stay lean and active."

5. Mediterranean Cuisine Is Good for You

What researchers call a "Mediterranean diet" is indeed good for your heart and may even lower your risk of cancer. For example, in a study that tracked roughly 75,000 women for 20 years, those with a high Mediterranean diet score had a 30 percent lower risk of heart disease and a 13 percent lower risk of stroke.[11]

But a Mediterranean diet isn't the pizza or lasagna you'd get at an Italian restaurant. "None of the current Mediterranean-type cuisines served in U.S. restaurants that come to mind are consistent with how scientists define a Mediterranean diet," says Alice Lichtenstein of Tufts University in Boston.

Most Italian restaurant dishes are loaded with cheese, meat, and white pasta or bread. Greek restaurants are heavy on the lamb, beef, white rice, white bread, and potatoes.

In contrast, researchers typically came up with Mediterranean diet scores by giving people one point each for higher-than-average intakes of vegetables (excluding potatoes), fruits, nuts, whole grains, legumes, and fish. People also got one point for each serving of alcohol, for eating at least as much monounsaturated as saturated fat, and for a less-than-average intake of red and processed meats.

"I'm sure you can find something that fits with a scientist's view of the Mediterranean diet in most restaurants," says Lichtenstein. "But it's more the exception than the rule."

The Mediterranean diet gained fame when the Seven Countries Study found a low risk of heart disease on the Greek island of Crete in the 1960s. But studies describing the diet on Crete don't mention whole grains or nuts (and do mention that white potatoes were a staple).[12]

"Scientists have defined a Mediterranean diet as whatever they thought would be an optimal dietary pattern," says Lichtenstein.

The answer, she suggests, is to forget labels. "It would be better to talk about fruits, vegetables, fish, beans, whole grains, and other foods rather than a Mediterranean diet."

6. You Only Need 20 Minutes of Exercise Three Days a Week

You can't blame people for being confused about how much exercise is enough. Years ago, experts promised that at least 20 minutes of aerobic exercise three times a week was enough for cardiovascular fitness.[13]

These days, the Centers for Disease Control and Prevention (CDC) recommends at least 150 minutes a week of brisk walking (or equivalent activity). Meanwhile, the National Academy of Sciences recommends at least 60 minutes a day.

"It's clear from many studies that 30 minutes of brisk walking five days a week is sufficient to lower the risk of many chronic diseases, such as heart disease, Type 2 diabetes, and certain types of cancer," says I-Min Lee of the Harvard School of Public Health. "But it might not be sufficient to control our weight, given the high number of calories we take in."

In Lee's recent study, women who gained less than 5 pounds over 13 years were active for about an hour a day.[14] "Most were walking," she explains. "If you do something more vigorous like running or jogging, swimming laps, or playing tennis, you can do 30 minutes a day."

Don't have an hour? Squeeze in a brisk 10-minute walk while you're on the cell phone. Use a treadmill or stationary bike while you watch TV or use your laptop computer. Anything is better than nothing.

"I don't want people to get discouraged and say 'I can't do the hour a day so therefore I'm not going to be physically active,'" says Lee. "Someone who gets 30 minutes a day of exercise is better off than someone who doesn't."

7. Aerobic Exercise Is Enough

We know we're supposed to get up off the couch and walk, run, bike, dance, swim, play tennis, whatever. But many people don't realize that aerobic exercise is just part of the equation.

The CDC recommends "muscle-strengthening activities on 2 or more days a week that work all major muscle groups (legs, hips, back, abdomen, chest, shoulders, and arms)."

That means exercising against a resistance, explains Ben Hurley, a professor of kinesiology at the University of Maryland at College Park (and husband of *Nutrition Action's* Jayne Hurley).

"The resistance could come from lifting' weights or from your own body weight-such as doing push ups or sliding your back up and down a wall from a squat to a standing position," notes Hurley.

Why do you need to strengthen muscles? "Without strength training, you start to lose muscle at age 40 if you're a woman and in your 50s if you're a man," says Hurley.

You also lose bone as you age. "The average postmenopausal woman loses about1 percent of her bone mineral density each year," he explains.

Strength training can stem the loss of bone and can rebuild some lost muscle.[15,16]

"The earlier you start, the better," says Hurley. "But there is no age limit for increasing strength."

His advice: "You should be able to do at least 8 and no more than 15 repetitions." If you can do more than 15, the load isn't heavy enough to build muscle and preserve bone.

8. Food Poisoning Is Just a Temporary Nuisance

A bout of food poisoning is bad enough. No one wants to go through the gut-wrenching vomiting and diarrhea that seems endless. But most people assume that they'll get over their food poisoning in a matter of hours or, at most, days.

Not always. In a small percentage of cases, food poisoning can lead to long-term consequences.[17]
Among them:

- **Guillain-Barré syndrome.** The terrifying disease starts as tingling in the arms and legs and progresses to paralysis that can lat for months.
- **Reactive arthritis.** It's an inflammation of the joints that's triggered by an infection, and it can last for years.
- **Kidney or nerve damage.** *E. coli* O157:H7 is the bacterium that contaminated Jack in the Box hamburgers in 1993 and fresh spinach in 2006. A small number of victims end up with permanent kidney or nerve damage, and some die.

9. Low-Fat Foods Are Best for Your Heart

Despite what many people think, "low fat" is not a yardstick that measures a food's impact on your risk of heart disease.

"Initially, when the nutrition community focused on low-fat foods, they were thinking of replacing full-fat dairy and meat, which have a fair amount of saturated fat," explains Tufts University's Alice Lichtenstein. "But the concept of low fat got distorted."

Some people assumed that they wouldn't gain weight if they ate low-fat cakes, cookies, and ice cream. "Some people ended up eating all low-fat foods with abandon, and they gained weight," says Lichtenstein. "But low fat doesn't always mean low calorie."

What's more, foods that are rich in unsaturated fats—like fatty fish, nuts, avocado, and most oils (like canola, soy, and olive)— protect your heart.

"If you squeeze out the healthy fats by eating too many sugars and refined grains, that's not good because triglycerides go up and HDL cholesterol goes down," says Lichtenstein.

What's the healthiest diet? It's a mix of some low-fat foods (vegetables, fruit, low-fat dairy, lower-fat poultry and meat) and some fattier foods (oils, fish, nuts, avocado), with surprisingly

little room for crabs like breads, rice, pasta, potatoes, and sweets. (See "What should I Eat?" October 2009, cover story.)

10. The Signs of a Heart Attack Are the Same in Men and Women

We've all seen what a heart attack looks like in movies and on TV. A man clutches his chest in severe pain and (in some cases) keels over. That's not how most heart attacks happen.

They're most likely to start slowly with milder pain in the chest. And instead of chest pain, some people report:

- **Pressure,** squeezing, or a sense of fullness in the chest. It usually lasts more than a few minutes, or it may go away and return.
- **Discomfort** or pain in one or both arms, the back, neck, jaw, or stomach.
- **Shortness of breath.**
- **Other signs** like breaking out in a cold sweat, nausea, or lightheadedness.

Women are more likely than men to experience nausea or vomiting, shortness of breath, or pain in the back or jaw.

In any case, the bottom line is the same for men and women: don't wait more than 5 minutes before calling 9-1-1. (Don't drive to the hospital yourself. You can get life-saving treatment in an ambulance, and you get there quicker.)

Notes

1. *Am. J. Clin. Nutr.* 88: 906, 2008.
2. *JAMA 292:* 927, 2004.
3. *N. Eng. J. Med.* 346: 393, 2002.
4. *Am. J. Clin. Nutr.* 83: 284, 2006.
5. *Am J. Clin. Nutr.* 76: 535, 2002.
6. *Am J. Clin. Nutr.* 73: 1019, 2001.
7. *Arch. Intern. Med.* 164: 2235, 2004
8. *Diabetes Care 25:* 417, 2002.
9. *J. Natl. Cancer Inst.* 102: 1, 2010.
10. *J. Natl. Cancer Inst.* 96: 1577, 2004.
11. *Circulation 119:* 1093, 2009.
12. *Am J. Clin. Nutr. 49:* 889, 1989.
13. *Med. Sci. Sports Exer. 10:* vii, 1978.
14. *JAMA 303:* 1173, 2010.
15. *J. Strength Cond. Res. 23:* 2627, 2009.
16. *Scand. J. Med. Sci. Sports 14:* 16, 2004.
17. *Emerg. Infect. Dis. 14:* 143, 2008.

Critical Thinking

1. Why aren't foods like pizza, lasagna, and other cheese, meat, refined pasta dishes considered part of what is referred to as the "Mediterranean diet?"
2. Why doesn't cutting 3,500 calories always equate to the loss of one pound of body fat for everyone?

From *Nutrition Action HealthLetter,* June 2010. Copyright © 2010 by Center for Science in the Public Interest. Reprinted by permission.

Eat Like a Greek

Want flavor plus good health? The Mediterranean style of dining has it all.

Diets are often doomed to fail because they focus more on what you can't eat than what you can. Don't eat bread. Don't eat sugar. Don't eat fat. On some diets, even certain fruits and vegetables are forbidden. After a few weeks of being told "no," our inner toddler throws a tantrum and runs screaming to Krispy Kreme.

That's what is so appealing about the Mediterranean diet, which isn't really a diet at all but a style of eating that focuses on an abundance of delicious, hearty, and nutritious food. Just looking at the pyramid at right, developed by Oldways Preservation Trust, a nonprofit organization that encourages healthy food choices, may be enough to make you look forward to the next meal.

"What I like about this approach to food is that it's very easy," says Sara Baer-Sinnott, executive vice president of Oldways. "It's not a fancy way of eating, but you'll never feel deprived because the foods have so much flavor."

The best part is that eating like a Greek not only satisfies your need to say yes to food, but has been scientifically proven to be good for your health. Decades of research has shown that traditional Mediterranean eating patterns are associated with a lower risk of several chronic diseases, including the big three—cancer, heart disease, and type 2 diabetes. Most recently, a systematic review of 146 observational studies and 43 randomized clinical trials published in the April 13, 2009, issue of the *Archives of Internal Medicine* found strong evidence that a Mediterranean diet protects against cardiovascular disease. Other recent research has linked the eating style to a lower risk of cognitive decline and dementia.

So, where do you start? Your next meal is as good a place as any. Just walk through our guide for menu planning.

Stepping into a Mediterranean Lifestyle

Although a trip to southern Italy or Greece would be nice, you needn't go farther than your local supermarket. If your menu planning usually begins with a meat entrée, then adds a starch and a vegetable side dish as an afterthought, you'll want to reprioritize your food choices. "Think about designing a plate where a good half of it is taken up with vegetables, another one-quarter is healthy grains—whole-grain pasta, rice, couscous, quinoa—and the remaining quarter is lean protein," says Katherine McManus, R.D., director of nutrition at Brigham and Women's Hospital in Boston and a consultant on the most recent version of the Mediterranean pyramid. "Of course, you needn't physically separate your foods in that fashion, but it gives you a good idea of the proportions to aim for."

STEP 1: Start with plant foods. Build your menus around an abundance of fruits and vegetables (yes, even potatoes); breads and grains (at least half of the servings should be whole grains); and beans, nuts, and seeds. To maximize the health benefits, emphasize a variety of minimally processed and locally grown foods.

STEP 2: Add some lean protein. The Mediterranean diet draws much of its protein from the sea, reflecting its coastal origins. Fish is not only low in saturated fat but can also be high in heart-healthy omega-3 fatty acids. Aim for two servings of fish a week, especially those, such as salmon and sardines, that are high in omega-3s but lower in mercury. You can also include moderate amounts of poultry and even eggs.

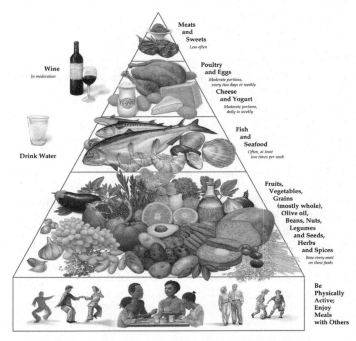

© 2009 Oldways Preservation Trust, www.oldwayspt.org

A Day in the Mediterranean Life

Breakfast

It's hard to go wrong with whole-grain cereal, fruit, and low-fat milk. Variations on the theme include low-fat yogurt with fresh berries and granola, or meaty steel-cut oats topped with fresh fruit, applesauce, whipped yogurt, or a sprinkle of nuts. Enjoy eggs? Try sautéing vegetables or greens in a bit of olive oil until soft and then scramble in a beaten egg. Go Greek with chopped olives and feta, or top with salsa and avocado for a Tex-Mex flair.

Lunch

Whether you're at home or brown-bagging, a Mediterranean lunch is tastier and healthier than drive-through fare and often faster and cheaper, too. Bagged salad greens provide a base for whatever you have on hand—fruit, vegetables, nuts, cheese, or a bit of leftover grilled chicken or fish. Consider topping it with a low-fat ranch dressing, an olive-oil vinaigrette, or just a drizzle of flavorful oil and a squeeze of fresh lemon. Or fill a whole-wheat pita pocket with hummus and as much fresh lettuce, peppers, cucumbers, and tomatoes as you can stuff in. If you're really pressed for time, heat up a can of low-sodium lentil, minestrone, or vegetable soup.

Snack Time

Keep a ready supply of fruit and veggies on hand so you'll grab them at snack time. Hummus, low-fat yogurt, and salad dressings pair nicely with them. If you don't want to invest the prep time, buy pre-cut. It's also a good idea to keep some nonperishable snacks at your desk or in your car—raisins or other dried fruit, nuts, and whole-grain crackers or pretzels.

Dinner

This is when many of us lose sight of nutrition goals because it's so easy after a long day to fall into old, comfortable habits. Fortunately, Mediterranean-style dining emphasizes simple foods and cooking methods.

While your pasta boils, for example, you can sauté a variety of vegetables in olive oil and garlic, then toss in a few shrimp and cook until they turn pink. Mix it all with a sprinkle of cheese, pour yourself a glass of wine, and you're sitting down to a relaxing dinner in less than 20 minutes.

In much the same manner, you can put together a quick stir-fry with slices of chicken breast, vegetables, and rice. Fresh fish is the simplest of entrées because it cooks quickly and doesn't take much dressing up. Spritz it with olive oil and your favorite seasonings and broil it, or coat it in bread crumbs and pan fry in a bit of olive oil. Squeeze on fresh lemon juice and adorn with parsley just before serving.

Two things you should have on hand for your evening meal: frozen vegetables, which are usually just as nutritious as fresh, and a plastic container of salad, preferably filled with a variety of greens. It's also a good idea to stock your crisper with seasonal fruit. A bowl of ripe berries, a chunk of melon, or a soft, farm-fresh peach is a delicious and satisfying end to any meal.

Oldways Preservation Trust, a nonprofit organization that promotes healthful eating, has more recipes and menu ideas on the two websites it sponsors: www.oldwayspt.org and www.mediterraneanmark.org.

Or substitute with vegetarian sources of protein, such as beans, nuts, or soy products. Limit red meat to a couple of servings a month, and minimize consumption of processed meats.

STEP 3: Say cheese. Include some milk, yogurt, or cheese in your daily meal. While low-fat versions are preferable, others are fine in small amounts. A sprinkle of high-quality Romano or Parmesan, for example, adds a spark to vegetables and pasta. Soy-based dairy products are fine, too, if you prefer them or are lactose intolerant.

STEP 4: Use oils high in "good" fats. Canola oil is a good choice, but many Mediterranean recipes call for olive oil. Both are high in unsaturated fat. Minimize artery-clogging saturated fat, which comes mainly from animal sources, and avoid the even more heart-harming trans fat, which comes from partially hydrogenated vegetable oil.

STEP 5: End meals with the sweetness of fruit. Make sugary and fatty desserts just an occasional indulgence.

STEP 6: Drink to your health. A moderate amount of alcohol—especially red wine—may help protect your heart. But balance that against the increased risks from drinking alcohol, including breast cancer in women. A moderate amount is one drink a day for women, two for men.

STEP 7: Step out. "The Mediterranean lifestyle is built around daily activity," McManus says. Go for a walk after dinner. And choose leisure activities that keep you moving.

Critical Thinking

1. Why do the authors support the use of the term Mediterranean lifestyle rather than Mediterranean diet?
2. Following a Mediterranean lifestyle has been associated with lower risk of several chronic diseases. What are five chronic diseases that are positively correlated with following the Mediterranean lifestyle?
3. An easy guide to Mediterranean meal planning is a meal of vegetables, whole grains, and lean protein. What proportions of the plate should each of these food groups make up in the meal?

Definition of the Mediterranean Diet Based on Bioactive Compounds

Antioxidant (polyphenols and carotenoids) and nonantioxidant (phytosterols) bioactive compounds and dietary fiber may have a significant role in health. The intake of these compounds is strongly linked with the high consumption of fruits, vegetables, and unrefined cereals. A whole-diet approach to these food constituents is intended to render the current definition of Mediterranean diet based on food consumption more comprehensive.

The Mediterranean dietary pattern can be characterized by the following four essential dietary indicators: 1) Monounsaturated to saturated fatty acid ratio (range: 1.6 to 2.0); 2) Intake of dietary fiber (41 to 62 g/person/day); 3) Antioxidant capacity of the whole diet (3500 to 5300 trolox equivalent/person/day); 4) Phytosterols intake (370 to 555 mg/person/day). The contribution of foods and beverages to these parameters is described. Spanish National Food Consumption Data for the years 2000 and 1964 were used to quantify the lowest and highest range values. The occurrence of these indicators in the Mediterranean diet has specific characteristics and there is sufficient scientific evidence to support the beneficial health effects.

FULGENCIO SAURA-CALIXTO AND ISABEL GOÑI

Introduction

Nowadays we possess a good understanding of metabolism and daily macronutrient and micronutrient requirements. But plant foods also contain hundreds of nonnutrient microconstituents with significant biological activity, generally called bioactive compounds or phytochemicals, which appear to play a role in the maintenance of human health. The main groups of these substances are polyphenolic compounds, carotenoids, and phytosterols. The current knowledge of their bioavailability, metabolism, and dietary intakes is incomplete or nonexistent, and there are consequently no recommended daily allowances for bioactive compounds. The traditional approach in this field has focused on the physiological properties associated with the ingestion of single compounds or specific food extracts, generally involving doses well in excess of those contained in common diets (Bjelakovic et al., 2004). This may be of only relative value as it is generally thought that what really produces an effect on human health is the synergistic and cumulative action of these substances in the diet. To assess the real significance of bioactive compounds for human health, the diet needs to be approached as a whole (Martinez-González et al., 2004). In adopting a whole-diet approach to bioactive compounds it may be useful to look at diets in connection with which observational and epidemiological studies have shown low rates of morbidity and morbidity by chronic disease. The Mediterranean diet (MD), the Japanese diet, or other specific diets rich in fruits and vegetables may all be good models. Here we focus on the Mediterranean dietary pattern.

Over 500 journal articles have addressed the Mediterranean diet in the last ten years; of these, 76 are clinical trials and 136 are reviews (MEDLINE, National Library of Medicine, Bethesda, MD). A systematic review of studies reveals a significant association between the MD and a lower rate of mortality from all causes, and favorable effects of the MD on lipoprotein levels, endothelium vasodilatation, insulin resistance, antioxidant capacity, and metabolic syndrome (Serra-Majem et al., 2006). Recent prospective investigations have reported that adherence to the MD was associated with lower arterial blood pressure, (Psaltopoulou et al., 2004), increased survival among older people (Trichopoulou et al., 2005; Knoops et al., 2004) and significantly lower total mortality, mortality from coronary heart disease, and mortality from cancer (Trichopoulou et al., 2003; Vincent-Baudry et al., 2005; Cottet, et al., 2005). Trichopoulou and Lagiou

(2001) and Trichopoulou et al., (2003) included in the commonly-reported definition of MD, the following nine components:

a. High monounsaturated-to-saturated lipid ratio (derived from high olive oil consumption)
b. Moderate ethanol consumption (mainly as wine)
c. High consumption of legumes
d. High consumption of cereals (mainly unrefined cereals and bread)
e. High consumption of fruits
f. High consumption of vegetables
g. Low consumption of meat and meat products
h. Moderate consumption of milk and dairy products
i. High consumption of fish and fish products

A health pyramid for the general adult population based on the Mediterranean dietary pattern provides a guide to the relative proportions and frequency of consumption of the respective food groups and it is used to give advice on healthy food choices. The Mediterranean dietary pattern is nowadays considered highly appropriate for public health objectives, and consumer trends globally indicate growth in demand for mediterranean products, (Regmi et al., 2004).

Mediterranean Diet: A New Complementary Definition

The definition of the MD is mainly based on consumption of foods. However, despite the robust inverse association between MD and mortality found in observational and epidemiological studies, no appreciable associations have been identified with any individual foods, including olive oil (Trichopoulou et al., 2003; Hu, 2003). The only single food item whose role in the beneficial effects of the MD is widely considered and discussed is olive oil. Trichopoulou et al. (2003) described inverse associations with mortality but only found in connection with high intakes of food groups rich in bioactive compounds, comprising dozens of individual foods such as fruits and vegetables (over 500 g/person day) or fruits and nuts (over 300 g/person day).

It is not yet clear which food constituents of the MD contribute most to its apparent health effects. The intake of energy and nutrients in the MD is similar to that in diets of North European countries where there is a higher prevalence of chronic diseases and an excess of total energy provided to a large extent by fat and protein at the expense of carbohydrates. However, there are differences between Mediterranean and Northern European countries in relation to fat consumption. Mediterraneans recorded high availability of olive oil and unprocessed red meat, while Central and Northern Europeans preferably consumed meat products (Naska et al., 2006).

As far as micronutrients are concerned, to our knowledge, clear significant differences in the intake of vitamins and minerals in Northern and Southern European countries have not been reported (Elmadfa et al., 2004), and therefore the role of bioactive compounds or phytochemicals as a key factor in the health effects of the MD is an attractive hypothesis. The plant foods in the MD, of which there is a considerable amount and variety, contribute a large proportion of the overall dietary intake of dietary fiber (DF) and bioactive compounds and a small proportion of the overall dietary intake of energy. In this connection, a complementary definition of the MD was recently proposed by Saura-Calixto and Goñi (2005), based on the following dietary indicators: monounsaturated/saturated lipid ratio, intake of DF, antioxidant capacity of the whole diet, and the intake of phytosterols. These indicators were selected for two reasons: first, there is sufficient scientific evidence to support their beneficial health effects, and second, their occurrence in the MD has specific characteristics (Table 1).

Monounsaturated to Saturated Fatty Acids Ratio (Derived from High Olive Oil Consumption)

There is general consensus among scientists as to the significant role of the monounsaturated to saturated fat ratio (MUFA/SFA) in disease etiology. This ratio is predictive of total mortality and is the first point in the definition of the MD (Trichopoulou et al., 2003; Gibney and Roche, 2001; Fernandez and West, 2005). A high MUFA/SFA ratio is a common feature in Mediterranean countries; it is much higher than in other parts of the world including northern Europe and North America (Naska et al., 2006).

Intake of Dietary Fiber (as Total Indigestible Fraction)

Nowadays the importance of DF in nutrition and health is well defined. Numerous clinical and epidemiological studies have addressed the role of DF in intestinal health, prevention of cardiovascular disease and cancer, obesity, and diabetes (Krichevsky and Bonfield, 1995; Cho and Dreher, 2001). The daily intake of DF is quantitatively similar in Mediterranean and non-Mediterranean European countries (around 20 g per capita) (Goñi, 2001; Elmadfa et al., 2005). However, there are qualitative differences arising from the fact that a large proportion of the DF intake in Mediterranean countries comes from fresh fruit and vegetables, while in Northern

Table 1 Essential dietary indicators in the Mediterranean diet

Indicator	Associated health effects	Diferential features in Mediterranean diet
Monounsaturated fatty acid to saturated fatty acid ratio	Inverse correlation with cardiovascular disease and total mortality	High ratio derived from consumption of olive oil (high) and animal fat (moderate)
Dietary fiber intake (as total indigestible fraction)	Prevention of coronary heart disease and colon cancer	High consumption of fresh fruit and vegetables (fiber with associated bioactive compounds)
Antioxidant capacity of the whole diet	High serum antioxidant capacity Prevention of oxidative damage	High variety of antioxidants from plant foods and beverages
Phytosterols intake	Lower total and LDL-cholesterol	High intake from vegetable oils

European countries it comes more from cereals (Saura-Calixto and Goñi, 1993; Goñi, 2001). This suggests that the composition and properties of the DF in the MD may have specific characteristics. Fruits and vegetables possess a higher soluble fiber to insoluble fiber ratio than cereals. On the other hand, it is well known that DF, especially from fruits and vegetables, is a carrier of bioactive compounds. DF transports a significant amount of polyphenols, carotenoids, and other bioactive compounds linked to the fiber matrix through the human gut. (Goñi et al., 2007; Saura-Calixto et al., 2007). A part of the postulated benefits of the Mediterranean diet might then be attributable to the intake of fiber. It is important to note at this point that the use of food DF data in nutrition may be subject to some limitations arising from the concept of DF itself and from the methodology used to determine DF in foods. The concept of DF was first developed 40 years ago. DF was defined as plant polysaccharides and lignin which are resistant to hydrolysis by the digestive enzymes of man (Trowell et al., 1976). However, knowledge has increased since then. On the basis of bacterial growth, it has been calculated that up to 60 g of carbohydrates have to reach the colon to maintain the bacterial cell turnover on a daily basis. Nevertheless, the intake of DF in European countries only accounts for 20 g of carbohydrate/day, which leaves what was called a "carbohydrate gap" of 40 g/d (Cumming and Macfarlane, 1991; Stephen, 1991). The general tendency among nutritionists nowadays is to extend the concept of DF to include all major food constituents that are resistant to hydrolysis by digestive enzymes.

In this context the American Association of Cereal Chemists (2001) recently defined DF as the edible part of plants or analogous carbohydrates that are resistant to digestion and absorption in the human small intestine with complete or partial fermentation in the large intestine. That includes polysaccharides, oligosaccharides, lignin, and associated plant substances. Nevertheless, the analytical methodology for determination of DF in food (Prosky et al., 1992) focused on non-starch polysaccharides and lignin has not been adapted to the new concept but is still widely used. Therefore, most DF values recorded in food composition tables and databases are defined by the traditional concept, which may cause errors in nutritional and epidemiological studies addressing the health effects of DF. In the same context, DF as total indigestible fraction was recently defined as the part of plant foods that is not digested or absorbed in the small intestine and reaches the colon, where it serves as a substrate for the fermentative microflora, (Saura-Calixto et al., 2000). As such, it comprises not only the non-starch polysaccharides plus lignin (traditional concept of DF), but also other compounds of proven resistance to the action of digestive enzymes such as a fraction of resistant starch, protein, certain polyphenols, and other associated compounds. A significant part of dietary starch, called resistant starch, is not digested in the human gut. The resistant starch fraction is a major component of the indigestible fraction of cereals. Resistant starch is an insoluble substrate largely fermented by the colonic bacteria (Asp et al., 1996). A specific methodology has been developed to determine DF as the total indigestible fraction (Saura-Calixto et al., 2000) which may provide data that reflect the amount of substrates available in the human colon more accurately than traditional DF values. A recent report (Saura-Calixto and Goñi, 2004) concluded that DF intake determined as traditional DF underestimates a major part of the dietary substrates that enter the colon, while DF intake determined as total indigestible fraction more closely matches the amount of substrates needed to maintain a typical human colonic microflora. Therefore, in order to avoid the limitations of the traditional DF data, we have used values of DF determined as total indigestible fraction as a dietary indicator of the Mediterranean dietary pattern, (Saura-Calixto and Goñi, 2004).

Antioxidant Capacity of the Whole Diet

Ongoing research aims to elucidate the role of dietary antioxidants in disease prevention. The main approach was based on the hypothesis that the chronic disorders common in many industrialized societies are related to cumulative oxidative damage to DNA, proteins, and lipids in body tissues. Even at very low concentrations, dietary antioxidants protect against oxidative damage and may also have a greater impact than realized hitherto on the regulation of gene expression, profoundly affecting metabolism (Beckman and Ames, 1998). Vitamins (C, E, and A), polyphenolic compounds, and carotenoids are recognized as the main groups of antioxidants present in beverages and plant foods. Vitamins are single molecules, but polyphenols (flavonoids, phenolic acids, stilbenes, tannins) and carotenoids (carotenes and xanthophylls) are made up of hundreds of compounds with a wide range of structures and molecular masses. Recent reviews have addressed the role of these bioactive compounds in nutrition and health, (Manach et al., 2005; Williamson and Manach, 2005; Tapiero et al., 2004; Cooper, 2004). There is abundant literature on the antioxidant capacity of single compounds and food extracts, but as mentioned earlier, there is a lack of comprehensive data on the antioxidant capacity of whole diets. The antioxidant capacity of a whole diet is derived from the accumulative and synergistic antioxidant power of vitamins, polyphenols, carotenoids, and other minor food constituents such as Maillard compounds and trace minerals. The fact that dietary antioxidants come from a wide variety of sources is a specific feature of the MD. The consumption of a large variety of fruits and vegetables, legumes, nuts, cereals, red wine, citrus juices, and other beverages supply the MD diet with a considerable range of lipophilic and hydrophilic antioxidants. The total antioxidant capacity of the MD is probably higher than in other countries with a higher incidence of chronic diseases, especially cardiovascular disease, such as Northern Europe and the United States.

There is growing scientific evidence that dietary antioxidants may be a critical mediator of the beneficial effects of the MD. There are a number of recent studies supporting this. The work of Pitsavos et al. (2005) on the effects of the MD on total antioxidant capacity, performed with a random sample of over 3000 adults, concluded that greater adherence to the MD is associated with high total antioxidant capacity levels in serum. Serafini et al. (2003) found that the dietary antioxidant intake, measured as total antioxidant capacity, was inversely associated with both cardia and distal cancer risk in a population based case control. Brighenti et al. (2005) reported that total antioxidant capacity is inversely and independently correlated with plasma concentration of highly sensitive C-reactive protein, and this could be one of the mechanisms whereby antioxidant rich foods protect against cardiovascular disease. On that basis we selected the total antioxidant capacity of the MD as a key parameter in their health effects. Total dietary antioxidant capacity (TDAC) can be defined as the antioxidant capacity of all plant foods and beverages (alcoholic and non alcoholic) consumed daily in a diet. This parameter provides an integrated measurement rather than a single sum of measurable antioxidants and may represent the amount of antioxidant units (trolox equivalents) present daily in the human gut (Saura-Calixto and Goñi, 2006).

Phytosterols Intake

Human clinical trials have established that plant sterols lower total and LDL cholesterol, since they competitively inhibit intestinal cholesterol uptake (Kritchevsky, 2005). Plant foods contain a large number of plant sterols (chiefly campesterol, ßsitosterol, stigmastanol and stigmasterol) as minor lipid components. The high phytosterol content in traditional Mediterranean food (olive oil, nuts, legumes) along with the fact that the bioavailability of these compounds is higher in oils than in cereals—the main dietary source of phytosterols in Northern Europe—suggests that dietary phytosterols may be a factor in the lower cardiovascular disease death rates in Mediterranean countries (Fito et al., 2007; Jiménez-Escrig et al., 2006). Most bioactive compounds have antioxidant capacity. Thus, dietary polyphenols, carotenoids, and other minor antioxidants contribute to TDAC values. But phytosterols exhibit no antioxidant activity, and a specific parameter for phytosterols is needed.

Dietary Indicators in the Spanish Mediterranean Diet

The essential dietary indicators were quantified in the Spanish diet on the basis of national food consumption data for the year 2000 (MAPA, Ministerio de Agricultura Pesca y Alimentación, 2001).

Monounsaturated to Saturated Lipid Ratio

The Spanish diet contains a high level of dietary fat, and that fat contains a high percentage of monounsaturated fatty acids (contributing 19% of energy; saturated fatty acids contribute 12% and polyunsaturated fats 6%). The MUFA/SFA was estimated at 1.6 (Saura-Calixto and Goñi, 2005).

Table 2 Intake of dietary fiber (DF) in the Spanish diet (Saura-Calixto and Goñi 2004)

	DF (indigestible fraction) (g/person/day)			DF (traditional) (g/person/day)		
Source	Total	Soluble	Insoluble	Total	Soluble	Insoluble
Cereals	22.25	5.47	16.78	7.28	1.95	5.33
Fruits	6.49	0.71	5.78	5.05	2.09	2.96
Vegetables	8.16	1.66	6.50	4.69	1.90	2.79
Legumes	3.92	0.50	3.42	0.75	0.23	0.52
Nuts	0.67	0.04	0.63	0.57	0.13	0.45
Total	41.49	8.38	33.11	18.35	6.30	12.05

Table 3 Total dietary antioxidant capacity (TDAC) in the Spanish diet (Saura-Calixto and Goñi, 2006)

Source	Antioxidant capacity (ABTS method) (µmol trolox equivalent)
Nuts	176.0
Fruits	342.0
Vegetables	272.0
Legumes	134.7
Cereals	33.4
Beverages	
Coffee	1581.7
Wine	616.6
Others	377.7
Vegetable oils	
Olive	12.8
Others	2.4
TDAC	3549.3

Antioxidant Capacity

TDAC of the Spanish diet was estimated at 3550 µmol trolox equivalent by ABTS method (free radical scavenging capacity), (Table 3). This represents the estimated amount of dietary antioxidants, expressed as trolox equivalent, that daily enters in the gut (Saura-Calixto and Goñi, 2006). It is generally thought that plant foods are the main source of antioxidants in the diet; however, the findings of these reports indicate that beverages are the largest source of antioxidants in the Spanish diet (72.6%—ABTS values—of TDAC). Fruits and vegetables contributed 17.3%, while the contribution of cereals and vegetable oils was very low; olive oil accounted for just 0.4%. Nuts and legumes contributed nearly 9% of TDAC.

Food items such as olive oil and wine are very important components of the Spanish diet. Olive oil has been shown to have a significant association with lower blood pressure, (Psaltopoulou et al., 2004) but not with lower mortality (Hu, 2003). The MUFA/SFA is the only item included in the definition of the MD that has been shown to have a significant association with low mortality from cardiovascular disease and overall mortality. Olive oil may produce its dietary health benefits by lowering blood pressure (Psaltopoulou et al., 2004)—a cardiovascular disease risk factor—and by contributing to a proper lipid intake in two ways: directly by increasing monounsaturated lipids, and indirectly by decreasing saturated lipids intake. It has also been widely suggested that the beneficial effects of olive oil derive not only from its high oleic content but also from the presence of polyphenolic antioxidants; however, other authors consider that the olive oil phenols intake in the MD is probably too low to produce a measurable effect on oxidation markers in humans (Vissers et al., 2004).

Regular, moderate consumption of wine is a feature of the MD. Wine consumption represents 17.4% of the

Dietary Fiber (as Total Indigestible Fraction)

The intake of DF as total indigestible fraction in the Spanish diet (41.5 g/person/day) was much higher than the total DF in-take measured as traditional DF (18.30 g/person/day), (Table 2), (Saura-Calixto and Goñi, 2004). Fresh fruits and vegetables are the main sources of DF: 53.1% of the total intake measured as traditional DF (Goñi, 2001) and 35.3% measured as indigestible fraction (Saura-Calixto and Goñi, 2004). The appreciable difference in the relative contribution of cereals to DF values (53.6% to indigestible fraction and 39.7% to traditional DF values) is due to the presence of resistant starch as a major constituent of the indigestible fraction. Resistant starch is not included in traditional DF values.

TDAC of the Spanish diet, but surprisingly, coffee was the single largest contributor (44.6%), (Saura-Calixto and Goñi, 2006). The high contribution of coffee to anti-oxidant intake in the Spanish diet had previously been reported (Pulido et al., 2003) and was again recently confirmed in a nationwide Norwegian survey (Svilaas et al., 2004). We know that the major antioxidants in coffee (chlorogenic acids) are less bioavailable than the major antioxidants in wine (flavonoids), but the health signifi-cance of high consumption of coffee antioxidants in west-ern countries remains to be elucidated.

With regard to food microconstituents, vitamins C and E account for only about 10% of TDAC in the Spanish Mediterranean diet, polyphenols being the major antioxi-dant (Saura-Calixto and Goñi, 2006). Determination of the TDAC may be a useful additional tool for interpreting some clinical and epidemiological results. Following is an account of two examples.

The MONICA epidemiological study (Renaud and Lorgeril, 1992) found the lowest coronary heart dis-ease mortality in the region of Toulouse, where a daily intake of 383 mL of wine was reported. If we assume that the antioxidant capacity of the Toulouse wine is comparable to that of Spanish red wine (Table 3), the antioxidant capacity from wine intake in Toulouse is equivalent to the TDAC of the whole Spanish diet (around 4000 μmol trolox equivalent, ABTS method). If we add the AC corresponding to the reported intake of 238 g of fruit and 306 g of vegetables, then the esti-mated TDAC in the Toulouse diet is very high and could be a key factor in the low coronary heart disease mortality in this region.

A prospective investigation in Greece of Tricho-poulou et al. (2003) showed that adherence to a MD was associated with significantly lower total mortal-ity, mortality from coronary heart disease, and mor-tality from cancer. However, despite a robust inverse association between the MD and mortality, no appre-ciable associations were found for most of the indi-vidual dietary components used to construct the score, including foods containing antioxidants such as olive oil, legumes, vegetables, cereals, nonalcoholic bev-erages, and juices. Only the intake of fruits plus nuts and the MUFA/SFA were predictive of total mortality. The introduction of the TDAC may contribute to a bet-ter understanding of these intriguing results (Saura-Calixto and Goñi, 2006). If we consider that fruits and nuts are the plant foods that exhibit the highest anti-oxidant capacity, and that the reported daily intake of these items (390 g) was higher than in the Spanish diet (272 g), it is not surprising that the intake of fruits and

Table 4 Phytosterols intake in the Spanish diet (Jimenez-Escrig et al., 2006)

Source	mg/person/day
Cereals	87.9
Fruits	38.4
Vegetables	24.0
Legumes	27.1
Nuts	8.3
Vegetable oils	188.5
Total	374.2

nuts was significantly associated with disease preven-tion. Probably fruits plus vegetables, as opposed to fruits plus nuts, would also exhibit a significant inverse association with mortality. The MD aside, numerous epidemiological studies have correlated the intake of fruits and vegetables with low incidence of cardiovas-cular diseases (Bazzano et al., 2002; Djoussé et al., 2004). The intake of antioxidant capacity derived from the consumption of the amount of fruits and vegetables reported in these studies, totalling over 500 g, is close to the total antioxidant capacity in the MD.

Phytosterols Intake

The per capita daily plant sterol intake in the Spanish diet was estimated at 374.2 mg, (Table 4). ß-sitosterol was the major contributor to the total intake. The main individual contributors are sunflower oil, olive oil, bread, oranges, chickpeas, lentils, and beans. Most of these are consid-ered typical Mediterranean foods (Jiménez-Escrig et al., 2006). Spanish intake of plant sterols is in the same range as other countries with higher mortality from cardiovas-cular disease such as Finland and the Netherlands (Val-sta et al., 2004; Normén et al., 2001). However, there are some qualitative differences in the plant sterol sources: cereals in the Northern diets versus vegetable oils in the Spanish diet. The intake from vegetable oils is especially important since the bioavailability of plant sterols is enhanced in oils.

A Complementary Definition of the Mediterranean Diet

A complementary definition based on the dietary indi-cators described above is useful to render the traditional definition based on food intakes more comprehensive. In this traditional definition the consumption of foods is assessed in imprecise terms such as "moderate" or "high," but not in concrete figures. Thus, in the Spanish diet 414 g/person/day of dairy products is moderate consumption, while 14 g/person/day of legumes is high and 179 g of meat and meat products is low.

The Spanish diet, an alimentary pattern that matches the defined characteristics of the MD, was used to quantify the dietary indicators. The traditional Spanish Diet is described as providing an abundance of plant foods (fruits, vegetables, bread, cereal products, legumes, nuts, and seeds), wine, and olive oil and favoring the consumption of locally grown, seasonally fresh, and minimally processed foods. It includes a wide variety of fish and modest amounts of foods from animal sources; this assures the necessary intake of macro- and micronutrients while keeping saturated lipids low.

During the Sixties the Spanish diet followed this traditional Mediterranean pattern, but since then the food consumption pattern has changed greatly (Table 5). It appears that consumption of meat, fruit, dairy products, and fish has increased while consumption of bread, potatoes, olive oil, and legumes has decreased. As a consequence, the contribution of fat and protein to the total energy intake is high while the contribution of carbohydrates is below the recommended levels. In spite of these changes, the present Spanish diet still falls within the pattern of the MD, mainly thanks to increased consumption of fruit and fish and a moderate decline in consumption of olive oil, wine, and legumes (Saura-Calixto and Goñi, 2005). These dietary indicators were at their highest in the 1960s and are lowest at present. The values of these indicators for current diet were determined by analytical determinations performed in foods collected in 2000. These values were extrapolated to food consumption in 1964 to estimate the dietary indicators at that date. 1964 was chosen because it was the first year in which National Surveys were conducted using the same methodology as nowadays. These data are obtained annually from daily budget questionnaires. Six thousand households are surveyed, along with 700 hotels and restaurants and 200 institutions such as schools, hospitals, and the armed forces (confidence level 95%; error range 2% in amount of food). Twenty-one food groups, which include 130 food items, are specified (MAPA Ministerio de Agricultura Pesca y Alimentación, 2001).

On this basis, the MD can be characterized by the following four essential dietary indicators:

1. MUFA/SFA between 1.6 and 2.0.
2. A daily intake of DF (as total indigestible fraction) of 41–62 g per capita.
3. A TDAC equivalent to a daily intake of 3500–3500 trolox equivalents per capita (measured by the ABTS method).
4. A daily phytosterols intake of 370–555 mg per capita.

Table 5 Intake of selected foods and nutritional parameters of the Spanish diet*

Food (g or mL/person/day)	1964	2000
Cereals (white bread)	436 (368)	222 (160)
Fruits	162	257
Vegetables (potatoes)	451 (300)	303 (132)
Legumes	41	14
Milk and dairy products	228	414
Fish	63	89
Meat and meat products	77	179
Olive oil	53	31
Wine	130	90
Total energy (Kcal)	3008	2795
Profile (%):		
Protein	11	14
Carbohydrates	58	40
Lipid	31	46
Monounsaturted fatty acids to saturated fatty acids ratio	1.98	1.58

*From the Spanish Ministry of Agriculture, Fisheries, and Food, and National Statistical Institute.

Table 6 Essential dietary indicators in the Mediterranean diet

Indicator	Range	Major contributors
Monounsaturated fatty acids/saturated fatty acids	1.6–2.0	Olive oil
Dietary fiber intake as indigestible fraction intake (g/person/day)	41–62	Cereals: white bread; pasta; rice Fruits: orange; apple; grape Nuts: walnut Vegetables: tomato; potato Legumes: dry beans; chickpeas
Antioxidant activity intake (µmol trolox equivalent/person/day)	3500–5300	Coffee; wine Fruits: Orange; apple; grape Vegetables: tomatoes; onions; capsicum; garlic Legumes
Phytosterols intake (mg/person/day)	370–555	Vegetable oils: Sunflower; olive Cereals: white bread Fruits: orange Legumes: chickpeas Vegetables: tomatoes

Bioactive compounds are integrated in the values of indicators 3 and 4, where they are the major or sole contributors, and partially in indicator 2 as a minor fraction associated with DF. Table 6 indicates the foods that contribute most to these dietary parameters. The majority are traditional Mediterranean foods.

Functional Foods and Healthy Diets

Nowadays, the market offers consumers a large variety of functional foods, dietary supplements, and traditional foods enriched with DF and bioactive compounds. The health claims of these products are often based on short-term studies conducted with doses which exceed the amounts consumed in common diets, while the real effects of long-term consumption are unknown. In order to avoid dietary disorders associated with uncontrolled consumption of functional foods and dietary supplements, it seems only prudent not to exceed the amounts historically ingested in human diets. The intake of bioactive compounds in recognized healthy diets such as the MD may serve as a benchmark until scientific knowledge in this field is sufficiently advanced to establish daily allowances.

A healthy diet, besides the required amounts of energy and nutrients, assures an adequate MUFA/SFA and a sufficient daily intake of DF and bioactive compounds to produce significant effects in the prevention of chronic diseases. Traditional mediterranean foods are rich in these compounds and the MD is a specific type of healthy diet.

References

American Association of Cereal Chemists (AACC). (2001). The definition of dietary fiber. *Cereal Foods World* 46:112–126.

Asp, N-G., van Amelsvoot, J. M. M., and Hautvast, J. G. A. J. (1996). Nutritional implications of resistant starch. *Nutr Res Rev.* 9:1–31.

Bazzano, L. A., He, J., Ogden, L. G., Loria, C. M., Vupputuri, S., Myers, L., and Whelton, P. K. (2002). Fruit and vegetable intake and risk of cardiovascular disease in US adults: the first National Health and Nutrition Examination Survey Epidemiologic Follow-up Study. *Am J Clin Nutr.* 76:93–99.

Beckman, K. B., and Ames, B. N. (1998). The free radical theory of ageing matures. *Physiol Rev.* 78:547–581.

Bjelakovic, G., Nikalova, D., Simonetti, R. G., and Gluud, Ch. (2004). Antioxidant supplements for prevention of gastrointestinal cancers: a systematic review and meta-analysis. *Lancet* 364:1219–1228.

Brighenti, F., Valtueña, S., Pellegrini, N., Ardigò, D., Del Rio, D., Salvatore, S., Piatti, P., Serafini, M., and Zavaroni, I. (2005). Total antioxidant capacity of the diet is inversely and independently related to plasma concentration of high-sensivity C-reactive protein in adult Italian subjects. *Br. J. Nutr.* 93:619–625.

Cho, S. S., and Dreher, M. L. Eds. (2001). Handbook of Dietary Fiber. Marcel Dekker Inc. New York.

Cooper, D. A. (2004). Carotenoids in health and disease: Recent scientific evaluation research, recommendations and the consumer. *J. Nutr.* 134:221S–224S.

Cottet, V., Bonithon-Kopp, C., Kronborg, O., Santos, L., Andreatta, R., Boutron-Ruault, M.-C., and Faivre, J. (2005). Dietary patterns and the risk of colorectal adenoma recurrence in a European intervention trial. *Eur. J. Cancer Prev.* 14(1):21–29.

Cumming, J. H., and Macfarlane, G. T. (1991). The control and consequences of bacterial fermentation in the human colon. *J Appli Bacterol.* 70:443–459.

Djoussé, L., Arnett, D. K., Coon, H., Province, M. A., Moore, L. L., and Ellison, R. C. (2004). Fruit and vegetable consumption and LDL cholesterol: the National Heart, Lung, and Blood Institute Family Heart Study. *Am. J. Clin. Nutr.* 79:213–217.

Elmadfa, I., Weichselbaum, E., König, J., Remaut de Winter, A.-M., Trolle, E., Haapala, I., Uusitalo, U., Mennen, L., Herberg, S., Wolfram, G., Trichopoulou, A., Naska, A., Benetou, V., Kritsellis, E., Rodler, I., Zajkás, G., Branca, F., D'Acapito, P., Klepp, K.-I., Ali-Madar, A., De Almaida, M. D. V., Alves, E., Rodrigues, S., Sarra-Majem, L., Roman, B., Sjöström, M., Poortvliet, E., and Margetts, B. (2005). *European nutrition and health report 2004.* Elmadfa, I., Weichselbaum, E. eds.. Forum of Nutrition. 58: Karger. Vienna, Austria.

Fernandez, M. L., and West, K. L. (2005). Mechanisms by which dietary fatty acids modulate plasma lipids. *J. Nutr.* 135(9):2075–2078.

Fitó, M., Guxens, M., Corella, D., Sáez, G., Estruch, R., De la Torre, R., Francés, F., Cabezas, C., López-Sabater, M. C., Marrugat, J., García-Arellano, A., Arós, F., Ruiz-Gutierrez, V., Ros, E., Salas-Salvadó, J., Fiol, M., Solá, R., and Covas, M. I. (2007). Effect of a traditional Mediterranean diet on lipoprotein oxidation: a randomized controlled trial. *Arch. Intern. Med.* 167:1195–1203.

Gibney, M. J., and Roche, H. M. (2001). Nutrition policy issues and further research on the Mediterranean diet: the importance of monounsaturated fatty acids. In: *The Mediterranean Diet: constituents and health promotion.* pp. 53–73. Matalas, A-L., Zampelas, A., Stavrinus, V., and Wolinsky, I. Eds., C. R. C. Press Modern Nutrition, Boca Raton, Fla. USA.

Goñi, I., Serrano, J., and Saura-Calixto, F. (2006). Bioaccessibility β-carotene, lutein and lycopene from fruits and vegetables. *J. Agric. Food Chem.* 54:5382–5387.

Goñi, I. (2001). Dietary fiber intake in Spain: Recommendations and actual consumption patterns. In: Handbook of dietary fiber. pp. 777–785. Cho, S.S., and Dreher, M. L. Eds. Marcel Dekker, New York.

Hu, F. B. (2003). The Mediterranean Diet and mortality olive oil and beyond. *N. Eng. J. Med.* 348(26):2595–2596.

Jiménez-Escrig, A., Santos-Hidalgo, A. B., and Saura-Calixto, F. (2006). Common sources and estimated intake of plant sterols in the Spanish diet. *J. Agric. Food Chem.* 54(9):3462–3471.

Knoops, K. T., de Groot, L. C., Kromhout, D., Perrin, A. E., Moreiras-Varela, O., Menotti, A., and van Staveren, W. A. (2004). Mediterranean Diet, lifestyle factors, and 10-year mortality in elderly European men and women: the HALE project. *JAMA.* 292(12):1490–1492.

Krichevsky, D., and Bonfield, Ch. Eds. (1995). Dietary fiber in health and disease. Eagan Press, St. Paul, MN. USA.

Kritchevsky, D., and Chen, S. C. (2005). Phytosterols health benefits and potential concerns: a review. *Nutr. Res.* **25**:413–428.

Manach, C., Williamson, Ch. M., Scalbert, A., and Rémésy, Ch. (2005). Bioavailability and bioefficacy of polyphenols in humans. I. Review of 97 bioavailability studies. *Am. J. Clin. Nutr.* **81**(S):230S–242S.

MAPA, Ministerio de Agricultura Pesca y Alimentación. (2001). La alimentación en España, 2000. Secretaría General de Agricultura y Alimentación, Madrid, Spain.

Martinez-González, M. A., and Estruch, R. (2004). Mediterranean Diet, antioxidants and cancer: the need for randomized trials. *Am. J. Cardiol.* **94**(10):1260–1267.

Naska, A., Fouskakis, D., Oikonomou, E., Almeida, M. D. V., Berg, M. A., Gedrich, K., Moreiras, O., Nelson, M., Trygg, K., Turrini, A., Remaut, A. M., Volatier, J. L., Trichopoulou, A., and DAFNE participants. (2006). Dietary patterns and their socio-demographic determinants in 10 European countries: data from the DAFNE databank. *Eur. J. Clin. Nutr.* **60** (2): 181–190.

Normén, A. L., Brants, H. A. M., Voorrips, L. E., Anderson, H. A., van den Brandt, P. A., and Goldbohm, R. A. (2001). Plant sterols intake and colorectal cancer risk in the Netherlands Cohort Study on diet and cancer. *Am. J. Clin. Nutr.* **74**:141–148.

Pitsavos, Ch., Panagiotakos, D. B., Tzima, N., Chrysohoou, Ch., Economou, M., Zampelas, A., and Stefanadis, Ch. (2005). Adherente to the Mediterranean Diet is associated with total antioxidant capacity in healthy adults: the ATTICA study. *Am. J. Clin. Nutr.* **82**:694–699.

Prosky, L., Asp, N-G., Schweizer, Y. F., De Vries, J., and Furda, I. (1992). Determination of insoluble and soluble dietary fiber in foods and food products: Collaborative study. *J. AOAC Int.* **75**(2):360–367.

Psaltopoulou, T., Naska, A., Orfanos, P., Trichopoulos, D., Mountokalakis, T., and Trichopoulou, A. (2004). Olive oil, the Mediterranean diet, and arterial blood pressure: the Greek European Prospective Investigation into Cancer and Nutrition (EPIC) study. *Am. J. Clin. Nutr.* **80**(4):1012–1018.

Pulido, R., Hernández-García, M., and Saura-Calixto, F. (2003). Contribution of beverages to the intake of lipophilic and hydrophilic antioxidants in the Spanish diet. *Eur. J. Clin. Nutr.* **57**:1275–1282.

Regmi, A., Ballenger, N., and Putnam, J. (2004). Globalisation and income growth promote the Mediterranean Diet. *Public Health Nutr.* **7**(7):977–983.

Renaud, S., and Lorgeril, M. (1992). Wine, alcohol, platelets, and the French paradox for coronary heart disease. *Lancet:*1532–1527.

Saura-Calixto, F., García-Alonso, A., Goñi, I., and Bravo, L. (2000). In vitro determination of the indigestible fraction in foods: an alternative to dietary fiber analysis. *J. Agric. Food Chem.* **48**:3342–3347.

Saura-Calixto, and F., Goñi, I. (2006). Antioxidant capacity of the Spanish Mediterranean diet. *Food Chem.* **94**:442–447.

Saura-Calixto, F., and Goñi, I. (1993). Dietary fiber intakes in Spain. In: Dietary fiber intakes in Europe. pp 67–75. Cummings, J. H., and Frolich, W. European Communities, Luxembourg.

Saura-Calixto, F., and Goñi, I. (2005). Fibra dietética y antioxidantes en la dieta española y en alimentos funcionales. In: Alimentos funcionales. pp.167–200. Fundación Española para la Ciencia y Tecnología (FECYT), Madrid, Spain.

Saura-Calixto, F., and Goñi, I. (2004). The intake of dietary indigestible fraction in the Spanish diet shows the limitations of dietary fibre data for nutritional studies. *Eur. J. Clin. Nutr.* **58**:1078–1082.

Saura-Calixto, F., Serrano, J., and Goñi, I. (2007). Intake and bioaccessibility of total polyphenols in a whole diet. *Food Chem.* **101**(2):492–501.

Serafini, M., Bellocco, R., Wolk, A., and Ekstrom, A. M. (2003). Total antioxidant potential of fruit and vegetables and risk of gastric cancer. *Gastroenterology* **124**(7):2006–2007.

Serra-Majem, L., Roman, B., and Estruch, R. (2006). Scientific evidence of interventions using the Mediterranean Diet: A systematic review. *Nutr Rev.* **64**(2):S27–S47.

Stephen, A. (1991). Starch and dietary fibre: their physiological and epidemiological interrelationships. *Can J Physiol Pharmacol.* **69**:116–120.

Svilaas, A., Sakhi, A. K., Andersen, L. F., Svilaas, T., Ström, E. C., Jacobs, D. R., Ose, L., and Blomhoff, R. (2004). Intakes of antioxidants in coffee, wine, and vegetables are correlated with plasma carotenoids in humans. *J. Nutr.* **134**:562–567.

Tapiero, H., Townsend, D. M., and Tew, K. D. (2004). The role of carotenoids in the prevention of human pathologies. *Biomed Pharacother.* **58**:100–110.

Trichopoulou, A., Costacou, T., Bamia, Ch., and Trichopoulos, D. (2003). Adherence to a Mediterranean Diet and survival in a Greek population. *N. Engl. J. Med.* **348**(26):2599–2608.

Trichopoulou, A., and Lagiou, P. (2001). The Mediterranean Diet: Definition, epidemiological aspects and current patterns. In: The Mediterranean Diet: constituents and health promotion. pp. 53–73. Matalas, A-L., Zampelas, A., Stavrinus, V., and Wolinsky, I., Eds. C. R. C. Press Modern Nutrition, Boca Raton, Fla. USA.

Trichopoulou, A., Orfanos, P., Norat, T., Bueno de Mesquita, B., Ocke, M. C., Peeters, P. H., van der Schouw, Y. T., Boeing, H., Hoffmann, K., Boffeta, P., Nagel, G., Masala, G., Krogh, V., Panico, S., Tumino, R., Vineis, P., Bamia, C., Naska, A., Benetou, V., Ferrari, P., Slimani, N., Pera, G., Martinez-García, C., Navarro, C., Rodriguez-Barranco, M., Dorronsoro, M., Spencer, E. A., Key, T. J., Bingham, S., Khaw, K. T., Kesse, E., Clavel-Chapelon, F., Boutron-Ruault, M. C., Berglund, G., Wirfalt, E., Hallmans, G., Johansson, I., Tjonneland, A., Olsen, A., Overvad, K., Hundborg, H. H., Riboli, E., and Trichopoulos, D. (2005). Modified Mediterranean Diet and survival: EPIC-elderly prospective cohort study. *Brit. Med. J.* **330**:991–994.

Trowell, H., Southgate, D. A. T., Wolever, T. M. S., Leeds, A. R., Gassull, M. A., and Jenkins, D. J. A. (1976). Dietary fiber redefined. *Lancet:***1**:967

Valsta, L. M., Lemströn, A., and Ovaskaimen, M.-L. (2004). Estimation of plant sterol and cholesterol intake in Finland: quality of new values and their effect on intake. *Br. J. Nutr.* **92**:671–678.

Vincent-Baudry, S., Defoort, C., Gerber, M., Bernard, M.-Ch., Verger, P., Helal, O., Portugal, H., Planells, R., Grolier, P., Amiot-Carlin,

M.-J., Vague, Ph., and Lairon, D. (2005). The Medi-RIVAGE study: reduction of cardiovascular disease risk factors after a 3-mo intervention with a Mediterranean-type Diet or a low-fat diet. *Am. J. Clin. Nutr.* **82**(5):964–971.

Vissers, M. N., Zock, P. L., and Katan, M. B. (2004). Bioavailability and antioxidant effects of olive oil phenols in humans: a review. *Eur. J. Clin. Nutr.* **58**:955–965.

Williamson, G., and Manach, C. (2005). Bioavailability and bioefficacy of polyphenols in humans. II. Review of 93 intervention studies. *Am. J. Clin. Nutr.* **81**(S): 243S–255S.

Critical Thinking

1. What are polyphenols and carotenoids? How do they function to protect human health?
2. What does the acronym TDAC stand for? What units are used in TDAC measurements?
3. How do plant sterols (phytosterols) lower cholesterol levels in the blood?

Acknowledgement—The authors thank the Spanish Ministerio de Ciencia e Innovación for financial support (Project AGL2005 04769).

Have a Coke and a Tax

The Economic Case against Soda Taxes

VERONIQUE DE RUGY

With the federal deficit reaching $.4 trillion and most state budgets deep in the red, policy makers are desperately searching for new sources of revenue that the tapped-out American public might support. They think they've found one at the corner store: a tax on carbonated beverages. Charging a few more cents for a soft drink, legislators claim, will not only refresh exhausted state and federal revenues; it will make us thinner.

Several versions of this year's health care bills included a soda tax to help offset new costs. In a September interview with *Men's Health,* President Barack Obama called it "an idea that we should be exploring" because "our kids drink way too much soda." The idea had been dropped from the health care legislation at press time but is expected to resurface next year.

The proposal is perennially popular on the state and local levels too. Thirty-three states tax the sale of soft drinks, at an average rate of 5.2 percent, and politicians in other jurisdictions are eager to jump on the bandwagon. After New York Gov. David A. Patterson floated the idea of a soda tax in December 2008, New York City Mayor Michael Bloomberg launched his own campaign to tax sugary drinks. "All the studies show that young kids drink an enormous amount of soda, and if they drink the sodas with all the sugar in it, it adds a great deal of weight to them," Bloomberg said in April.

The economic literature tells a different story. The rationale behind a tax on soft drinks, or any sin tax, is that when the government raises prices on a certain good, it will become so expensive that consumers will give it up. Having been forced to eschew that sin because of the high monetary price, consumers will reap the moral and/ or physical benefits of not indulging, thereby bettering themselves and society.

The story sounds plausible. The trouble is that sin taxers don't appreciate human creativity: Consumers have a knack for replacing one sin with another. When the price of a "sinful" good increases, people often substitute an equally "bad" good in its place.

The trouble is that sin taxers don't appreciate human creativity: Consumers have a knack for replacing one sin with another.

A 1998 study by William N. Evans, an economist at the University of Notre Dame du Lac, and Matthew C. Farrelly, a public health researcher at RTI International, found that smokers in high-tax states tend to consume cigarettes that are longer and higher in tar and nicotine than smokers in low-tax states. This effect is especially pronounced among 18-to-24-year-olds because they are more responsive to tax changes than older smokers. They have less money, so they want more bang for their bucks.

A 1992 study by University of Michigan economist John E. DiNardo and University of British Columbia economist Thomas Lemieux found that when states raised beer taxes or increased the minimum drinking age, teen marijuana consumption increased. A 1994 study by University of Illinois economist Frank Chaloupka and Chulalongkorn University economist Adit Laixuthai replicated those results—and also found that beer consumption declined in states that decriminalized marijuana.

Are soda lovers likely to do something similar? Richard Williams and Katelyn Christ, two economists at the Mercatus Center (where I work), argue that soda drinkers would. In a 2009 study, they wrote: "The assumption is that this sin tax would reduce caloric intake because consumers would stop drinking high-calorie drinks and/ or switch to lower-calorie drinks. However . . . if consumers respond to the proposed sin tax on sodas and sports drinks by switching to some of the potential substitute drinks [see table], their caloric intake would either remain the same or actually increase."

In a 2008 working paper, Emory University economists Jason Fletcher, David Frisvold and Nathan Tefft examined the impact that changes in states' taxation rates from 1990 to 2006 had on body mass index and obesity. They concluded that soft drink taxes have a vanishingly small impact on weight because, even when untaxed, soft drinks represent only 7 percent of the average soda drinker's total calorie intake.

Yet in a recent *New England Journal of Medicine* article, Arkansas' surgeon general, New York City's health commissioner, and five experts on health and economics insisted that a penny-per-ounce tax on sugared beverages could lead the average consumer to reduce soda consumption by about 10 percent and lose two pounds. The authors argue that the soda tax would

Table 1 Calories Per Cup of Popular Drinks

Drink	Calories Per Cup
Gatorade	63
Coca Cola	97
Orange Juice	105
Apple Juice (unsweetened)	117
2% Milk	120
Homemade Cocoa w/Skim Milk	135
Sweetened Lemonade	131
Whole Chocolate Milk (4%)	208
Red Table Wine	200

Source: Richard Williams and Katelyn Christ, "Taxing Sin," *Mercatus On Policy,* August 18, 2009, online at mercatus.org/PublicationDetails. aspx?id=27916.

be effective at reducing the number of soda drinkers because the federal cigarette tax, which amounts on average to $1.34 per cigarette pack, has been effective at reducing the number of smokers. Yet several widely reported studies found that the tax on cigarettes as a whole has reduced smoking in adults by just 2 percent and in teens by 7 percent.

So the soda tax won't do much to help us lose weight. But does it raise much revenue? Supporters say yes, but there's a problem here too. If the tax is effective at discouraging soda consumption, it won't raise much money because people won't be buying soda. Which does the government actually prefer? Skinnier citizens or fatter coffers?

Last July the Congressional Budget Office estimated that a federal three-cent-per-12-ounce soft drink tax would generate $24 billion over the next four years. Needless to say, that won't fix the current budget crisis, but the *NEJM* authors argue that

it could have an effect on obesity rates in America. They propose using any money raised by the tax for child nutrition and obesity prevention programs. That way, the thinking goes, even if people still drink soda the tax will help the fight against fat.

If that does happen, the government won't be able to use the funds to reduce the deficit, subsidize health insurance, or fulfill the other hopes politicians have for the money. But there's a fair chance it wouldn't happen in the first place. Governments don't always spend sin tax money the way they promise. Money from the Master Settlement Agreement, the deal that ended state litigation against the major tobacco companies, was supposed to fund smoking cessation programs and defray the costs that smoking imposes on public health systems. Once they had the money, though, states used it as a giant slush fund, diverting it to schools, roads, and various pet projects. They even invested some of it in tobacco stocks.

Americans may be fat, but the federal budget is morbidly obese; our hunger for chips and soda is nothing compared to the feds' hunger for our money. If I had to choose between putting the average citizen or the government on a diet, I know which would be better for our fiscal health.

Critical Thinking

1. Other than an easy revenue stream, why are taxes on soda being considered by federal, state, and local governments?
2. What type of health related programs is the government proposing to fund with the revenue from the soda tax?
3. What is the opinion of the economist who wrote this article on the overall effectiveness of "sin taxes"?

Contributing Editor VERONIQUE DE RUGY is a senior research fellow at the Mercatus Center at George Mason University.

Pepsi Brings in the Health Police

The snack food behemoth has hired a team of idealistic scientists to find alternatives to Doritos.

NANETTE BYRNES

In February 2007, when Derek Yach, a former executive director of the World Health Organization and an expert on nutrition, took a new job with PepsiCo, his mother worried that he'd lost his mind. "You are aware they sell soda and chips, and these things cause you to get unhealthy and fat?" she asked him. Yach's former colleagues in public health circles murmured similar concerns.

Yes, he said, he knew what Pepsi made. But he wanted to help guide the $43 billion snack food multinational toward a more balanced product menu. The company describes its current portfolio of "healthy" fare as a $10 billion business—a figure CEO Indra Nooyi says she wants to see jump to $30 billion over the next decade.

The question is, will Yach, now senior vice-president for global health policy, really have the influence his boss has promised? If he does, will Pepsi's strategy prove profitable? Can its growing team of health advocates—who in times past might have seen Pepsi as the enemy—come up with an apple treat that tastes as good as a deep-fried Lay's potato chip?

Over the past two years, Pepsi has hired a dozen physicians and PhDs, many of whom built their reputations at the Mayo Clinic, WHO, and like-minded institutions. Some researched diabetes and heart disease, the sort of ailments that can result in part from eating too much of what Pepsi sells.

Yach and his comrades aren't subversives. The goal, says Mehmood Kahn, Pepsi's first-ever chief scientific officer, is to create healthy options while making the bad stuff less bad. "It's O.K. to have a slice of birthday cake on your birthday," says Kahn, formerly a practicing physician specializing in nutrition who did a stint at the Mayo Clinic. "Would you eat it every day of the week? That's a different question." At Pepsi, he and the other scientists "can say we can actually make an impact on what is available for consumers."

Flight From Junk Food

Khan hunts for benign ingredients that can go into multiple products. Last year, technological improvements to an all-natural zero-calorie sweetener derived from a plant called stevia allowed Pepsi to devise several fast-growing brands, including Trop50, a variation on its Tropicana orange juice that has half the calories of the breakfast standby. Introduced in March, Trop50 has become a $100 million brand. Two Trop50 line extensions are hitting the shelves: Pomegranate Blueberry and Pineapple Mango.

Chief Executive Nooyi says she has no choice but to move in healthier directions. For more than 15 years, consumers have gradually defected from the carbonated soft drinks that once comprised 90% of Pepsi's beverage business. Many switched to bottled water. Meanwhile, the cloud of criticism shadowing Pepsi's largest business, oil- and salt-laden Frito Lay snacks, grew steadily. The company acquired Quaker Oats and other wholesome brands but until recently didn't emphasize research. Nooyi, who took over in 2006, is changing that. She has increased the R&D budget 38% over three years, to $388 million in 2008.

"Society, people, and lifestyles have changed," Nooyi says. "The R&D needs for this new world are also different." Her goal of expanding healthy products to $30 billion in sales would require annual growth in those lines of more than 10%, twice the company's overall historical average.

> ## Society, people, and lifestyles have changed. The R&D needs for this new world are also different.

Coming off a tough 2009, during which once high-flying brands such as Gatorade slipped, Pepsi hasn't convinced Wall Street that Nooyi's plans will pay off. The company trades at a significant discount to its rival, Coca-Cola. While securities analysts say that healthier foods look like a good long-term market, for now, the slowdown in the company's far larger traditional snack-and-soda portfolio cannot be ignored. "The consumer can move to baked chips, or pretzels, or Sun Chips, but they're not yet giving up their chips for an apple or carrot stick," says Bill Pecoriello, CEO of Consumer Edge Research, an independent stock-research firm in Stamford, Conn.

Pepsi built its empire on the manufacture and distribution of instantly recognizable products. It could get a bag of Lay's or a can of Mountain Dew to customers practically anywhere in the world. So far, healthier options have produced only modest hits, including TrueNorth nut snacks and SoBe Life-water. "We're not building Pepsi again," Nooyi says. She aims to sell a wider variety of products to meet all kinds of consumer demands.

Pepsi's health push includes a controversial plan to sell new products to undernourished people in India and other developing countries. This isn't charity, notes Nooyi, herself a native of India. The goal is to make money. As one of its exploratory ventures, Pepsi is supporting a nonprofit operation in Nigeria that distributes a protein-rich peanut-based paste. Khan says that once the company has figured out what's needed most, Pepsi will shift to for-profit production of nutritionally beneficial processed foods.

One potential hazard of marketing in the developing world is that Pepsi could be accused of trading on misfortune and not serving the overall dietary needs of the poor—a criticism that has haunted sellers of infant formula. Kelly D. Brownell, director of the Yale University Rudd Center for Food Policy & Obesity, says Pepsi's developing-nations initiative deserves scrutiny. But Brownell, an industry critic, praises Pepsi for improvements in its mainstream products, such as removing bad fats from its chips. "They're the most progressive player in the industry," he says.

Critical Thinking

1. What are some of the changes that have been made to improve Pepsi's image as a soda and snack food company?

2. What three products have been developed as healthier versions of processed foods/beverages?

3. How much money is Pepsi expecting to earn from healthy products by the year 2020?

From *Bloomberg BusinessWeek,* January 25, 2010, pp. 50–51. Copyright © 2010 by Bloomberg BusinessWeek. Reprinted by permission of Bloomberg LP.

Calorie Posting in Chain Restaurants

SARAH H. WRIGHT

Nutrition labeling on packaged food has been mandatory in the United States since the early 1990s, and printing tiny lists on cans and bags has long been accepted practice. Yet, in spite of this improvement in providing information, the share of Americans who are obese has continued to rise, increasing from 15.9 percent in 1995 to 26.6 percent in 2008.

The fraction of calories consumed in restaurants also has risen in recent years. In 2008, New York City extended nutrition labeling to chain restaurants, requiring them to post clearly the number of calories in every one of their foods and beverages. In March 2010, new federal health care legislation mandated calorie posting for chain restaurants nationwide beginning in 2011. Will these point-of-purchase postings have any public health effect? Could menus with "350 calories" printed beside "eight grain roll" drive a consumer to buy a banana (100 calories) instead?

In **Calorie Posting in Chain Restaurants** (NBER Working Paper No. 15648), study authors **Bryan Bollinger, Phillip Leslie,** and **Alan Sorensen** ask whether mandatory calorie posting influences consumers' purchase decisions. They use detailed data from Starbucks stores in New York City, where calories are posted; from Starbucks in Boston and Philadelphia, where calories are not posted; and from Starbucks stores throughout the nation. The researchers find that mandatory calorie posting influenced consumer behavior at Starbucks in New York City, causing average calories per transaction to drop by 6 percent (from 247 to 232 calories). They also find that these effects are long lasting: after the posting began, the calorie reduction persisted for at least 10 months (the duration of the sample period). There is also evidence of persistent learning effects: commuters who lowered their calories per transaction on weekdays in New York City also lowered them in transactions at Starbucks outside the city, where calories were not posted.

Mandatory calorie posting influenced consumer behavior at Starbucks in New York City, causing average calories per transaction to drop by 6 percent.

The researchers also find that almost all of the calorie-reduction effects in Starbucks are related to food—not beverage—purchases. Following calorie posting, average food calories per transaction fell by 14 percent. The effect is larger for high-calorie consumers: individuals who averaged more than 250 calories per transaction reacted to calorie posting by decreasing calories per transaction by 26 percent—dramatically more than the 6 percent average reduction for all consumers.

Beverage consumption was largely unaffected by calorie posting. Consumers tended to underestimate the calories contained in Starbucks' food and bakery items, but they overestimated the calories contained in Starbucks beverages. According to the researchers, consumers who discovered by calorie posting that an Iced Cafe Latte contains just 130 calories were pleasantly surprised—continued buying.

Noting that calorie reductions on the order of 6 percent at chain restaurants would yield only modest decreases in body weight, the researchers suggest that the direct effect of calorie posting on U.S. obesity may be small. The most meaningful effect of the calorie posting law may be its long-run impact on menu choices, as restaurants will have an economic incentive to offer low-calorie options. The new policy may also benefit public health as consumers grow accustomed to counting calories and choose or demand healthier foods.

The study also explores how calorie posting affected corporate profits. The authors find that it did not cause any significant change in Starbucks' overall revenue. At Starbucks stores located within 100 meters of a Dunkin Donuts store, revenue actually increased by 3 percent—suggesting that calorie posting may have caused some consumers to substitute away from Dunkin Donuts toward Starbucks.

Critical Thinking

1. What year will mandatory calorie posting be enforced for chain restaurants?

2. How did calorie posting affect consumer behavior of Starbucks customers?

3. What will be the long-term impact on a restaurant's menu offering a likely increased demand for lower-calorie items?

A Burger and Fries (Hold the Trans Fats)

Restaurants respond to demand for healthier oils.

Several cities have already put a ban on trans fats. Even if yours isn't one of them, you can still help your patients avoid the danger of these artery-clogging oils.

LINDSEY GETZ

Restaurants across the United States have been slowly making progress toward eliminating trans fats from their menus. Cities such as New York, Philadelphia, and Boston have already placed a ban on the use of these fats in restaurants, while California recently became the first to introduce a statewide ban. It's expected that such bans will continue across the country as consumers begin to recognize the importance of eliminating dangerous trans fats from their diets and demand a change in what restaurants are serving up.

"When California's Gov. Schwarzenegger signed the bill banning trans fats as of January 1, 2010, I think restaurants got the message loud and clear that this change will most likely spread nationwide quickly," suggests Joanne "Dr. Jo" Lichten, PhD, RD, creator of *Dr. Jo's Eat Out & Lose Weight Plan.*

Trans fats are formed when liquid oils are converted into solid fat through hydrogenation. Consuming trans fats can lead to heart disease by raising LDL cholesterol and simultaneously lowering HDL cholesterol. A study published in *The New England Journal of Medicine* in 2006 estimated that approximately 228,000 coronary heart disease occurrences could be avoided by reducing trans fat consumption or eliminating these fats from the American diet. Unfortunately, many popular foods contain them, and many Americans consume these foods in excess. The FDA estimates that the average American consumes approximately 4.7 pounds of trans fats every year.

Trans fats are especially common in baked goods, as they aid with preservation. "I tell my clients that trans fats are essentially a man-made fat," says Sara Shama, RD, director of nutrition for Kingley Health in New Jersey. "It helps Twinkies stay on the shelf for six years without going bad. Baked goods are supposed to go bad!"

Stephanie Dean, RD, LD, coauthor of the book *Fit to Serve,* adds, "While trans fats were created to increase the shelf life of foods, consumers can increase their own 'shelf life' by eliminating trans fats from their diets."

A Change for the Better

Fortunately, many restaurants and chains across the country are making changes—even if they aren't located in a city with a ban. The Cheesecake Factory was one of the leaders pioneering these changes in the industry. "Nearly two years ago, our management team and kitchen staff began partnering with our foodservice manufacturers to work toward the elimination of trans fats from our menu," says Mark Mears, senior vice president and chief of marketing for the company.

The restaurants of Passion Food Hospitality, including DC Coast, TenPenh, Ceiba, and Acadiana, located in Washington, D.C., decided to seek alternatives to trans fats about two years ago. Since losing 125 pounds, chef/owner Jeff Tunks decided to prepare his light dishes even lighter and healthier by eliminating trans fats. "I am the first to admit I would eat a fried shrimp po'boy every day if I could," he says. "But when I take that first bite, it surely sets me at ease to know there is not trans fat in the oil."

Fast-food restaurants, which are one of the biggest culprits of foods high in trans fats, have been quick to follow. Chains such as Burger King, McDonald's, and Hardee's have announced a switch to zero trans fat oils for their cooking. Subway, a chain that had very little trans fats in its food in the first place, has completely eliminated it from its core menu as well. "We always look for ways to improve our products," says Les Winograd, a Subway spokesman. "We have a reputation for offering healthy alternatives to traditional, fatty fast foods. Eliminating even the small amount of trans fats we had was just another way of improving."

Even hotels are recognizing the importance of switching to a healthier alternative. Last year, Carlson Hotels Worldwide announced plans to eliminate shortening containing trans fats at the majority of its hotels. The Radisson Fort McDowell Resort & Casino in Scottsdale, Ariz., was one of the hotels that participated in the pilot program. The resort's restaurant, the Ahnala Mesquite Room, successfully eliminated trans fats from its menu in October 2006 and found that guests actually preferred the flavor of its healthier alternatives and appreciated the restaurant's effort to emphasize good health.

Many restaurants have reported no change in taste after switching to a healthier alternative. Of course, each restaurant has its own alternative formula. McDonald's, for instance, uses a canola oil cooking blend for its fried items, such as French fries, chicken, and its Filet-O-Fish sandwiches. The Cheesecake Factory reports using a blend of olive and canola oils to replace the oils previously used for cooking. "In making the switch to trans fat-free cooking oils, our guests have reported no discernable taste differences to our unique menu items," says Mears, who adds that the switch has not affected menu pricing.

The public has responded positively to increased healthy options—especially those with no trans fat. "Our customers rave about the freshness and selection of ingredients," says Thomas DuBois, CEO and founder of Tomato Tamoto, a new made-to-order salad bar restaurant that recently opened in Plano, Tex.

Of course, that's not to say there haven't been any complaints since these bans first took effect. Much of the initial resistance was due to the high cost of trans fat-free oils, says Lichten. "But as more and more restaurants switch over, this has increased the availability from the oil companies," she adds. "Many restaurants have found that the trans fat-free oils are the same price or even lower."

Some in the restaurant industry have also complained that it's not the government or any other agency's place to ban these fats. Dan Fleshler, a spokesman for the National Restaurant Association, was quoted in 2006 (when New York City's Board of Health voted to make it the nation's first city to ban trans fats) as saying, "We don't think that a municipal health agency has any business banning a product that the Food and Drug Administration has already approved."

However, most restaurants have willingly complied—or even made changes without being placed under a ban—and the general public has been happy with the changes. And dietitians surely agree it's been a change for the better. "Even though it's each person's individual right to choose what they want to consume, as a nation, I believe we should be looking out for the well-being of our people," says Shama. "Everyone's lives are busy and everyone is on the go, and there are times they have to rely on fast or convenient foods. They should be comforted in knowing that whatever they do pick up is something that's not going to give them heart disease because of having trans fats. We have to give people choice, but we still need to look out for their best interest."

Helping Your Patients

Regardless of whether your city has a ban, there seems to be a lot of confusion surrounding trans fats, especially since it's become such a hot news item in the last couple of years. Shama says her patients ask her many questions, but she tries to make it simple. "I call them the artery-clogging, heart disease-causing fats," she says. "That makes it pretty clear."

Elaine Pelc, RD, LDN, of Baltimore, gives patients a visual picture to help them get the point. "I tell my patients to

think about what bacon grease does when it cools: It solidifies," she explains. "I tell them that trans fats do the same thing in your arteries. And when they solidify, they clog up the arteries."

Dietitians can help their patients make wiser choices when dining out, regardless of whether they reside in a city with a trans fat ban. Shama tells clients to check up on places where they plan to eat. "If they know where they're going to eat, they can look up the menu online," she says. "If they take the time to check out the menu beforehand and get a sense of what some of the healthier options are, they'll be less likely to opt for the colossal cheese-burger with fries."

"There are no health benefits of trans fats, and no level is considered to be safe," adds Janel Ovrut, MS, RD, LDN, who is based in Boston. "I tell my clients that when it comes to how much trans fats are in their diet, they should stick to zero."

Ovrut says that Boston's ban on trans fats has taken the guesswork out of which restaurant foods contain them. "Now we can all rest assured that the answer is 'none,'" she says. "I think that Boston residents take pride in the fact that we're part of a health initiative that will hopefully guide other cities and towns to make the same changes. The ban has also created more buzz about the harmful effects of trans fats, and consumers are starting to realize the negative impact after a unanimous vote that forbid trans fats from dining establishments. Consumers take notice and are hopefully making changes in their at-home eating habits as well."

Consumer habits are certainly an issue. Even if people live in an area where a ban is in place, they still may be consuming trans fats at home. That's why it's important to help clients be more proactive about their nutrition, not only when dining out but also when purchasing groceries.

"I advise my clients to read the ingredient list on foods," says Ovrut. "Just because a package says 'zero trans fats' per serving doesn't mean the product is completely void of partially hydrogenated oil. Products can be promoted as trans fat-free as long as there is less than 0.5 grams per serving. But once you consume more than one serving of a product—which is easy to do with packaged snacks or baked goods—you're creeping up toward 1 gram or more of trans fats. Some food manufacturers are even decreasing the listed serving size of their product so that it meets the trans fat-free guidelines. Consumers are hungry for more and often eat double or triple the serving size."

However, as a result of consumers' interest in trans fat-free products, some manufacturers—just like many restaurants—have decided to eliminate it, says Lichten. "But remember, trans fat-free still does not mean fewer calories. Most trans fat-free products have exactly the same amount of fat and calories as the original," she notes.

A Balanced Diet

Even without reading the ingredient list, patients can have a good idea of which foods might contain trans fat. These include premade desserts, butter spreads, convenience foods, and fried items, says Dean. These are the types of foods that clients should avoid in general.

They also tend to be the products that have a long list of ingredients, adds Stella Lucia Volpe, PhD, RD, LDN, FACSM, an associate professor and the Miriam Stirl Term Endowed Chair of Nutrition at the University of Pennsylvania School of Nursing in Philadelphia. "If you look at a packaged product and it has an extremely long list of ingredients, chances are it's probably not very good for you and may contain trans fats," she explains. "I advise clients to try to make pure food choices. Natural, unprocessed foods like lean meat, fish, fruits, or vegetables are always the best option."

While the increased awareness surrounding the dangers of trans fat has been wonderful, one potential problem with the focus on switching to "healthier alternatives" is that consumers may start to believe that certain foods are healthy just because they don't have trans fat. With or without trans fats, French fries are not a healthy choice. Clients need to know that trans fat-free items may be better for you than those with the dangerous fat, but they still aren't necessarily healthy. "It's important to make healthy choices in general," says Pelc. "People should be limiting their intake of these foods anyway in order to maintain a healthy lifestyle. Choosing trans fat-free foods does not mean that you are choosing healthy foods. It's important for clients to remember that removing trans fat from a food does not necessarily make it a healthy choice."

Most restaurants have willingly complied— or even made changes without being placed under a ban—and the general public has been happy with the changes.

"Just because it says they have zero trans fat still doesn't mean those potato chips or French fries were the best option on the menu," adds Volpe. "I typically try to work on portion control with my clients. If they really love something like potato chips and won't give them up, we can at least work on limiting their portion."

The bottom line? Getting clients to eat a healthy, well-balanced diet may not happen overnight, but helping them eliminate or even simply cut down on trans fat is definitely a step in the right direction.

Critical Thinking

1. Identify three cities and one state that have banned the use of trans fats in restaurants. Do you think this is a good idea? Explain your answer.

2. Why did food scientists create trans fats?

3. Why are trans fats considered a "bad fat"? How can you best avoid trans fats in your diet?

LINDSEY GETZ is a freelance writer based in Royersford, Pa.

The Potential of Farm-to-College Programs

Colleges and universities across the United States are increasingly sourcing the food for their dining halls from local farms through farm-to-college (FTC) programs. Although participation in FTC programs may increase the visibility of the school to prospective students and parents, support the local economy, and introduce new options into campus eateries, FTC programs face a number of operational barriers. Inadequate student support, institutional procurement policies, and seasonality limit the reach of FTC efforts. This article discusses these barriers in detail through the perspective of New England higher education institutions and uses Tufts University as a case study in the challenges and potential for FTC programs to become mainstream in college and university food service.

KATHLEEN A. MERRIGAN, PhD AND MELISSA BAILEY, MS

The demand for local food has been stimulated, among other things, by Michael Pollan's best-selling book *Omnivore's Dilemma,* food safety scares, and advocacy organizations seeking to support family farms. As a result, the share of food spending that US consumers put toward the purchase of local farm products is increasing as individual households, K-12 school systems, and, more recently, university and college dining halls join the "buy local" food movement.[1] Many institutions of higher education now have procurement managers and food service directors who specifically work toward connecting the consumer (the students frequenting their dining facilities) to the producer of the food served (local farmers) through what are called "farm-to-college" (FTC) programs. The implementation of FTC programs is meant to support the goals of the broader buy-local movement. These include preservation of farmland from development pressure by keeping farmers in business, support of local economies within a community via retention of dollars spent at local farms and grocers, improved freshness and flavor through minimizing food travel time, and reductions in energy used in trucking and shipping to transport foods to their destination.[2]

Regardless of the specific goals that a given FTC program strives to meet, it is often the implementation of the FTC program itself that proves difficult for both farmers and universities. These difficulties can be further complicated in the northeastern United States because of its short farm season and relatively small agricultural base. This article uses Tufts University as a case study to demonstrate the barriers faced by New England higher educational institutions in their journey to start and maintain a successful FTC effort. Data from the National FTC Survey conducted by the Community Food Security Coalition (CFSC) confirm that the Tufts experience is common to many New England universities and colleges and that food service providers in the Northeast share similar motivations, barriers, and opportunities while participating in the FTC movement.

What Motivates the Creation of FTC Programs?

Each college that participates in FTC programs has different operational characteristics that influence its ability to adopt the practice of local food sourcing. In the case of Tufts University, the main campus, which is located in Medford, Massachusetts, has 2 main dining halls that serve an undergraduate population of 4,900 students. In a sense, Tufts has a "captured" consumer who must purchase from the dining facilities because all freshmen and sophomores at Tufts are required to participate in a meal plan, although it is optional for juniors and seniors. In general, Tufts' meal plans combine dining hall meals with "Dining Dollars" that can be used elsewhere on campus (eg, vending machines) or at a number of other on-campus eateries (eg, grab-n-go service, campus convenience store). Graduate students, staff, and faculty also use the various on-campus eateries, although far less frequently than do the undergraduate students. All of the eateries are self-operated by Tufts University Dining Services (TUDS). Food suppliers/vendors are in a contractual relationship for their services with the university.

The FTC program at Tufts began in 1994, prompted by a graduate student project that brought together students and

TUDS staff to investigate the potential of substituting apples sourced from New England orchards for those imported from Washington State. In this case, the FTC program succeeded because of student involvement and demand for produce from local farms. In fact, from 1994 through 2007, the amount of FTC programming undertaken by TUDS ebbed and flowed with the falling and rising student interest in having such a program. For a number of years, Tufts' FTC efforts were minimal because of the lack of student inquiries requesting more locally sourced foods. This experience highlights what we consider to be the most important factor motivating and enabling FTC programs to succeed: student support and demand. It is reasonable to think of the university's dining service as a business and the students as its clientele who drive the current and future direction of the business. Unless the clientele request a service such as FTC and support it through their spending habits, it is less likely for a self-operating dining service to take on the added logistical and financial burden of sourcing from local farms.

Student support and demand for the program are essential.

Although student demand may be the strongest motivator for a university dining service to implement a FTC program in its daily operations, there are a number of alternate rationales that engage food service in higher education institutions to work toward sourcing more of their food supply locally. These motivators range from philosophical reasons (eg, a college wants to be a good citizen) to reasons that are grounded in business strategy, institutional policy, and government incentives. As can be demonstrated from the Tufts experience and evidence from local universities, it is often a convergence of these motivators, combined with student interest, that prime higher education institutions for FTC programs.

Tufts has a strong history of citizen action and public service. By establishing a university-wide environmental policy and a Dining Services policy that embraces sustainability, Tufts has set a goal of being an environmentally responsible institution. Because of the need to work toward these goals, Tufts became ripe for embracing changes in facilities and operations, such as the implementation of a FTC program. However, in the case of business strategy, Tufts has not capitalized on implementing a FTC program as a way to add value in its marketing approaches to attract new students. A well-positioned public relations campaign on the successes of Tufts' FTC program to date may stand out and draw new students and their parents to Tufts as a progressive competitor in elite higher education. In contrast, Yale University appears to have used its position as an early innovator of a FTC approach, which includes a vegetable farm and a hugely popular dining hall that uses only local ingredients as a marketing tool to gain some degree of competitive advantage in the Ivy League marketplace.

Various local, state, and federal agencies that mandate or encourage education institutions to source local foods have proliferated in recent years, providing yet another motivator for establishing FTC programs. At the federal level, a partnership between the US Department of Defense and the US Department of Agriculture allows a portion of purchases under the National School Lunch Program in K-12 schools to go toward provision of locally produced fruits and vegetables. This ability to source local foods for school food service was further emphasized in the 2002 Farm Bill, which directed the Secretary of Agriculture to encourage institutions in the school lunch and breakfast programs to purchase locally produced foods for school meal programs, to the maximum extent practicable and appropriate.[3,4] Federal action has not yet begun, however, to influence FTC programs because directives have been limited to public K-12 school systems via required nationwide school lunch and breakfast programs.

In contrast, regulations at the state level have been relevant to higher education. The Massachusetts legislature, for example, passed a local purchasing provision in 2006 as part of an economic stimulus package, directing purchasing agents of the Commonwealth, including agents at state colleges and universities, to give preference to sourcing local agricultural products:

> To effectuate the preference for those products of agriculture grown or produced using locally grown products, the state purchasing agent responsible for procuring the products on behalf of a state agency or authority shall: (1) in advertising for bids, contracts, or otherwise procuring products of agriculture, *make reasonable efforts to facilitate the purchase of such products of agriculture grown or produced using products grown in the commonwealth;* and (2) *purchase the products of agriculture grown or produced using products grown in the commonwealth,* unless the price of the goods exceeds, by more than 10 percent, the price of products of agriculture grown or produced using products grown outside of the commonwealth (emphasis added).[5]

Farm-to-college programs may be good publicity for participating colleges.

Similar efforts are under way in other states to allow preferential purchasing of agricultural goods in public education institutions, both K-12 and state-funded universities.[6] These kinds of regulations can serve as stimuli for state colleges and universities to establish and grow FTC programs. The Massachusetts procurement provision, coupled with a strong local farm economy in western Massachusetts, for example, has enabled the University of Massachusetts in Amherst to expand its FTC effort. The university established a goal of purchasing 30% of its food from local farms in the 2007–2008 academic year; this is a 5% increase in local farm product purchases from the last academic year (Ken Toong, e-mail communication, October 15, 2007).

Understanding the Barriers to Successful Implementation

FTC programs face varying challenges given the differing operational structures in which they function (eg, "all you can eat" vs "pay as you go" dining halls). However, data from a recent FTC survey effort show that there are commonalities, especially when regional/geographical differences such as those in the Northeast are taken into account. In 2004, the CFSC began collecting data on FTC programs around the United States via a self-administered Web survey.[7] A senior member of the Dining Services staff of each college or university was targeted to fill out a survey that included information on how their FTC program started, the degree of student involvement, the percentage of the overall dining budget allocated for local purchases, and the barriers and solutions faced in implementing their program. As of May 2007, a total of 117 self-selected surveys have been submitted to this database since the fall of 2004. Overall, the CFSC survey identified coordination and seasonality as the most significant barriers to FTC programs nationally. However, the CFSC analysis does not break down respondents by region to look for any differences in the barriers faced by FTC programs in New England as compared to the national survey results.

To understand the context and challenges faced by FTC programs in New England, publicly available data from CFSC were aggregated by the authors to include only respondents from New England institutions. Of the 117 surveys available when the CFSC database was accessed, a total of 20 surveys sent in by New England institutions were included in this aggregate. This aggregate provides a good summary of the challenges and barriers faced by FTC programs in the northeastern United States.

As shown in Figure 1, the coordination of purchasing and delivery for procuring from local farms was identified by 11 of the 20 New England schools as a key challenge. Practical examples from Tufts' FTC program confirm this sentiment. If the university is to purchase directly from a farmer (which gives the farmer the highest proportion of each dollar in sales as profit), then a new vendor relationship must be established through the purchasing system. This requires an adaptation of the ordering software, a relatively easy accommodation. More significantly, it means that the farmer must have a certain amount of liability insurance to be eligible to enter into an agreement as a vendor with the university, but many farmers do not. College administrators are also leery of heavy truck traffic on campus. Direct farmer deliveries mean increasing traffic on loading docks and complicating the timing of staffing to help unload trucks and stock supplies. Furthermore, it means increased traffic where students expect to stroll and enjoy the beauty of campus with little regard to vehicular interference.

Direct buying from the farmer has been fraught with inventory problems. Managers of dining halls place orders in anticipation of receiving the goods they specified to meet the large volume and quick turnover of meals in their facilities. In a number of instances, farmers will substitute items when they run short. This is not because these farmers are poor planners or irresponsible, but because the nature of farming itself is unpredictable. Farmers may deliver different vegetables from

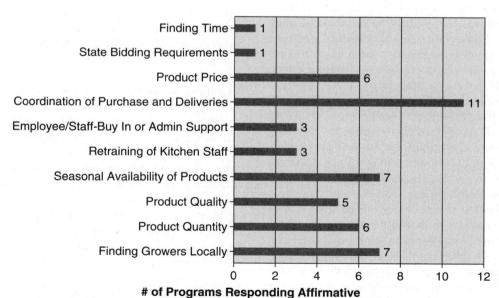

Figure 1   Barriers in 20 Farm-to-college programs in New England.   Most frequently cited barriers by New England farm-to-college (FTC) programs. Data from the following Community Food Security Coalition FTC survey respondents: Colby College, Bates College, Bowdoin College, Clark University, College of the Atlantic, Dartmouth College, Harvard University, Massachusetts Institute of Technology, Middlebury College, St Joseph's College (Maine), St Joseph's College (Connecticut), Smith College, Sterling College, Trinity College, Tufts University, University of Connecticut, University of Massachusetts, University of New Hampshire, Williams College, and Yale University.

what was ordered because bad weather delayed maturation of the desired vegetable (whereas a distributor would simply fill the order with the desired vegetable from a different region). This has had negative consequences. The dining manager must revise the meal for that particular day, if possible, and if the substituted vegetable requires unexpected processing (eg, peeling, chopping), labor must be found to undertake the task. Such a situation leaves the manager frustrated with the ordering and receiving process and cites lack of time to "deal with" coordinating an FTC program.

One way to ease these problems is to work with produce distributors who are able to serve as the middleman between local farms and the institution. The advantage from an institutional perspective is that many of these distributors are already vendors with contracts and liability coverage with the university. Another option is to work with dining hall managers over the years, securing a great deal of "relationship capital." This approach, however, does have its own coordination problems similar to those when buying direct from farmers. For example, a box of apples may arrive with the expectation that they have been sourced from a local Massachusetts orchard only to discover that the apples are from Washington state. In this scenario, dining hall managers are not as frustrated as with farmer substitutions because, in a sense, they have the same product (ie, do not have to adjust the menu for the day). However, representing to students that the university buys local and then serving apples with stickers declaring "Grown in Washington State" easily erode the spirit of the FTC program. With improved tracking and traceability throughout local supply chains and a better understanding between distributors and dining staff, this kind of mix-up could be avoided, making the use of distributors a feasible approach in institutional sourcing of local foods. Conversely, some distributors may place demands on the institution, imposing contractual terms that establish themselves as sole distributor of certain products, thus preventing FTC programs altogether.

Another major barrier to FTC programs in New England is the seasonal availability of local products. Figure 1 shows that almost half of CFSC survey participants from the New England region identified this as a challenge for their dining operations; this is similar to the national survey results. Currently, Tufts' regular purchases of locally grown produce are limited to apples, pumpkin, squash, pears, peaches, nectarines, Swiss chard, and tomatoes. The tomatoes are sourced from a Maine farm that uses greenhouses to extend their vegetable season. Special events featuring local foods do bring more variety (eg, locally raised beef). Despite significant effort, however, Tufts' purchases of local produce account for about $85,000—less than 2% of what is spent on all food procurement at the university (Julie Lampie, e-mail communication, October 15, 2007). This accounts only for Tufts' produce purchases and does not include the amount spent on other local farm products (eg, dairy); there is much more potential to be realized.

One reason why most purchasing goes to nonlocal fruits and vegetables is a mismatch in the academic year (September–June) with the New England peak harvest season (June–September). For example, stone fruits from local orchards

would be a great alternative to the usual offering of bananas and apples in the dining halls; however, Tufts can only catch the tail end of local peach, plum, and pear production when the fall semester kicks off. One way to address this is through an annual "Summer Fruit Extravaganza" at the start of the academic year, but this 1-day event does not translate into huge economic benefits for the farmers and may not be worth their time for a 1-day sale. Cold storage could extend the season for these locally grown products. But most farmers need to sell their product within days of harvest because they lack cold storage facilities to maintain product quality for extended periods. Universities typically face the same constraint, so there is limited ability to keep food on-site for more than a few days. To add to these challenges, dining staff and students are largely unaware of production regions and seasons for fresh produce because they, along with the general population, have grown accustomed to an international flow of goods that has erased these previously known food facts. This lack of sensitivity translates in low expectations for farm fresh food.

Dining room consumers are not always knowledgeable about local sources.

Finding local growers is a significant barrier identified in the New England aggregate of the CFSC survey. Oftentimes, the burden of locating good sources for locally produced products falls upon a dining service staff member who has embraced the FTC program as a pet project. This means that there is little time to devote to seeking out the best quality and pricing that will truly fit the institution's needs. Quantity is a challenge in New England, where typical farms are small and diversified. This may make a distributor who is able to consolidate product from various farms attractive. However, the bundling of products from various farms may create problems of uniformity, as one farmer may grow Roma tomatoes while his neighbor grows Brandywine. Large-scale farming operations may provide some processing before delivery to the distributor or institution, meaning less labor for dining staff. For example, most large producers of California lettuce harvest, wash, and bag lettuce before distribution, whereas small New England growers do not. To overcome some of these barriers, a small working group was established at Tufts to help find new sources of goods from local farmers and facilitate conversation. Similarly, others have recognized the need for a "matching service" of sorts to connect farmers with institutions. A new online program, for example, Farm Fresh Rhode Island, allows farmers to post what will be harvested soon, allowing colleges to order in advance to fulfill their dining hall needs.[8]

A Strategy to Increase Student Demand

The most critical barrier to implementing a FTC program is not an operational characteristic but rather the drive of current students to demand and support the FTC effort. This was not mentioned explicitly in the barriers section of the CFCS survey; however, it has been voiced repeatedly by FTC leaders in New England at buy-local and related meetings. As discussed, the "good citizen" mission of our university has enabled the development of a modest FTC effort on campus. However, this "do good" motivator only goes so far and cannot compensate for the lack in student support for a buy-local program. Recognizing this reality, advocates of FTC programs have refocused their efforts on educating and mobilizing the student body. Activities have included developing a Web site on food options and sustainability initiatives, establishing an annual 1-day farmers' market on campus, serving an all locally grown menu during freshmen orientation events for subpopulations of likely supporters (eg, fitness club orientation), and a poster campaign.

The series of fun posters may be the most innovative effort. The posters display students endorsing alternative food choices, specifically locally grown, organic, and fair trade options. Students were chosen to be poster celebrities, with a calculation for diversity (eg, different academic majors, years, sex, ethnicity, sports, and club interests). In one, a senior biochemical engineering student juggles local fruits and vegetables and comments on why he supports buying local foods. In another example, a junior international relations major holds homemade pizza made from local ingredients. These and other posters are a new intervention, and the extent to which they have succeeded in raising awareness is unknown.

It may be prudent for FTC champions at colleges and universities to take a step back and reflect on the kind of student body and culture evident at their school. Campaigns should be tailored based on this information. The predominant undergraduate major at Tufts is international relations. Given this, events such as "Multicultural Night" should be targeted for FTC education. The university also has an immigrant farmer training program, providing the school an opportunity to feature ethnic dishes in dining halls made with items such as locally grown bitter melon and Chinese broccoli grown on satellite farms.

The Future of FTC Programs in New England

Institutional purchasing direct from farmers is catching on. According to CFSC, more than 768 school districts in 34 states have farm-to-school programs.[9] Regional supermarkets such as Hannaford Brothers and national retailers, ranging from "natural food" stores such as Whole Foods to the largest retailer in the world, Wal-Mart, have instituted varying degrees of buy-local in their operations. Healthcare management companies (eg, Kaiser Permanente) are beginning to partner with local hospitals to bring farmers markets and local produce to medical institutions. And now, more than 100 colleges and universities have begun or are seriously considering FTC programs.

But direct farm purchasing programs require serious effort. A solid foundation for FTC programs in the Northeast has been set, but much more must be done to ensure their success. The next steps range from revising institutional policies (eg, making terms of payment for direct purchases from farmers less than the 90 days and more in line with their needs of 30-day terms) to inspiring students to demand local products in their dining halls.

References

1. Shartin E. Movement toward more sustainable food systems is growing. *Boston Globe,* third edition. July 26, 2006:E2.
2. Hinrichs CC. The practice and politics of food system localization. *J Rural Stud.* 2003; 19:33–45.
3. The Public Health and Welfare. School lunch programs. Chapter 13. 42 USC §1758.
4. Caplan R. Memo to the Harrison Institute for Public Law on Preemption of Geographic Preferences in School Food Procurement. http://www.foodsecurity.org/HarrisonPreemptionAnalysis.doc. Accessed September 30, 2007.
5. Section 23B of Massachusetts General Law. Mass Stat Chap 7 §23B.
6. Section 5-60.4 of Oklahoma Statues. Oklahoma Stat Title 2 §5-60.4 on the development of nutrition plans using locally grown farm-fresh products in state school districts.
7. Community Food Security Coalition. http://www.farmtocollege.org/survey.htm. Accessed May 14, 2007.
8. Farm Fresh Rhode Island. RI fresh Network. http://www.farmfreshri.org/about/freshnetwork.php. Accessed October 15, 2007.
9. Community Food Security Coalition. National Farm to School program Web site. http://www.farmtoschool.org/. Accessed October 22, 2007.

Critical Thinking

1. What are the benefits of establishing a farm-to-college program at your college/university?

KATHLEEN A. MERRIGAN, PhD, is an assistant professor and director of the Agriculture, Food, and Environment Program at the Friedman School of Nutrition Science and Policy at Tufts University. MELISSA BAILEY, MS, is a PhD candidate in the Agriculture, Food, and Environment Program at the Friedman School of Nutrition Science and Policy at Tufts University.

UNIT 2
Nutrients

Unit Selections

Learning Outcomes

After reading this unit, you should be able to

- Identify foods that you eat that are naturally dark orange, red, yellow, green, and purple.

- Determine ways that you can improve the color quality, and therefore nutrient quality, of your diet.

- Identify the four groups that should pay particular attention to sodium content of foods and consume no more than 1,500 mg of sodium per day, as recommended in the Dietary Guidelines for Americans.

- List the benefits of consuming docosahexaenoic acid and identify the best food sources for this long-chain omega-3 fatty acid.

- Identify the three "bad fats" and food sources of each.

- Describe the health benefits of consuming monounsaturated and omega-3 fatty acids.

- Explain why some individuals prefer to consume supplements rather than getting their nutrients from foods.

- List the four nutrients that function as antioxidants. Identify the best food sources of these nutrients in foods that you commonly eat.

Student Website

www.mhhe.com/cls

Internet References

Dietary Supplement Fact Sheet: Vitamin D
http://ods.od.nih.gov/factsheets/vitamind.asp

Food and Nutrition Information Center
www.nal.usda.gov/fnic

Nutritionalsupplements.com
www.nutritionalsupplements.com

Office of Dietary Supplements: Health Information
http://ods.od.nih.gov/Health_Information/Health_Information.aspx

U.S. National Library of Medicine
www.nlm.nih.gov

Nutrition is a young and evolving science. Early research into nutrients began in the mid 18th century with investigations into how the body requires and uses calories from the macronutrients (carbohydrates, protein, and fats). It wasn't until the early 20th century that scientists began to discover, investigate, and identify the micronutrients and their affect on human health. The fundamentals of nutrition were discovered just over 100 years ago. From a perspective of scientifically confirming results, this is a short amount of time. A vast amount of knowledge about nutrients has been discovered and scientists continue to investigate the best way for these nutrients to be provided—safely and in proper amounts to facilitate optimal functioning of the human body.

The articles of this unit have been selected to present current knowledge about macronutrients and micronutrients, with particular interest in the four nutrients of concern as indicated in the 2010 U.S. Dietary Guidelines: vitamin D, calcium, potassium, and fiber. Decreasing overall intake of sodium and increasing the amount of "good fats" consumed are also important points that are included in the dietary guidelines.

The USDA and HHS are now recommending that all American adults strive to consume 1,500 mg of sodium rather than the previously recommended 2,300 mg. The reasoning for lowering the recommended amount across the board is that over 70% of the population fits into groups that are at high risk for developing hypertension, stroke, and heart disease. The challenge with meeting this guideline is that it will be difficult to consume processed foods or eat in restaurants in the United States. "Keeping a Lid on Salt: Not So Easy" by Nanci Hellmich covers many of these challenges with restricting sodium in the current U.S. food environment.

The beneficial effects of naturally occurring fibers on cardiovascular disease, diabetes, colon cancer, obesity, and overall gastrointestinal health have been documented. The food industry is responding to consumer demand by adding isolated fiber in foods that do not naturally contain fiber even though there is scant evidence of beneficial effects of this form of fiber on degenerative disease. The most important question to consider when thinking of fiber is whether it is soluble or insoluble fiber, as these two fibers work differently in the human body. Both types of fiber are beneficial; however, the mode of action and benefit of the fibers is dramatically different. "Fiber Free-for-All" from *Nutrition Action Healthletter* addresses the benefits and sources of these different types of fiber.

Another topic of current interest is omega-3 fatty acids, especially the best and safest sources for these beneficial fats. A great deal of information has been published regarding the imbalance of the polyunsaturated fatty acids, omega-6 and omega-3, in the typical American diet. The vast use of corn, vegetable, and soybean oil in the western diet has led to an unhealthy proportion of fats from omega-6 fatty acids. This imbalance of omega-6 to omega-3 fatty acids has been implicated in atherosclerosis, heart attack, and stroke. Demand for supplements and fortified foods containing omega-3s has culminated in a number of products on the market. Since the metabolic pathways of these PUFAs are complex, there is a great deal of confusion when information is presented on the label and/or in the media. The most beneficial of these omega-3s is docosahexaenoic acid (DHA) found in cold water fatty fish (salmon, halibut, swordfish, tilefish, shark, tuna), which are frequently high in heavy metals and other toxins. The current recommendation from the Dietary Guidelines for Americans is to vary types and sources of fish that you consume. Future research to address the problem of how to consume safe sources of DHA will strengthen, with particular attention to improving fish farming techniques.

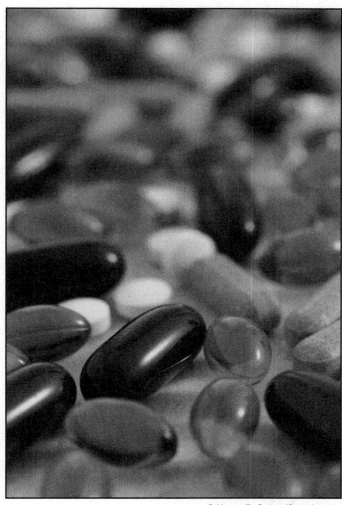

© Nancy R. Cohen/Getty Images

One of the main health messages elicited in the 1990s was "fat is bad." The next decade ushered in the "carbs are bad" era, and thankfully, we now consider the nutrient density or quality of a food rather than just eliminating an entire macronutrient group. "The Fairest Fats of Them All" by Sharon Palmer addresses the difference in bad fats and good fats and provides an Oil Primer that reviews the different oils available in the U.S. market, their fatty acid components, and practical information about the oils that will help you add the healthier oils to your diet.

Historically, the health benefits of foods have been explained by vitamins, minerals, fiber, and protein. Research on other bioactive food components, such as phytochemicals, provides yet another aspect to the benefit of eating a variety of natural colors from plant-based foods, as described by Julian Schaeffer in "Color Me Healthy: Eating for a Rainbow of Benefits." "Antioxidants: Fruitful Research and Recommendations" by Pamela Brummit discusses antioxidants and the best food sources for these naturally occurring promoters of health.

Color Me Healthy
Eating for a Rainbow of Benefits

Got the blues? Not your mood, your food! While you're at it, make sure you also have reds, yellows, and other bright colors on your plate.

JULIANN SCHAEFFER

Beige may be a mainstay in many wardrobes because of its versatility, but when it relates to diet, simply beige is all the rage for all the wrong reasons. Americans' affinity for all that is quick, cheap, and convenient is directing many to the cracker, cereal, and cookie aisles, leading to a high-fat and highly processed "beige diet" that is nutrient impaired.

According to Susan Bowerman, MS, RD, CSSD, a lecturer in the department of food science and nutrition at Cal Poly San Luis Obispo and coauthor of *What Color Is Your Diet?* a purely beige diet may fill Americans up now, but it could cost them later.

"We eat foods primarily based on their taste, their cost, and how convenient they are," she notes. "The food manufacturers have done a great job of creating many foods that are easy to eat, inexpensive, and rich in sugar, fat, and salt so that they taste good. Starches, fats, and sweets are the least expensive foods in the diet, so it's easy to see why we lean toward these 'brown/beige' foods. They fill us up for very little monetary cost, but there are significant health costs to a diet that is so high in refined carbohydrates and devoid of the vitamins, minerals, fiber, and phytochemicals that are so abundant in plant foods."

Americans' fondness for foods lacking color also reflects a metaphor of what else is lacking in processed foods: phytochemicals. While some processed foods may reincorporate key nutrients during processing, "Many of the flavonoids, tannins, etc are not replaced during processing," says Susan Kasik-Miller, MS, RD, CNSC, a clinical dietitian at Sacred Heart Hospital in Eau Claire, Wis. "The metaphor also holds for the look of our diet. Literature references bland beige swill as the only food offered to suffering people. A colorful, balanced diet is associated with good health and prosperity."

Phytochemical-Filled Produce

So what does color have to do with diet anyway? One word: phytochemicals. These substances occur naturally only in plants and may provide health benefits beyond those that essential nutrients provide. Color, such as what makes a blueberry so blue, can indicate some of these substances, which are thought to work synergistically with vitamins, minerals, and fiber (all present in fruits and vegetables) in whole foods to promote good health and lower disease risk.

According to information from the Produce for Better Health Foundation (PBH), phytochemicals may act as antioxidants, protect and regenerate essential nutrients, and/or work to deactivate cancer-causing substances. And while research has not yet determined exactly how these substances work together or which combination offers specific benefits, including a rainbow of colored foods in a diet plan ensures a variety of those nutrients and phytochemicals.

"Plant products are sources for phytochemicals of which there are thousands that have been identified," explains Kasik-Miller. "These chemicals are known to have disease-preventing properties, but the color of a food does not necessarily mean it contains one particular phytochemical class. Foods contain multiple phytochemicals, as well as vitamins and minerals, and it is not known how many other phytochemicals await to be identified and what functions they have with health."

Kathy Hoy, EdD, RD, nutrition research manager for the PBH, says eating a variety of foods helps ensure the intake of an assortment of nutrients and other healthful substances in food, such as phytochemicals, noting that color can be a helpful guide for consumers. "Nutrients and phytochemicals appear to work synergistically, so maintaining a varied, colorful diet with healthful whole foods is a pragmatic approach to optimal nutrition."

"Tomatoes help support the health of prostate and breast tissue," adds Bowerman.

And although some nutrients, such as vitamin C, are diminished with the introduction of heat, Hoy says, "The benefits of eating produce are not dependent on eating raw foods. In fact, cooking enhances the activity of some phytochemicals, such as lycopene. Obtaining optimal benefit from the nutrients in food, especially produce, depends on proper selection, storage, and cooking of the produce."

Cooked tomato sauces are associated with greater health benefits compared with the uncooked version because the heating process allows all carotenoids, including lycopene, to be more easily absorbed by the body, according to information from the PBH.

"In addition to vitamin C and folate, red fruits and vegetables are also sources of flavonoids, which reduce inflammation and have antioxidant properties. Cranberries, another red fruit [whose color is due to anthocyanins, not lycopene], are also a good source of tannins, which prevent bacteria from attaching to cells," says Kasik-Miller of more reasons to relish red.

Examples: Tomatoes and tomato products, watermelon, pink grapefruit, guava, cranberries.

Yellow/Orange

Behind the color: "We had an orange/yellow group representing beta-cryptoxanthin and vitamin C," says Bowerman. "Our orange group foods are also rich in beta-carotene, which are particularly good antioxidants."

Beta-cryptoxanthin, beta-carotene, and alpha-carotene are all orange-friendly carotenoids and can be converted in the body to vitamin A, a nutrient integral for vision and immune function, as well as skin and bone health, according to information from the PBH.

"These foods are commonly considered the eyesight foods because they contain vitamin A. Beta-carotene, which can be converted into vitamin A, is a component of these foods as well. In addition, they may have high levels of vitamin C, and some contain omega-3 fatty acids," says Kasik-Miller.

Since eyesight is dependent on the presence of vitamin A, Kasik-Miller notes that it is considered the "vision vitamin." "Other [phyto]chemicals typically found in yellow/orange fruits and vegetables protect our eyes from cataracts and have anti-inflammatory properties. They also help with blood sugar regulation," she adds.

Tsang notes that the beta-carotenes in some orange fruits and vegetables may also play a part in preventing cancer, particularly of the lung, esophagus, and stomach. "They may also reduce the risk of heart disease and improve immune function," she says.

Examples: Carrots, mangos, cantaloupe, winter squash, sweet potatoes, pumpkins, apricots.

No Color? No Problem

While color can give clients a general idea about what lies beneath eggplant's exterior, a food's hue does not tell all, and it is certainly not an exclusive indicator of phytochemical content. While some phytochemicals are pigments that give color, others are colorless.

"The largest class of phytochemicals are the flavonoids, which for the most part are colorless," explains Bowerman. "Flavonoids are powerful antioxidants, and these help the body

---

Menu

Breakfast
Cereal with dried fruit and low-fat milk
Glass of 100% fruit juice
Whole grain toast with fruit spread

Lunch
Vegetable soup
Sandwich with lettuce, tomato, peppers, and olives
Fresh fruit in season (or canned fruit in juice)
Low-fat milk

Snack
Fruit muffin, dried fruit, or whole wheat bagel with peanut butter

Dinner
Black bean burritos with avocado slices and lettuce
Brown rice with tomatoes Fruit salad

—Menu Provided By Susan Kasik-Miller, MS, RD, CNSC.

---

to counteract free-radical formation. When free-radical damage goes unchecked, it can cause significant damage to body cells and tissues."

There are more than 4,000 different flavonoids, and according to information from the PBH, they are classified into the following categories:

- flavonols:
  -myricetin (in berries, grapes, parsley, and spinach);
  -quercetin (in onions, apples, broccoli, cranberries, and grapes);
- flavones:
  -apigenin (in celery, lettuce, and parsley);
  -luteolin (in beets, bell peppers, and Brussels sprouts);
- flavanones:
  -hesperetin and naringenin (both in citrus fruits and juices);
- flavan-3-ols:
  -catechin (in tea, red wine, and dark chocolate);
  -epicatechin, gallate, epigallocatechin, and epigallocatechin gallate (in teas, fruits, and legumes); and
- anthocyanidins (in blue/purple and red fruits and vegetables).

Although not enough research has been conducted to definitively match specific phytochemicals with particular benefits, researchers are currently investigating flavonoids' effect on lowering the risk of cardiovascular disease and several types of cancer and their role in promoting lung health and protecting against asthma.

Eat Your Colors

The concept of suggesting that clients eat a certain color ratio of foods may be premature, but Hoy says the take-away message is that including a variety of colors in one's diet seems to equal better overall health, especially in relation to produce. "Epidemio-logical research suggests that food patterns that include fruits and vegetables are associated with lower risk for some diseases, and a recent article suggested that more variety in fruit and vegetable intake was associated with a lower risk for pharyngeal and laryngeal cancers, suggesting that variety may also be another important factor to consider. However, it is not known if there is an optimal ratio of colors to be consumed or what that is," says Hoy.[2,3]

Kasik-Miller agrees: "At this time, scientists are not sure what proportion of phytochemicals is the right balance for disease prevention. There have been studies where specific antioxidants were given and there was an increase in the disease rate. To make recommendations to eat a specific number of servings of beets or blueberries is premature; eat what looks good and you can afford. Foods of the same color do not necessarily contain the same vitamins, minerals, or phytochemicals, so recommendations to eat specific amounts of colored foods is impossible."

And considering that the majority of individuals are not meeting current recommendations for fruit and vegetable intake, encouraging consumers to use color as a guide for increasing produce consumption is a good strategy, Hoy says.[1]

What's the best way to convey this message to clients? Instead of delving into a complex and complicated conversation about phytochemicals, Molly Morgan, RD, CDN, owner of Creative Nutrition Solutions, says the more matters idea can easily be tweaked to more color matters. "I believe consumers can do better by consciously trying to include many different colors in their eating plan rather than getting stuck on what colors do what. Each color provides various health benefits and no one color is superior to another, which is why I believe a balance of all colors is most important," she says.

"I think the color approach that we used in *What Color Is Your Diet?* resonated well with people because intuitively they knew that colors equal health and that the more colors that were eaten, the better it probably was to overall health," says Bowerman of getting this message out to the masses. "Educating people as to the health benefits is a start, but they also have to be willing to try new foods or new varieties of foods—or maybe to prepare unfamiliar foods in a way that will make them taste good—so that they will be willing to add more plant foods to their diet."

Once people are aware of this dietary color concept, Hoy says creativity can go a long way. "Creatively including fruits and vegetables at meals will help them to include a wide range of different foods. In addition to simple things like adding fruits or vegetables to casseroles, cereal, or sandwiches, being open to trying new foods, recipes, or meal patterns will help to increase variety," she says. "Other ways to increase variety would include making fruits and vegetables more center of the plate when planning meals, including a fruit and/or vegetable at every eating occasion, adding an extra fruit and/or vegetable side dish to meals, and substituting fruits, vegetables, and beans for other ingredients such as meat in recipes."

Planning ahead is Morgan's mantra, and she recommends challenging clients to take notice of color when grocery shopping. She says to tell clients, "Challenge yourself to look at your cart when leaving the produce section, and if you have all red items, head back and swap something out for another color. For example, if you had strawberries, watermelon, and tomatoes, swap the strawberries for some oranges."

And since winter is fast approaching and the season is swinging away from some of the colorful foods familiar to consumers, such as blueberries and strawberries, Kasik-Miller says a trip to the farmers' market may be warranted. "Also, people need to get into the habit of cooking at home," she says. "If you are not sure about what to do with a colorful food or are looking for a new way to eat it, go to the grower's association Web site to get recipes and new ways to eat foods. I think people need to be more creative with how they prepare foods. People know they need lots of color in their diet but find it hard to change food habits. They need to make small changes over a period of time to achieve success."

While there may not be much to compare between dinner and Dior, it seems this much is true: There appears to be more reason to eat the spectrum of colors than to wear them.

Notes

1. Cook AJ, Friday JE. *Pyramid Servings Intakes in the United States 1999–2002, 1 Day.* Beltsville, Md.: USDA, Agricultural Research Service, Community Nutrition Research Group. 2005. Available at: http://www.ars.usda.gov/sp2UserFiles/Place/12355000/foodlink/ts_3-0.pdf

2. Garavello W, Giordano L, Bosetti C, et al. Diet diversity and the risk of oral and pharyngeal cancer. *Eur J Nutr.* 2008;47(5):280–284.

3. Garavello W, Lucenteforte E, Bosetti C, et al. Diet diversity and the risk of laryngeal cancer: A case-control study from Italy and Switzerland. *Oral Oncol.* 2008; Epub ahead of print.

Resource

Produce for Better Health Foundation:
www.pbhfoundation.org, www.fruitsandveggiesmorematters.org

Critical Thinking

1. How can a person improve the color quality (therefore improving the nutrient quality) of their diet?

JULIANN SCHAEFFER is an editorial assistant at *Today's Dietitian.*

Keeping a Lid on Salt: Not So Easy

Known as a silent killer, it's part of how we live.

NANCI HELLMICH

For years, Americans have been advised to consume less sodium, and they've taken that advice with a grain of salt.

Even many health-conscious consumers figured it was the least of their worries, especially compared with limiting their intake of calories, saturated fat, trans fat, cholesterol and sugar.

All that changed last week when a report from the Institute of Medicine urged the government to gradually reduce the maximum amount of sodium that manufacturers and restaurants can add to foods, beverages and meals. The report put a spotlight on what doctors and nutritionists have argued is a major contributor to heart disease and stroke.

More than half of Americans have either high blood pressure or pre-hypertension, says cardiologist Clyde Yancy, president of the American Heart Association and medical director at the Baylor Heart and Vascular Institute in Dallas.

"That puts a lot of us in the bucket of people who need to be on a lower sodium diet. Sodium contributes to most people's high blood pressure, and for some it may be the primary driver."

Cutting back on sodium could save thousands of people from early deaths caused by heart attacks and strokes each year, and it could save billions of dollars in health care costs, he says.

Others second that. "Salt is the single most harmful element in our food supply, silently killing about 100,000 people each year," says Michael Jacobson, executive director of the Washington, D.C.-based Center for Science in the Public Interest. "That's like a crowded jetliner crashing every single day. But the food industry has fended off government action for more than three decades."

Now salt has our attention.

But reducing it in the American diet is easier said than done. "We have, in essence, ignored the advice because we are driven by convenience, and sodium makes a fast-food lifestyle very easy," Yancy says. "To change, we would need to live and eat differently."

Very differently.

Americans now consume an average of about 3,400 milligrams of sodium a day, or about 1½ teaspoons, government data show. Men consume more than women.

But most adults—including those with high blood pressure, African Americans, the middle-aged and the elderly—should consume no more than 1,500 milligrams a day, according to the dietary guidelines from the U.S. Department of Agriculture. Others should consume less than 2,300 milligrams, or less than a teaspoon, the guidelines say.

And yet it's virtually impossible to limit yourself to such amounts if you often eat processed foods, prepared foods or restaurant fare, including fast food. Most Americans' sodium intake comes from those sources, not the salt shaker on the table.

Some restaurant entrees have 2,000 milligrams or more in one dish. Fast-food burgers can have more than 1,000 milligrams. Many soups are chock-full of sodium. So are many spaghetti sauces, broths, lunch meats, salad dressings, cheeses, crackers and frozen foods.

Can't see it, can't taste it.

Salt serves many functions in products. Besides adding to a food's taste, it is a preservative. "You can't see it," Yancy says. "You can't even taste it because you are so accustomed to it. If you want the freedom to make healthy choices, you are limited by today's foods. That's a problem."

To change that, food companies and restaurants will have to come up with new ways to formulate products and recipes to help consumers gradually lower their salt levels, which would wean them off the taste.

That's a huge challenge, but nutritionists and public health specialists say it can be done and will be worth it. "There is no health benefit to a high-sodium diet, and there is considerable risk," says Linda Van Horn, a professor of preventive medicine at Northwestern University Feinberg School of Medicine.

Even those whose blood pressure is in the normal range should watch their intake, Yancy says. "Here's a wake-up call: Every American who is age 50 or older has a 90% chance of developing hypertension. That increases the risk of heart disease and stroke. This is a preventable process, and it's preventable with sodium reduction, weight control and physical activity."

Why It Can Be Harmful

There are several theories for why sodium increases blood pressure, Yancy says, "but the most obvious one is that it makes us retain fluids, and that retention elevates blood pressure," which injures blood vessels and leads to heart disease and stroke. "It's a connect-the-dots phenomenon."

Some people, especially some African Americans, are more salt-sensitive than others, Yancy says.

"When they are exposed to sodium, they retain more fluid, and because of the way their kidneys handle sodium, they may have a greater proportional rise in blood pressure," he says.

The cost of this damage? An analysis by the Rand Corp. found that if the average sodium intake of Americans was reduced to 2,300 milligrams a day, it might decrease the cases of high blood pressure by 11 million, improve quality of life for millions of people and save about $18 billion in annual health care costs.

The estimated value of improved quality of life and living healthier longer: $32 billion a year. Greater reductions in sodium consumption in the population would save more lives and money, says Roland Sturm, a senior economist with Rand.

Yancy says the country doesn't just need health care reform, "we need health reform. If we don't adjust the demand part of the equation, no system will work. Remarkably, people might be overall healthier by simply reducing sodium."

But Yancy says people need to keep in mind that sodium is just one of the factors that increase the risk of heart disease and stroke. Others include obesity, consuming too much sugar and too few fruits and vegetables, lack of physical activity and smoking.

Salt Industry Disagrees

Leaders in the salt industry say their product is being unfairly maligned. The Institute of Medicine report and the government "are focusing on one small aspect of health, which is a small increase in blood pressure in a small segment of population," says Lori Roman, president of the Salt Institute, an industry group.

Some of the research that ties salt to health risks is based on faulty assumptions and extrapolations, Roman says. She says a recent worldwide study indicated there is no country where people eat an average of less than 1,500 milligrams a day. "That's way below the normal range," Roman says. The Italians eat more sodium than Americans, but their cardiovascular health is better than Americans', and the reason is they eat a lot of fruits and vegetables, she says.

"This is the real story that the government is missing," Roman says. "It is the secret to good health."

She says people may end up following a less healthy diet if they cut back on sodium. "Have you ever bought a can of low-sodium string beans and then tried to season it to taste good? It's impossible," Roman says. "Here's one of the unintended consequences of this recommendation: People will eat fewer vegetables, and by eating fewer vegetables, they will be less healthy."

Yancy says the first step for many people is making the decision to cut back on salt intake. He knows from experience that it can be done.

An African American, Yancy, 52, has high blood pressure and a family history of heart disease and stroke. He's lean and exercises for an hour a day, but still he has to take medication for hypertension. Before he started watching his sodium intake a few years ago, Yancy says, he was consuming more than 4,000 milligrams a day, partly because he grew up in southern Louisiana and was used to a salty, high-fat diet.

But he has weaned himself off the taste. He doesn't have a salt shaker in his house, and he reads the labels on grocery store items and doesn't buy any that have more than 100 milligrams of sodium in a serving.

"I taste the salt in items and put them aside. I find it difficult to enjoy prepared soups. I can taste the salt in prepared meals. I've learned to make my own soups."

When he eats out, he orders salads and asks for his fish and meat to be grilled. "Typically, I eat fish with lemon juice and pepper."

Even so, he believes his sodium intake is probably higher than it should be because he often eats in restaurants and cafeterias, and many foods have hidden sodium.

Changes in food products need to be made over time as the Institute of Medicine report suggests, says Van Horn, a research nutritionist at Northwestern. "If we drop the sodium overnight, people will be desperately seeking salt shakers."

So how hard is it going to be to reduce the salt in processed and prepared foods?

"We've been trying to reduce the sodium in foods for more than 30 years. If this were easy, it would have been accomplished," says Roger Clemens, a professor of pharmacology at the University of Southern California and a spokesman for the Institute of Food Technologists.

The primary dietary source of sodium is sodium chloride, also known as table salt, he says. There are other sodium salts, such as sodium bicarbonate (baking soda) in baking and sodium benzoate (preservative) in bread and beverages. And there are potassium salts that are used in foods—as emulsifiers in cheese and buffers in beverages, he says.

"Salt is a natural preservative. It has been used in the food supply to ensure food safety for centuries," Clemens says. "It's critical for preserving bacon, olives, lunch meats, fish and poultry".

"Some foods, such as cheese, can only be produced with salt. No other compound allows the proteins to knit together to become cheese."

If It Doesn't Taste Good...

To make cheese that is lower in sodium, foodmakers must put the cheese through a special procedure that basically extracts some of the sodium. "It's a very long, tedious process," he says.

Salt also is crucial for making most breads. To get dough to rise, manufacturers use sodium chloride and sodium bicarbonate, Clemens says. "If you were to eat a sodium-free product, the texture and flavor would be markedly different. It would be more compressed. I don't think you'd like it at first."

He says some manufacturers have experimented with low-sodium items, and in some cases consumers have turned up their noses. "If it doesn't taste good, consumers won't buy it."

Melissa Musiker, a nutrition spokeswoman for the Grocery Manufacturers Association, agrees. "You can't get ahead of consumers," she says. "You work on the recipes, test them, see how consumers respond and go back and tweak."

There is no one single alternative for replacing it in various foods, she says. "It has to be replaced on an ingredient-by-ingredient basis."

Clemens says food companies will continue to try to develop new technologies to lower the sodium.

"It has taken us 30 years to get this far, and it will probably take us another decade to get a significant difference in the intake. If we can lower sodium in our diet, we'll have a huge health impact on generations to come."

Critical Thinking

1. Which groups of people should consume less than 1,500 mg of sodium per day, as recommended in the Dietary Guidelines for Americans?

2. What is the largest source of sodium in the typical western diet?

3. How does dietary sodium increase blood pressure in someone who is salt sensitive?

Fiber Free-for-All

Not all fibers are equal.

How much fiber do you need?

According to food labels, 25 grams is a day's worth. That's right for women 50 and under, but men of the same age need 38 grams, says the National Academy of Sciences. And the targets drop to 21 grams for women and 30 grams for men over 50.

It's not that people need fiber less as they get older. "The advice is to get 14 grams of fiber per 1,000 calories, and older people need fewer calories," explains Thomas Wolever, a fiber researcher and professor of nutritional sciences at the University of Toronto.

Most Americans consume half the recommended levels. A typical woman gets about 13 grams of fiber a day, while the average man hovers around 17 grams.

What's the harm in falling short of the target? Here's a rundown of the key links between fiber and health.

Fiber was big in the mid-1980s, when President Ronald Reagan was diagnosed with colon cancer and Kellogg ran TV commercials saying that high-fiber foods like All-Bran could "reduce the risk of some cancers."

But the fiber boomlet was soon eclipsed by the (much bigger) oat bran craze, followed by the low-carb bubble, and, most recently, the whole-grain movement (with scattered minifads in between).

Now things have come full circle. Fiber is back. Foods that never had any (yogurt, ice cream, water, juice) sometimes have some, and foods that always had some (cereals, breads, pasta) often have more. Why?

Fiber is showing up in foods because, well, companies have figured out how to put it there. And they know that if they pump up the fiber, people will pull out their pocketbooks.

Here's what you need to know about fiber and where to get the kinds that matter.

Heart Disease

The daily fiber targets "are based on data that fiber prevents cardiovascular disease," notes Joanne Slavin, a University of Minnesota researcher who served on the National Academy of Sciences Panel on the Definition of Dietary Fiber.

The NAS relied heavily on studies that found a lower risk of heart disease in people who reported eating the most fiber (about 29 grams a day for men and 23 grams a day for women).[1,2] In each of those studies, the fiber that seemed to protect the heart came from cereals, breads, and other grains, not from fruits or vegetables.

But it was never absolutely clear that it was the fiber that mattered. Several inconsistencies have always troubled scientists:

Fiber or whole grains? It's hard for researchers to know if it's the fiber, or something else in whole grains, that matters.

"Whole grains also have phytoestrogens, antioxidants, lignans, vitamins, and minerals, so a lot comes along with the fiber package," says Slavin.

Soluble or insoluble? The kind of fiber that's linked to a lower risk of heart disease isn't the kind that lowers cholesterol.

Although all fruits, vegetables, and grains have both soluble and insoluble fiber, most grains, like wheat, are richer in *insoluble* fiber, which is not broken down by digestive enzymes or by bacteria in the gut.

In contrast, a few grains (oats and barley, for example) are richer in viscous (gummy) *soluble* fibers, which *are* broken down by bacteria in the gut.

"When researchers feed people viscous soluble fiber, it lowers cholesterol, but insoluble fiber doesn't," notes Wolever.

Yet in the large studies that the National Academy of Sciences relied on, a lower risk of heart disease was linked to foods rich in either kind of fiber, not just soluble. "It's a disconnect," says Wolever.

One possibility: even though the mostly insoluble fiber from grains doesn't lower cholesterol, it may protect the heart by reducing blood pressure or the risk of blood clots.

"Insoluble fiber may prevent heart attacks by reducing inflammation," says Wolever. "We don't know how the heck it works."

Fiber or fiber eaters? Researchers can't be sure if it's fiber, or something else about people who eat high-fiber diets, that lowers their risk of heart disease.

"We just don't have a lot of people who eat high-fiber, whole-grain diets and are out there smoking," says Slavin. "Eating fiber goes together with other healthy behaviors."

Researchers typically adjust for smoking, weight, exercise, education, alcohol, saturated fat, and other factors that influence heart disease risk, but they could still miss something.

Those inconsistencies didn't matter so much as long as people were getting their fiber from whole grains, fruits, and vegetables, rather than from purified fibers added to foods like ice cream.

"That's why we have always encouraged people to eat fiber from foods like whole grains," says Slavin. That way they're getting both soluble and insoluble fiber and the whole "fiber package."

Diabetes

"There's moderately strong evidence that fiber is linked to a reduced risk of diabetes, and it's based on whole foods like vegetables, fruits, and whole grains," says JoAnn Manson, professor of medicine at Harvard Medical School and chief of preventive medicine at Brigham and Women's Hospital in Boston.

The evidence that fiber prevents diabetes parallels the evidence that it prevents heart disease, as do the inconsistencies.

In two studies—on roughly 65,000 women and 43,000 men—those who reported eating the most fiber *from grains* (8 grams a day) had about a 30 percent lower risk of diabetes than those who reported eating the least fiber from grains (3 grams a day).[3,4]

As with heart disease, it could always be something else about fiber eaters, or something other than the fiber in grains, that matters. "We don't have large-scale trials showing that fiber prevents diabetes," cautions Manson.

But in short-term clinical studies, the gummy *soluble* fibers (in foods like oats and barley) keep a lid on blood sugar.

"There's good evidence that fiber slows the absorption of the carbohydrate in foods, which leads to a less marked increase in blood sugar and less demand for insulin," explains Manson.

If those studies had lasted longer, researchers might have found that *insoluble* fiber also lowered blood sugar.

"When we fed insulin-resistant women a cereal high in insoluble fiber for a year, nothing happened for six months," says Wolever. Then the bacteria in the colon started to change, and the women became more sensitive to insulin.

How? "We think that bacteria in the colon affect gut hormones, which could keep beta-cells in the pancreas from dying," he speculates. Beta-cells produce insulin.

Much of that evidence is preliminary, cautions Wolever. What fiber does to bacteria in the colon "is still pretty much a black box."

Colon Cancer

In the mid-1980s, the evidence made it seem like a slam-dunk that fiber could prevent colon cancer. Then in April 2000, two large studies released unexpected news.

In a three-year trial, roughly 700 people who were told to eat 13 ½ grams of wheat bran a day had no fewer new precancerous colon polyps than 700 others who were told to eat only 2 grams a day.[5]

The Bottom Line

- Whole-grain breads and cereals, which are naturally rich in fiber, are linked to a lower risk of **heart disease** and **diabetes**.
- Foods rich in insoluble fibers, like wheat bran, help prevent **constipation** and possibly **diverticular disease**.
- The evidence that high-fiber foods lower the risk of **colon cancer** is inconclusive.
- Eating fruits, vegetables, and other high-fiber, lower-calorie foods may help slow **weight gain**.
- Isolated inulin, polydextrose, and maltodextrin are soluble fibers but they're not gummy, so they probably don't lower **blood cholesterol** or **blood sugar**.
- Isolated oat fiber and soy fiber are insoluble, so they may help keep you **regular**. Polydextrose may also help, but inulin and maltodextrin don't seem to.

And in a four-year trial, roughly 1,000 people who were told to eat a lower-fat diet rich in fiber (36 grams a day) from fruits, vegetables, and whole grains had no fewer polyps than 1,000 others who were told to eat their usual diet.[6]

"The trials are not ambiguous," says John Baron, a professor of medicine at Dartmouth Medical School who has conducted trials testing calcium and folic acid on the risk of precancerous colon polyps. "They have shown no effect."

Despite the two disappointing trials, the American Institute for Cancer Research concluded last year that fiber-rich foods "probably" prevent colon cancer. Its evidence: studies like the European Investigation into Cancer and Nutrition (EPIC), which tracked more than 500,000 people in 10 countries for five years. EPIC found a 40 percent lower risk of colon cancer in people who reported eating more fiber-rich foods.[7]

So why did the two trials strike out? Maybe it's not fiber, but something else about fiber eaters, that cuts their risk of cancer.

Or maybe the trials found nothing because they looked at polyps, not cancers.

"If fiber keeps polyps from progressing to colon cancer but has no effect at earlier stages, you may not see a connection between fiber and polyps in these trials," offers Manson.

The bottom line: "The jury is still out for fiber lowering the risk of colorectal cancer," says Manson. "The evidence is stronger for coronary heart disease and diabetes than for cancer."

Baron is less optimistic. "The jury may still be out, but it's polling eight-to-four against."

Obesity

Can fiber help keep you slim by slowing the rate at which food exits your stomach, which could make you feel full for longer?

"Fiber might help maintain weight," says the University of Toronto's Thomas Wolever. "But it's not magic. It's not a strong effect."

In a study of roughly 75,000 women, those who boosted their fiber intake by 12 grams a day curbed their weight gain

Bulk Delivery

Here's a sampling of foods that are rich in intact fiber (along with a few lower-fiber foods for comparison). Whole wheat is mostly insoluble fiber, but most fruits, vegetables, beans, and nuts have a mix of soluble and insoluble fiber.

Fruits & Juices	Fiber *(grams)*
Blackberries *(1 cup)*	8
Pear *(1)*	5
Apple or Orange *(1)*	4
Figs, dried *(2)*	4
Kiwi *(2)*	4
Apricots, dried *(5)*	3
Banana *(1)* or Raisins *(¼ cup)*	3
Blueberries or Strawberries *(1 cup)*	3
Prunes *(5)* or Prune juice *(1 cup)*	3
Peach *(1)*, Avocado *(⅕)*, or Grapefruit *(½)*	2
Cantaloupe *(¼)* or Grapes *(1½ cups)*	1
Orange juice *(1 cup)*	0.5

Vegetables *(cooked, unless noted)*	
Peas *(½ cup)*	5
Sweet potato, baked, with skin *(1)*	4
Broccoli *(½ cup)* or Green beans *(⅔ cup)*	3
Green pepper, raw *(1)*	3
Potato, baked, with skin *(1)*	3
Asparagus *(6 spears)*	2
Carrot, raw *(1)*	2
Cauliflower *(⅔ cup)* or Corn *(½ cup)*	2
Romaine lettuce *(1¾ cups shredded)*	2
Spinach, Kale, or Brussels sprouts *(½ cup)*	2
Tomato *(1)*	2

Grains & Pasta *(cooked)*	
Bulgur *(¾ cup)*	6
Pasta, whole wheat *(1 cup)*	6
Popcorn, air-popped *(4 cups popped)*	4
Pasta, regular *(1 cup)*	3
Rice, brown *(¾ cup)*	3
Rice, white *(¾ cup)*	0.5

Nuts *(number closest to 1 oz., unless noted)*	Fiber *(grams)*
Almonds *(24)*	4
Peanuts *(28)* or Peanut butter *(2 Tbs.)*	2
Cashews *(18)*	1

Beans *(½ cup cooked, unless noted)*	
Black beans or Split peas	8
Kidney beans	7
Lentils	7
Chickpeas or Pinto beans, canned	6
Hummus *(2 Tbs.)* or Tofu *(3 oz.)*	2

Bread & Crackers	
Finn Crisp Thin Crisps, Original *(4)*	6
Whole wheat bread *(2 slices)*	6
Nabisco Triscuits *(6)*	3
White bread *(2 slices)*	1

Hot Cereal *(1 cup cooked)*	
Oat bran	6
Wheatena	5
Oatmeal	4
Cream of wheat	1

Cold Cereal	
Kellogg's All-Bran, Original *(½ cup)*	10
Post Shredded Wheat 'n Bran *(1¼ cups)*	8
Kellogg's Raisin Bran *(1 cup)*	7
Post Grape-Nuts *(½ cup)*	7
Post Shredded Wheat *(2 biscuits)*	6
Post Bran Flakes *(¾ cup)*	5
General Mills Wheaties *(¾ cup)*	3
Kellogg's Corn Flakes *(1 cup)*	1
Special K *(1 cup)*	1

Note: numbers below 1 rounded to the nearest 0.5 gram.
Sources: company information and USDA.
Table compiled by Amy Johnson.

by 8 pounds over the next 12 years.[8] And in a study that tracked 22,000 men for 8 years, those who upped their fiber by 20 grams a day cut their weight gain by 12 pounds.[9]

"We saw less weight gain in women who consumed a higher-fiber diet," says Manson, who was a co-author of the study on women. "It's plausible that fiber leads to satiety and a less calorie-dense diet, but long-term trials are needed."

Of course, if high-fiber foods curb weight gain because people are eating high-fiber, lower-calorie foods like fruits and vegetables, that wouldn't apply to high-fiber, *not*-low-calorie bars, crackers, cereals, and ice cream.

Regularity

A few studies have suggested that people who eat more insoluble fiber have a lower risk of diverticular disease (small pouches that bulge out through weak spots in the large intestine, sometimes becoming inflamed or infected).[10]

But fiber's starring role in the GI tract is in the stool department. Insoluble fiber tends to help "laxation" by adding bulk to stool.

"We know that insoluble fibers like wheat bran are good for stool weight and laxation and soluble fibers like pectin aren't," explains the University of Minnesota's Joanne Slavin.

After dozens of studies, researchers have even estimated how much you can expect stool weight to increase for each gram of fiber you eat. (That's 5.4 grams for wheatbran fiber, 4.9 grams for fruit and vegetable fiber, 3 grams for isolated cellulose, and 1.3 grams for isolated pectin, in case you were wondering.)[11]

Insoluble fiber from bran helps prevent constipation because it bulks up the stool. "The bran fiber is still there at the end of the GI tract, where it binds water, so it's going to increase stool weight," explains Slavin.

In contrast, most soluble fibers, like the pectin in fruits and vegetables, are digested by bacteria in the gut, "so there's nothing left at the end of the GI tract."

But it's not just a question of insoluble vs. soluble. For example, psyllium, the (mostly) soluble fiber in Metamucil, is a laxative. And wheat bran has a bigger impact than cellulose—its purified cousin—even though both are insoluble.

"If you pulverize wheat bran, it has less effect on stool weight," notes Slavin. "The size of the particles or structure of the food may make a difference in how much survives the digestive tract."

Isolated vs. Intact

Companies are now adding a host of isolated fibers—like inulin, maltodextrin, oat fiber, and polydextrose—to foods. And their ads and labels imply that those fibers are equal to the intact, naturally occurring fiber in foods.

But the evidence on isolated fibers is much skimpier. "There's not much out there," says Slavin.

Researchers can divide the new fibers into soluble and insoluble, but that's not enough. To lower LDL ("bad") cholesterol, for example, fiber has to be soluble *and* viscous.

"Inulin, polydextrose, and maltodextrin are soluble fiber, but they're not viscous at all, so they absolutely don't lower cholesterol," says Slavin.

Isolated viscous fibers—like those from oats, barley, or guar gum—would make foods like ice cream and yogurt too gummy. "They'd be almost impossible to consume," explains Slavin.

The new isolated fibers aren't gummy at all, she adds. "That's why you can put them in so many foods."

Each fiber's impact on regularity also goes beyond soluble vs. insoluble. For example, you wouldn't expect inulin to do much for regularity because gut bacteria gobble most of it up.

In contrast, polydextrose might help keep your GI tract moving, at least according to one industry-sponsored study done in China.[12] "It would be nice to have more evidence," notes Slavin.

Unfortunately, both inulin and polydextrose have a downside in large doses.

"Inulin may cause gas or other GI problems at doses above 15 grams a day," says Slavin. "For some people, the gas isn't a big issue, but others are really sensitive."

And foods that contain more than 15 grams of polydextrose per serving must warn consumers that "sensitive individuals may experience a laxative effect from excessive consumption of this product."

On the other hand, "some modified starches have no GI effects at 50 grams a day," adds Slavin.

And yet, despite all the differences among isolated fibers—and between isolated and intact fiber—they all look the same on a food's Nutrition Facts panel.

"On the label, it all looks like good stuff," says Slavin. "But fiber does not equal fiber," she adds.

"If you eat five fiber-fortified yogurts a day, you can meet your fiber goal. But that's not the message we want people to get. It's not the same as getting 25 grams of fiber from a variety of fruits, vegetables, and whole grains."

It won't hurt to eat yogurt, ice cream, or other foods with added fiber . . . unless it becomes an excuse to eat fiber-rich cookies instead of bran cereal.

"I wouldn't want people to feel that they don't have to eat fruits, vegetables, and whole grains any more because they're eating ice cream with inulin," says Wolever, "especially if it means that instead of one serving of ice cream, they'll have two servings because they think it's healthy."

Notes

1. *JAMA 275:* 447, 1996.
2. *JAMA 281:* 1998, 1999.
3. *JAMA 277:* 472, 1997.
4. *Diabetes Care 20:* 545, 1997.
5. *N. Engl. J. Med. 342:* 1156, 2000.
6. *N. Engl. J. Med. 342:* 1149, 2000.
7. *Lancet 361:* 1496, 2003.
8. *Am. J. Clin. Nutr. 78:* 920, 2003.
9. *Am. J. Clin. Nutr. 80:* 1237, 2004.
10. *J. Nutr. 128:* 714, 1998.
11. *Spiller, GA, ed., CRC Handbook of Dietary Fiber in Human Nutrition* (Boca Raton, FL: CRC Press, 1993), 263–349.
12. *Am. J. Clin. Nutr. 72:* 1503, 2000.

Critical Thinking

1. How much fiber do a typical male and female living in the United States consume?
2. Differentiate between the health benefits and food sources of soluble and insoluble fiber.
3. If you need 2000 calories per day to maintain your body weight, how many grams of fiber should you consume in a day?
4. Explain why isolated fibers such as inulin, polydextros, and maltodextrin do not have the same effect on lowering LDL cholesterol as intact soluble fibers from foods.

Seafood Showdown: Fatty Acids vs. Heavy Metals

JULIE HANUS

Ever feel like we've just totally screwed ourselves with the oceans? I'm not even talking about BP's gushing well: It's this recent report from the *Telegraph* that U.K. nutritionists are now advising pregnant women to eat more fish.

Fish, of course, contains mercury, a heavy metal pollutant that comes from human industry (and, to be fair, from some natural sources like volcano eruptions). Pregnant women, children, the elderly—nutritional convention has been to watch how much you eat. Except seafood also is a rich source of omega-3s, and nutritionists now say that the fatty-acid benefits, especially for pregnant women, could outweigh the heavy-metal risks.

What benefits, you say? The star of the omega-3 cast is docosahexaenoic acid (DHA), and as *The Economist* tidily explains:

DHA is a component of brains, particularly the synaptic junctions between nerve cells, and its displacement from modern diets by the omega-6 acids in cooking oils such as soya, maize and rape is a cause of worry.

Many researchers think this shift—and the change in brain chemistry that it causes—explains the growth in recent times of depression, manic-depression, memory loss, schizophrenia and attention-deficit disorder. It may also be responsible for rising levels of obesity and thus the heart disease which often accompanies being overweight.

Stateside nutritionists are also changing their minds. A group has petitioned the Food and Drug Administration to adjust its stance on pregnant women's diets, and the Department of Defense plans to launch a program to augment soldiers' diets with omega-3s, *The Economist* reports. Low levels of DHA are a suicide risk factor for people in the service.

So here's the positive take-away, if there is one: Should you wish to get more fish-based omega-3s into your diet, eating lower on the fish food chain is the best way to make that happen, keep mercury levels low, and, oh yeah, stop straining the ocean's ecosystems by gobbling up big predators like tuna, swordfish, and grouper. (For what it's worth, there are also plant-based sources of omega-3s, although there have been studies that shed doubt on whether they are as beneficial as the fish-based ones.)

For some excellent reading about eating lower on the fish food chain, follow the link to an excerpt from Taras Grescoe's book *Bottomfeeder,* which is one of the most illuminating studies I've read on how to eat fish ethically. (And he's a big fan of the omega-3s.)

Critical Thinking

1. What type of fatty acid is docosahexaenoic acid (DHA)? Identify the fish that are the best sources of DHA.

2. What are the health benefits of consuming DHA?

3. Soybean oil, corn oil, and rapeseed (canola) oil are examples of what type of fat?

The Fairest Fats of Them All (and Those to Avoid)

The science on fats is changing as rapidly as today's fashions. So work hard to know your fats—from bad to good.

SHARON PALMER, RD

Think you're in step with the latest in fat science? If you're still preaching low fat to your patients, perhaps you need to brush up on your fat knowledge. Low fat is as out of fashion as shoulder pads. Today's nutrition advice should be all about healthy fats.

"I think the fat phobia of the '90s is old school now. Dietitians need to keep up with the research. We should not really be recommending low fat anymore. There is tremendous value in olive oil. Dietitians need to know this concept and to recommend that their patients consume good fats. People can have an enjoyable diet with food that tastes great. Dietitians need to be aware of these issues and incorporate them in their work," says Janet Bond Brill, PhD, RD, LDN, a nutrition and fitness consultant and the author of *Cholesterol Down: 10 Simple Steps to Lower Your Cholesterol in 4 Weeks—Without Prescription Drugs.*

If keeping up with research on fat is challenging for nutrition professionals, you can imagine how confusing it is for the public. First it was low fat, then zero trans fat, and now it's a push toward monounsaturated fatty acids (MUFAs). "Absolutely, there is confusion in the public over fats," says Brill. And it's time to set them straight.

"There is general agreement that about 30% of total calories should come from fat," says Joyce Nettleton, DSc, editor of the *Fats of Life* newsletter and *PUFA Newsletters*. The American Heart Association (AHA) suggests that 25% to 35% of total calories should come from fat. Brill reports that within the total fat intake, 7% of calories or less should come from saturated fats, less than 1% should come from trans fats, at least 10% and up to 20% of calories should come from MUFAs, and the remaining amount (up to 10%) should come from polyunsaturated fatty acids (PUFAs).

Fats to Beware

"The message needs to be made loud and clear that saturated fats, cholesterol, and trans fats need to be avoided. These are the three things that contribute to heart disease, which is our No. 1 killer among men and women," says Brill.

Suggestions for limiting dietary cholesterol and saturated fats have existed for decades. We know that saturated fats increase low-density lipoprotein (LDL) cholesterol levels, thus increasing the risk of heart disease. And during the past few years, the public has been hit over the head with the message that trans fats are the bad guys, since trans fats raise LDL cholesterol and may lower high-density lipoprotein cholesterol.

While saturated fats may not be totally eliminated from the diet because they are found in foods that provide important nutrients, such as animal and dairy products, artificial trans fats can be phased out. Naturally occurring trans fats are found in very small amounts in animal products, but most of the trans fats people consume are found in processed and restaurant foods, which can be produced using healthier oil formulations.

Nettleton points out that food manufacturers and restaurants have made great strides in ridding the food supply of trans fats; however, there are still areas for improvement. Many products, from deep-fried fast foods to microwave popcorns, are still chock full of trans fats, and manufacturers may still list "0 grams" of trans fat on food labels when products contain less than 0.5 grams of trans fat per serving.[1]

"Hopefully, we are getting trans fats out of the food supply. We need legislation like Denmark, where it is banned in the entire country. California state legislation against trans fats is a great step," says Brill, who advises her clients to look for and then avoid sources of hydrogenated oils on all ingredient lists before choosing foods.

Today, we face new challenges with upholding the strategy of lowering saturated fats. The elimination of trans fats from food production has reintroduced saturated fats as a functional solution to food processing. Even home cooks are turning more frequently to butter as a baking alternative in an attempt to avoid trans fats. And although the high-protein diet has lost its initial gloss, it promoted a lingering notion that eating larger portions of animal protein, with their accompanying contribution of saturated fat, is a "lean" way of eating.

The solutions to these issues are not always clear. For example, Nettleton reports that palm oil, an increasingly common fat that food manufacturers use to replace trans fat, is rich in palmitic acid, which for the most part has no effect on blood cholesterol levels. But many experts still recommend avoiding palm oil because it is a source of saturated fat. And when people are reaching for a suitable fat for their favorite chocolate chip cookie recipe, which presents the lesser evil: saturated fat in butter or trans fat in stick margarine?

Navigating these challenges may be best accomplished by analyzing individual lifestyles and making recommendations accordingly—something at which dietitians are skilled. The "budget" approach to saturated fats is an option. How do you want to spend your saturated fat allotment for the day: on really good cheese, filet mignon, or homemade cookies? Trans fat may be a nonissue for someone who enjoys cooking and eating at home, but it can pose difficulties for people who regularly eat out of food packages and from fast-food drive-throughs. "It depends on people's food habits. It comes down to individual food choices and everything in moderation," says Nettleton.

The new shift in fat science focuses on the fact that the Western diet is flooded with the omega-6 fatty acid linoleic acid and is low in omega-3 fatty acids, an eating style that appears to be proinflammatory and conducive to chronic disease. As people were urged to increase their intake of polyunsaturated vegetable oils to reduce blood cholesterol levels in decades past, there was a tremendous increase in the agricultural production of oil seed crops, primarily soybean. Estimates indicate that 20% of the calories in the American diet come from soybean oil alone. The vast majority of liquid vegetable oils used in food processing, such as soybean, corn, and safflower oils, are high in omega-6 fatty acids. "We need to get our omega-6 fatty acids way down. Right now, they are at a ratio of 20 to 30:1 omega-6 to omega-3 fatty acids, and they need to be at a ratio of 4:1 or lower," says Brill.

"At the same time that we need to decrease omega-6, we need to increase long-chain omega-3 fatty acids. Epidemiological studies show overall heart health with high PUFAs, but we need higher levels of long-chain omega-3 fatty acids to offset the high levels of omega-6. If we didn't have such low levels of long-chain omega-3 fatty acids, the high omega-6 intake wouldn't be so problematic," adds Nettleton.

Good Fats to the Rescue

To achieve a healthier fat lineup, the secret is to focus on healthier MUFAs and omega-3 fatty acids. According to the AHA, adding healthy MUFAs and omega-3s can help provide antioxidants such as vitamin E and selenium; foster absorption of important nutrients in fruits and vegetables; prevent and treat

diabetes, heart disease, cancer, obesity, musculoskeletal pain, and inflammatory conditions; positively affect cholesterol, blood pressure, blood clotting, and inflammation; and support brain growth and development.[1]

"The best strategy for getting a more positive ratio of omega-6 to omega-3 fatty acids is to eat less linoleic acid and increase omega-3 fatty acids. We need to replace these oils with olive oil as the main fat, which is part one. The No. 1 oil for home use should be olive oil; it can be used in salad dressings and cooking. For baking, canola oil is a good choice," says Brill, who also notes that extra-virgin olive oil is an even better choice than regular olive oil because it has not been treated with excessive heat or solvents. Thus, it offers an added bonus of polyphenols and antioxidants.

> **"The best strategy for getting a more positive ratio of omega-6 to omega-3 fatty acids is to eat less linoleic acid and increase omega-3 fatty acids."**
> —Janet Bond Brill, PhD, RD, LDN

MUFAs are found in canola, olive, peanut, and sunflower oils, as well as avocados, seeds, and nuts. But it's difficult to find MUFAs as the main source of fat in processed foods, so focusing on whole foods and cooking at home is paramount. "There should be an emphasis on monounsaturated fats in cooking use, such as canola oil and olive oil. Minimize the use of corn, soybean, and safflower oils, as you'll get mostly linoleic acid," adds Nettleton.

"Part two is bumping up omega-3 fatty acids by getting daily doses of plant omega-3 fatty acids such as flax and walnuts and marine sources of omega-3 fatty acids, DHA [docosahexaenoic acid] and EPA [eicosapentaenoic acid], by eating fatty fish at least two to three times per week. This shifts the physical environment away from a high omega-6 ratio, which promotes a proinflammatory situation conducive to blood clotting and chronic disease," says Brill. Unfortunately, the conversion of the plant form of omega-3 fatty acids, alpha-linolenic acid (ALA), to long-chain omega-3 fatty acids is modest at best. "Plant sources of omega-3 fatty acids are not equivalent to the long-chain omega-3 fatty acids DHA and EPA. People should target 500 milligrams per day of long-chain omega-3s," says Nettleton.

A growing body of evidence is linking increased intakes of long-chain omega-3 fatty acids found in fish and fish oil to decreased risk of cardiovascular disease, arrhythmias that can lead to sudden cardiac death, and thrombosis that can prompt myocardial infarction or stroke; decreased levels of triglycerides; slower growth of atherosclerotic plaque; improved vascular endothelial function; modest blood pressure lowering; and decreased inflammation. The omega-3 fatty acid ALA has benefits of its own, including reduced coronary heart disease risk.[2]

Oil Primer

"It's time for an oil change in this country," says Janet Bond Brill, PhD, RD, LDN, a nutrition and fitness consultant. Check out this profile on popular cooking oils to see how they rate for their fat ratios and cooking properties.

Oil	Fat Lineup	Properties
Olive	77% mono, 9% poly, 14% saturated	Rich olive taste, low smoke point. Best in dressings, marinades, sauces, sautés, pastas, casseroles, stir-fries, soups, and meat dishes.
Hazelnut	76% mono, 14% poly, 10% saturated	Brown colored with hazelnut flavor, high smoke point. Best used to bring out flavor in baked desserts, dressings, and meats.
Avocado	70% mono, 10% poly, 20% saturated	Light avocado flavor, high smoke point. Best in salad dressings and marinades, sautés, casseroles, pastas, and meats.
Canola	62% mono, 32% poly, 6% saturated	Light color and flavor, moderately high smoke point. Best for baking or in dishes that require a mild flavor.
Peanut	49% mono, 33% poly, 18% saturated	Peanut flavor and aroma, high smoke point. Best in foods that benefit from peanut flavor, such as Asian stir-fries, noodles, rice, and salads.
Sesame	40% mono, 46% poly, 14% saturated	Light and mild sesame flavor, moderately high smoke point. Best in Asian stir-fries, noodles, rice, and salads.
Palm	38% mono, 10% poly, 52% saturated	Red-orange color and unique flavor, high smoke point. May bring out the flavor in Caribbean and South American dishes but is moderately high in saturated fat.
Corn	25% mono, 62% poly, 13% saturated	Light and mild flavor, high smoke point. Best used in baking or deep-frying but is high in linoleic acid.
Soybean	24% mono, 61% poly, 15% saturated	Slightly heavy flavor, high smoke point. Best used in baking or deep-frying but is high in linoleic acid.
Sunflower	20% mono, 69% poly, 11% saturated	Light and flavorless, high smoke point. Best used in baking but is high in linoleic acid.
Walnut	19% mono, 67% poly, 14% saturated	Rich walnut flavor, moderately high smoke point. Best used to bring out flavor in baked desserts, dressings, and meats. High in alpha-linolenic acid.
Grape seed	17% mono, 71% poly, 12% saturated	Mild flavor, high smoke point. Best in sautéing or frying but is high in linoleic acid.
Safflower	13% mono, 77% poly, 10% saturated	Light color and flavor, high smoke point. Best for searing meats, baking desserts, and deep-frying foods but is high in linoleic acid.
Coconut	6% mono, 2% poly, 92% saturated	Solid at room temperature, buttery texture, low smoke point. Popular in Southeast Asian dishes but is high in saturated fats.

Note: Sorted in descending order of monounsaturated fat level. Fat levels and smoke points may vary depending on variety and oil refinement process.
Adapted from RecipeTips.com. Oils and fats nutritional facts, Available at: www.recipetips.com/kitchen-tips/t-153-1194/oils-and-fats-nutritional-facts.asp; The Nibble, Culinary oils glossary, Available at: www.thenibble.com/reviews/main/oils/culinary-oil-glossary.asp; What's Cooking America, Questions & Answers—Smoking points of various oils. Available at: http://whatscookingamerica.net/Q-A/SmokePointOil.htm

"There is significant research pointing out that ALA has tremendous health benefits. Even though the conversion rate to long-chain omega-3 fatty acids is low, I say get it in the diet anyway. These plant sources of ALA are very healthy foods, and we haven't fully discovered yet how they provide such great value to health. Perhaps there is some other mechanism other than conversion by which they provide benefits," says Brill.

Nettleton points out that ALA can help redress the balance of omega-6 to omega-3. But if people rely on ALA exclusively, they will not get the tremendous benefits specifically linked with long-chain omega-3s.

In the end, it seems dietitians have their work cut out for them trying to simplify the complicated science on fats for the public's easy digestion. But it looks like the stars are aligned for doing so. Chefs are warbling their praise for extra-virgin olive oil, the Mediterranean Diet is as hot as ever, and there seems to be a newfound respect for healthy food that tastes great.

"The public is slowly but surely realizing the value of adding healthy fats to the diet. You can see it in the popularity of the Mediterranean Diet, and the American Heart Association is no longer concentrating on low fat but on healthy fats," says Brill.

Notes

1. American Heart Association. Face the fats. Available at: www.americanheart.org/presenter.jhtml?identifier= 3046074
2. Linus Pauling Institute. Essential fatty acids. Available at: http://lpi.oregonstate.edu/infocenter/othernuts/omega3fa/index .html

Critical Thinking

1. What are the health benefits of consuming monounsaturated and omega-3 fatty acids?
2. Identify the three "bad fats" and food sources of each.
3. What effects do saturated fat and trans fats have on LDL (bad cholesterol)?
4. How many grams of trans fats per serving can a food product contain that has "0 trans fat" on the nutrition label?

SHARON PALMER, RD, is a contributing editor at *Today's Dietitian* and a freelance food and nutrition writer in southern California.

Vitamins, Supplements

New Evidence Shows They Can't Compete with Mother Nature

Americans want to believe in vitamin and mineral pills: We spent an estimated $10 billion on them in 2008, according to the Nutrition Business Journal. But recent studies undertaken to assess their benefits have delivered a flurry of disappointing results. The supplements failed to prevent Alzheimer's disease, cancer, heart attacks, strokes, type 2 diabetes, and premature death.

"We have yet to see well-conducted research that categorically supports the use of vitamin and mineral supplements," says Linda Van Horn, PhD, a professor of preventive medicine at Northwestern University's Feinberg School of Medicine in Chicago. "Most studies show no benefit, or actual harm."

The Power of Food

While some people may need supplements at certain stages of their lives, nutritional deficiencies are uncommon in the U.S. "Almost all of us get or can get the vitamins and minerals we need from our diet," says Paul M. Coates, PhD., director of the Office of Dietary Supplements at the National Institutes of Health (NIH).

Major health organizations for cancer, diabetes, and heart disease all advise against supplements in favor of a healthful diet rich in fruits, vegetables, whole grains, and legumes. Unlike pills, those foods contain fiber plus thousands of health-protective substances that seem to work together more powerfully than any single ingredient can work alone. "That's why it's dangerous to say, 'I know I don't eat well, but if I pop my vitamins, I'm covered,'" says Karen Collins, RD, nutrition adviser to the American Institute for Cancer Research. "We now know that you're not covered."

Too Much Can Harm

Another concern is that some vitamin pills can be toxic if taken in high doses for a long time. Studies show that beta-carotene pills, for example, can increase the risk of lung cancer in smokers, and a 2008 review suggests that the pills, plus supplemental doses of the vitamins A and E, may increase the risk of premature death. In addition, a government survey found that more than 11 percent of adults take at least 400 international units of vitamin E a day, a dose that has been linked to heart failure, strokes, and an increased risk of death.

People are also apt to combine vitamin tablets and fortified foods, which can cause problems. For instance, too much folic acid—added to wheat products in this country—can mask vitamin B12 deficiency. Untreated, that can lead to irreversible nerve damage. In addition, high doses of folic acid may be associated with an increased risk of precancerous colon polyps, according to a trial of some 1,000 people at risk for them. "We're getting several alarming signals that more may not be better," says Susan T. Mayne, PhD., a professor of epidemiology at the Yale School of Public Health.

Yet despite the unfavorable results, vitamin and mineral pills are widely used to fend off diseases. Read on to find our review of the latest evidence on their effects.

Critical Thinking

1. If people choose to consume their nutrient requirements by taking supplements, what nutrients are they not consuming?

2. What type of cancer has been linked to excess intake of folic acid?

3. What nutrient in supplement form has been shown to increase the risk for smokers developing lung cancer?

Antioxidants: Fruitful Research and Recommendations

PAMELA S. BRUMMIT, MA, RD/LD

Free radicals, which are produced during food metabolism and by external factors such as radiation and smog, can damage cells and may contribute to some diseases—notably heart disease and cancer—and many experts believe antioxidants can help prevent this damage.

The body's immune system helps defend against oxidative stress. As we age, this defense becomes less effective, which contributes to poor health. Clinical studies hypothesize that when we consume antioxidants, we provide our bodies with protection and health benefits.

Antioxidants Defined

The USDA identifies beta-carotene (vitamin A), selenium, vitamin C, vitamin E, lutein, and lycopene as antioxidant substances.

Lycopene is a pigment that gives vegetables and fruits such as tomatoes, pink grapefruit, and watermelon their red hue. Several studies suggest that consuming foods rich in lycopene is associated with a lower risk of prostate cancer and cardiovascular disease. Lycopene is better absorbed when consumed in processed tomato products rather than in fresh tomatoes.

Selenium is a trace mineral that is essential to good health but required only in small amounts. Its antioxidant properties help prevent cellular damage from free radicals. Plant foods are the major dietary sources of selenium, but the content in a particular food depends on the selenium content of the soil where it's grown. Soils in the high plains of northern Nebraska and the Dakotas have very high levels of selenium.

Lutein is found in large amounts in the lens and retina of our eyes and is recognized for its eye health benefits. It may also protect against damage caused by UVB light and is a critical component to overall skin health. Lutein is found naturally in foods such as dark green, leafy vegetables and egg yolks.

The antioxidant function of beta-carotene (precursor to vitamin A) is its ability to reduce free radicals and protect the cell membrane lipids from the harmful effects of oxidation.

In addition, beta-carotene may provide some synergism to vitamin E.

As a water-soluble antioxidant, vitamin C reduces free radicals before they can damage the lipids. These antioxidant properties fight free radicals that can promote wrinkles, age spots, cataracts, and arthritis. Also, the antioxidants in vitamin C have been found to fight free radicals that prey on organs and blood vessels.

As an antioxidant, vitamin E may help prevent or delay cardiovascular disease and cancer and has been shown to play a role in immune function. DNA repair, and other metabolic processes.

Fruits and vegetables, nuts, grains, poultry, and fish are major sources of antioxidants.

Research

Researchers have studied antioxidants and disease processes for years. Some studies have found that an increased intake of beta-carotene is associated with decreased cardiovascular mortality in older adult populations. Studies on the effects of vitamin E on aging have shown potential relationships between the vitamin and the prevention of atherosclerosis, cancer, cataracts, arthritis, central nervous system disorders such as Parkinson's disease, Alzheimer's disease, and impaired glucose tolerance. Studies on vitamin C suggest that it may help protect against vascular dementia, and studies on selenium point to its potential role in cancer prevention.[1–3] Beta-carotene, vitamin C, and vitamin E showed a positive improvement in muscle strength and may improve physical performance in older adults.[4]

One lycopene study found that eating 10 or more servings per week of tomato products was associated with up to a 35% reduced risk of prostate cancer. Another study suggested that men who had the highest amount of lycopene in their body fat were one half as likely to suffer a heart attack as those with the least amount. Numerous studies correlate a high intake of lycopene-containing foods or high lycopene serum levels with reduced incidence of cancer, cardiovascular disease, and macular degeneration. However, estimates of lycopene consumption have been based on reported tomato intake, not on the use of lycopene supplements. Since tomatoes are sources of other nutrients, including vitamin C, folate, and potassium, it is unclear whether lycopene itself is beneficial.[5–7]

Some researchers suggest that eliminating free radicals may actually interfere with a natural defense mechanism within the body. Large doses of antioxidants may keep immune systems from fighting off invading pathogens.

Three out of four intervention trials using high-dose beta-carotene supplements did not show protective effects against cancer or cardiovascular disease. Rather, the high-risk population (smokers and asbestos workers) showed an increase in cancer and angina cases. It appears that beta-carotene can promote health when taken at dietary levels but may have adverse effects when taken in high doses by subjects who smoke or who have been exposed to asbestos.[8]

Results from one study indicate that antioxidant supplementation may not be beneficial for disease prevention. This study showed no consistent, clear evidence for health effects. However, the preliminary studies suggest antioxidants may block the heart-damaging effects of oxygen on arteries and the cell damage that might encourage some kinds of cancer.[9]

There remains a lack of knowledge regarding the safety of long-term mega-doses of vitamins. Research continues to be inconclusive and the data incomplete. Research has not been able to validate a link between oxidative stress and chronic disease. As with all research, the studies have been too diverse to provide conclusions.

Recommendations

The American Dietetic Association and the American Heart Association (AHA) recommend that people eat a variety of nutrient-rich foods from all of the food groups on a daily basis because this provides necessary nutrients, including antioxidants. Some researchers believe antioxidants are effective only when they are consumed in foods that contain them.

The recognized beneficial roles that fruits and vegetables play in the reduced risk of disease has led health organizations to develop programs encouraging consumers to eat more antioxidant-rich fruits and vegetables. The AHA and the American Cancer Society recommend that healthy adults eat five or more servings per day. The World Cancer Research Fund and the American Institute for Cancer Research report that "evidence of dietary protection against cancer is strongest and most consistent for diets high in vegetables and fruits."

Given the high degree of scientific consensus regarding the benefits of a diet high in fruits and vegetables—particularly those that contain dietary fiber and vitamins A and C—the FDA released a health claim for fruits and vegetables in relation to cancer. Food packages that meet FDA criteria may now carry the claim, "Diets low in fat and high in fruits

and vegetables may reduce the risk of some cancers." The FDA also released a dietary guidance message for consumers: "Diets rich in fruits and vegetables may reduce the risk of some types of cancer and other chronic diseases." The 2005 Dietary Guidelines for Americans states, "Increased intakes of fruits, vegetables, whole grains, and fat-free or low-fat milk and milk products are likely to have important health benefits for most Americans."

Antioxidant research continues to grow and emerge as researchers discover new, beneficial components of food. Reinforced by current research, the message remains that antioxidants obtained from food sources, including fruits, vegetables, and whole grains, may reduce disease risk and can benefit human health.

Using the latest research technologies, USDA nutrition scientists measured the antioxidant levels in more than 100 different foods, including fruits, vegetables, nuts, dried fruits, spices, and cereals. The top 20 ranked foods that interfere with or prevent damage from free radicals are artichokes (cooked), black beans, black plums, blackberries, cranberries, cultivated blueberries, Gala apples, Granny Smith apples, pecans, pinto beans, plums, prunes, raspberries, Red Delicious apples, red kidney beans, Russet potatoes (cooked), small red beans, strawberries, sweet cherries, and wild blueberries.

How can we encourage older adults to eat more fruits and vegetables, especially those high in antioxidants? Share this helpful list with your older adult clients and patients.

1. Try one new fruit or vegetable per week. Variety is key!
2. Keep washed, ready-to-eat fruits and vegetables on hand and easily accessible. On the run? Take a bag of fruits or vegetables with you to munch on.
3. Serve fruits and vegetables with other favorite foods.
4. Add vegetables to casseroles, stews, and soups and puréed fruits and vegetables to sauces. Include vegetables in sandwiches and pastas.
5. Sprinkle vegetables with Parmesan cheese or top with melted low-fat cheese or white sauce made with low-fat milk.
6. Experiment with different methods of cooking fruits and vegetables.
7. Enjoy vegetables with low-fat dip for a snack.
8. Try commercial prepackaged salads and stir-fry mixes to save time.
9. Drink 100% fruit juice instead of fruit-flavored drinks or soda.
10. Serve fruit for dessert.
11. Keep a bowl of apples, bananas, and/or oranges on the dining room table.
12. Choose a side salad made with a variety of leafy greens.
13. Bake with raisin, date, or prune purée to reduce fat intake and increase fiber consumption.
14. Order vegetable toppings on your pizza.

15. Sip fruit smoothies for breakfast or snacks. Blend papaya with pineapple for a cool afternoon treat, or sip on a glass of fresh tomato juice at dinner.

16. Make a fruit salad to try many different types of fruit at once.

17. Learn to recognize a serving of fruits and vegetables: a medium-sized piece of fruit or ½ cup of most fresh, canned, or cooked fruits and vegetables.

18. Start your day with fruit. For example, add fruit to cereal or yogurt or pile on waffles. Or add vegetables—tomatoes, onions, potatoes—to an omelet or scrambled eggs.

19. Top meat and fish with salsa made from tomatoes, onions, corn, mangos, or other fruits and vegetables.

20. Try vegetarian choices: Vegetable stir fry, bean burrito, etc.

Critical Thinking

1. What diseases have been linked to free radical damage? What is the relationship of free radicals and antioxidants?

2. Identify three vitamins, one mineral, and two bioactive compounds that function as antioxidants.

3. Classify the top 20 foods that prevent damage from free radicals by food group (fruit, vegetable, or legumes).

PAMELA S. BRUMMIT, MA, RD/LD, is the founder and president of Brummit & Associates, Inc, a dietary consulting firm. She has held more than 20 board positions in local, state, and national dietetic associations and is past chair of Consultant Dietitians in Health Care Facilities dietetic practice group.

UNIT 3
Diet and Disease

Unit Selections

Learning Outcomes

After reading this unit, you should be able to

- Illustrate the link between the consumption of high-fructose corn sweeteners and increased risk for heart disease, metabolic syndrome, type 2 diabetes, gout, and accumulation of visceral fat.

- Define discretionary calories. Identify the recommended amount of discretionary calories for an average male and female.

- Describe the DASH diet. Identify how many servings of fruits and vegetables and how much sodium is recommended per day with the DASH diet.

- Discuss why it is more challenging for older adults to lose or maintain their body weight.

- Define mindful eating. Discuss why these principles are beneficial in eating disorders treatment, lowering cardiac disease risk, and weight loss in the overweight/obese.

- Explain why a high-fiber, low-fat (where most fats are from monounsaturated and omega-3 fats) diet is the best overall long-term diet advice for a person with type 2 diabetes.

Student Website
www.mhhe.com/cls

Internet References

American Cancer Society
www.cancer.org
American Diabetes Association
www.diabetes.org
American Heart Association (AHA)
www.americanheart.org
The Center for Mindful Eating
www.tcme.org
The Food Allergy and Anaphylaxis Network
www.foodallergy.org
LaLeche League International
www.lalecheleague.org
National Eating Disorders Association
www.nationaleatingdisorders.org

Research that focuses on the connection between diet and disease has unraveled the role of many nutrients in the delay of onset of certain diseases, prevention of diseases, and in some instances disease reversal. The challenging aspect of releasing findings from nutrition research is communicating this information in a manner that is not controversial or contradictory to previously released messages. With the increasing interest in health and disease prevention among Americans, media outlets publish scientific findings prematurely and without the physiological context in which the message should be conveyed. Scientific research takes time to answer the questions about health, nutrition, disease, and medicine, whereas consumers want answers to these questions much quicker than scientifically possible.

Medical and nutrition research has changed since the mapping of the human genome. We have come to better understand the role of genetics in the expression of disease and its role in how we respond to dietary change. In addition, research about diet and disease has enabled us to understand the importance and uniqueness of the individual (age, gender, ethnicity, and genetics) and his or her particular response to dietary interventions. Individualizing one's diet to prevent disease and promote health is a new concept that we will see developing in the future.

The prevalence of diet and lifestyle related diseases in the United States is astronomical. Heart disease, type 2 diabetes, obesity, stroke, high blood pressure, osteoporosis, and certain cancers are diet-and lifestyle-related conditions that affect millions of Americans. Proper nutrition plays a vital role in these diseases. Components of foods such as saturated fats, trans fats, sodium, and added sugars continue to be highlighted as the premier culprits of these diseases.

The American Institute for Cancer Research estimates that 45 percent of colon cancers, 38 percent of breast cancers, and 69 percent of esophageal cancers would be prevented if Americans ate better, weighed less, and exercised more. One of the articles in this unit describes in detail why a Western diet, obesity, and physical inactivity all contribute to a higher risk for cancer and discusses the importance of lifestyle changes on decreasing the incidence of these diseases.

The number one concern of the health of the United States is the prevalence of overweight and obesity. Although much of the attention is centered on childhood obesity and tactics to prevent or curtail it, there is also an ongoing problem with overweight or obesity as our population ages. On average, Americans in their sixties are 10 pounds heavier than they were just a decade ago. A typical woman in her 40s weighs 168 pounds, compared to 143 pounds in the 1960s. People used to start midlife at a lower weight and lose weight when they reached their 50s. Humans need fewer calories as they age because of slower metabolism and the tendency to lose muscle mass and gain fat, especially abdominal fat. Since muscle burns more calories than fat, it is challenging to lose weight in older years and maintain weight while eating the usual intake. Staying lean and eating right can delay onset or prevent certain diseases that plague older Americans, such as osteoporosis, heart disease, hypertension, insulin resistance, memory loss, arthritis, and some cancers.

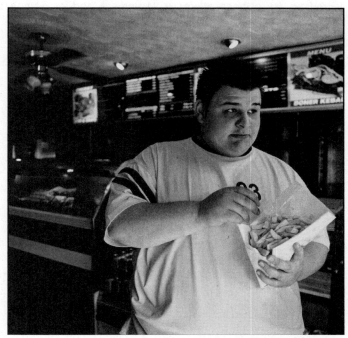
© Photodisc/Getty Images

The link between sodium intake and high blood pressure has been well defined with many research studies; however, the question of salt sensitivity is a lesser known principle. Currently there is no diagnostic test for sodium sensitivity, although several research groups are actively trying to discover a valid indicator. For now, we address sodium sensitivity by groups that are considered at higher risk. The current recommendation is for all Americans to cut back on sodium in their diet, with particular attention to those populations that are more likely to have increased blood pressure related to their sodium intake.

One of the latest areas of concern is the degree of added sugars that are consumed by Americans. The average American consumes 350 to 475 grams of added sugars each day. The most commonly consumed form of added sugars is high-fructose corn syrup, but other forms of sugar such as table sugar, honey, and cane juice are considered to be "added sugar" too. As more research explores the negative effects of high-fructose corn syrup on human health, food companies are developing products using other forms of sugar. These "natural sugars" still provide empty calories in the diet that may lead to weight gain if consumed in excess and not balanced by physical activity. Discretionary calories (calories consumed after nutrient needs are met from healthy food and beverage sources) are an effective way to think about the calories that you consume in relation to the calories needed to provide adequate nutrient intakes. The USDA recommends discretionary calories of approximately 100 calories for women and 150 calories for men. Individual recommendations for discretionary calorie allowances can be calculated using mypyramid.gov.

High-fructose sweeteners have been linked to greater risk for heart disease, metabolic syndrome, type 2 diabetes, gout, and accumulation of visceral fat. The link may be secondary to increased triglycerides and uric acid in the bloodstream secondary to the way fructose is metabolized. The Nurse's Health Study found that drinking 12 oz of regular soda correlates with increased risk of heart attack by 24 percent, and 24 or more ounces correlates to a risk of greater than 35 percent. Liquid calories from sugar sweetened beverages are not only empty calories, but also promote increased calorie intake at meals, possibly through suppression of leptin, a hormone that triggers you to stop eating.

An approach aiming to change our perspective of food and possibly help people who have trouble controlling their food intake is referred to as mindful eating. The busy lifestyle of Americans has changed our perception of food. We have desensitized ourselves of the normal homeostatic regulation of hunger cues and have a detached view of our food sources. Mindful eating is a new concept that has proven beneficial in eating disorders treatment, lowering cardiac disease risk, and weight loss in the overweight/obese. "Food for Thought: Exploring the Potential of Mindful Eating" by Sharon Palmer introduces the concept of mindful eating and gives tips on how to slow down, appreciate, and change your view of food.

We Will Be What We Eat

When it comes to staving off the problems of aging, from bone and muscle loss to high blood pressure and heart disease, your diet is your friend—or enemy.

MERYL DAVIDS LANDAU

If your mental image of an older person is someone frail and thin, it may be time for an update. For the generation currently moving through middle age and beyond, a new concern is, well, growing: obesity. "We're already seeing a large number of obese elderly, and if we don't do something, that figure is sure to rise," laments David Kessler, former commissioner of the Food and Drug Administration and author of *The End of Overeating*. Government figures show that Americans in their 60s today are about 10 pounds heavier than their counterparts of just a decade ago. And an even more worrisome bulge is coming: A typical woman in her 40s now weighs 168 pounds, versus 143 pounds in the 1960s. "People used to start midlife [at a lower weight] and then lose weight when they got into their 50s, but that doesn't happen as much anymore," Kessler says.

People used to start midlife at a lower weight than they do now and then lose weight in their 50s, but not anymore.

If you're entering that danger zone now, be aware that it's not going to get any easier to lose weight, because people need fewer calories as they age. Blame slowing metabolism and the body's tendency starting in midlife to lose muscle mass—a process known as sarcopenia—and gain fat, especially around the abdomen. (Fat burns fewer calories than does muscle.) "All that conspires to make it harder for people to maintain the same body weight when they eat their usual diets," says Alice Lichtenstein, director of the Cardiovascular Nutrition Laboratory at Tufts University. "People have fewer discretionary calories to play with, so they need to make better food choices."

Why do those choices matter? First, carrying an extra 20 or 30 pounds with you into old age doesn't bode well for attempts to head off the myriad diseases that strike in midlife and later and are linked to weight—including diabetes, arthritis, heart disease, and some forms of cancer. (It's probably not a coincidence that one recent study finds that people in their 60s have more disabilities than in years past.)

But paying attention to what you eat isn't only about controlling weight; the need for certain vitamins and minerals increases with age. One is calcium, necessary to protect bones. Another is B$_{12}$, since some older adults make less of the stomach acid required to absorb the vitamin. More vitamin D also is required. "The skin gets less efficient at converting sunlight into this vitamin, so more is needed from other sources," Lichtenstein says. Fewer than 7 percent of Americans between 50 and 70 get enough vitamin D from the foods they eat, and fewer than 26 percent get enough calcium.

Staying lean and eating right are both crucial for maintaining health through the years. (Kessler recalls a fellow researcher at Yale who, upon realizing the panoply of diseases linked to body weight, promptly lost 30 pounds.) If weight is a problem, it is especially important to cut back on the processed foods that combine sugar and fat. Studies with rats indicate that when the two are added to chow, animals can't easily stop eating, says Kessler. This happens in humans, too, he says, and food manufacturers have taken note and added sugar and fat to many products.

So what should people eat? A healthful diet at midlife is the same as for younger adults—it's just that the stakes may be higher. The focus should be on fruit, vegetables, whole grains, low- and nonfat dairy, legumes, lean meats, and fish. For someone whose current diet is far from this ideal, Lichtenstein suggests starting small: Swap dark-green lettuce for iceberg, load more veggies on the dinner plate, eat more skinless chicken or beans in place of hamburger. And exercise. Walking briskly for at least 30 minutes every day makes it easier to get away with the occasional cookie. With some further fine-tuning of that basic healthful eating plan, you can greatly improve your odds of staving off the major barriers to a vital old age:

Bone Loss

No nutrient can stop bones from losing mass over time, but consuming sufficient calcium and vitamin D can slow the deterioration, says Felicia Cosman, an osteoporosis specialist at Helen Hayes Hospital in West Haverstraw, N.Y., and clinical director of the National Osteoporosis Foundation. Once a person reaches age 50, calcium requirements jump from 1,000 mg to 1,200 mg per day. Cosman recommends adding up the number of servings consumed in a typical day of dairy products and foods that are highly calcium-fortified, such as orange juice and cereal, and multiplying that by the 300 mg each most likely supplies. Add 200 to 300 mg for the combined trace amounts in leafy green vegetables, nuts, and other sources. Then get the remainder in a supplement. By midlife, adults also need at least 800 to 1,000 IU of vitamin D to help the body absorb calcium and, possibly, prevent other diseases, according to the NOF. Sources include fatty fish such as salmon (also important for heart health), egg yolks, and fortified foods, but most people need to supplement.

Heart Disease

By now, every American surely knows the roll call of foods that affect your heart, for better and for worse. Good for the ticker: monounsaturated fats like olive oil and the omega-3 fatty acids found in such cold-water fish as salmon and herring and in flaxseed and walnuts. Harmful: too much red meat and full-fat dairy, because of their saturated fat content, and margarine and baked goods, because of the trans fats they contain.

But expunging troublesome foods from your daily fare can be surprisingly difficult. "Although many supermarket products have removed the trans fats, they're hardly history. Restaurants, especially, continue to use them," cautions Robert Eckel, former president of the American Heart Association and a professor at the University of Colorado-Denver. Some food manufacturers, moreover, have simply swapped out their trans fats for saturated fat, which is equally problematic, Eckel says. Saturated fat should total no more than 7 percent of daily energy intake— about 16 grams for the average 2,000-calorie diet.

Recent research points to another potential heart danger. It's not fat; it's high-fructose corn syrup, commonly found in soda. The decades-long, 88,000-woman Nurses' Health Study found that, even controlling for weight and other unhealthful habits, drinking one 12-ounce can of regular soda daily boosts a woman's risk of later having a heart attack by 24 percent; two or more servings raise the risk by 35 percent. "We don't know exactly why this is, but fructose does increase uric acid and triglycerides in the blood, which are known contributors to hypertension and heart disease," says study coauthor Teresa Fung, associate professor of nutrition at Simmons College in Boston.

Hypertension

Lowering high blood pressure before it contributes to the development of heart disease is vital for people in midlife. It can be accomplished with an eating plan known as the DASH (Dietary Approaches to Stop Hypertension) diet. "The DASH diet has the same effect as taking a blood-pressure-lowering medication," Eckel says. The DASH-Sodium version, which subtracts salt, works as well as up to two medications. The plan is rich in fruits and vegetables (eight to 10 servings a day for someone on a 2,000-calorie diet), grains (six to eight servings daily, with most being whole grains), and low-fat protein sources. And it's low in saturated fats and added sugars. The biggest difference from standard healthful eating advice is DASH's focus on lowering sodium, which can damage artery walls in people sensitive to the nutrient. The diet limits sodium to 2,300 mg a day, while DASH-Sodium slashes it to 1,500 mg—just two thirds of a teaspoon. It's not enough to go easier on the salt shaker; the National Institutes of Health recommends looking for low- or no-salt labels, limiting high-sodium foods like bacon and sauerkraut, and rinsing canned foods. (A one-day sample menu of a DASH eating plan is available on the *U.S. News* website at *www.usnews.com/dash*.)

Insulin Resistance

Research has repeatedly demonstrated that type 2 diabetes and insulin resistance (a precursor to the disease in which the body begins to respond less well to the hormone that clears glucose from the blood stream) can often be prevented or postponed with a healthful diet, exercise, and weight loss. That three-part combination, in fact, actually has been shown to be more effective than medication. An eating plan aimed at minimizing the risk of insulin resistance does not have to be complex. "I coach people to mentally divide their lunch and dinner plate into thirds, with one third protein, one third nonstarchy vegetables, and the final third a starch like brown rice, whole-wheat pasta, potatoes, or corn," says Nora Saul, a dietitian and diabetes educator at Harvard's Joslin Diabetes Center in Boston. It's also a good idea to get serious about cutting back on sugar and white flour, both of which have a high glycemic index and can spike blood glucose levels.

Memory Problems

Alas, there's no magic bullet that will guarantee protection from dementia. But researchers are finding that a Mediterranean diet—similar to a conventional healthful diet but with an emphasis on fish and olive oil—seems to lower the odds of developing cognitive problems. Scientists at Columbia University followed more than 1,300 people for up to 16 years; those most closely adhering to this diet developed Alzheimer's at half the rate of those who didn't. One caveat: Alcohol (particularly in the form of wine), one element of the Mediterranean Diet that has been suggested to enhance memory function, has not been proved to do so, says Gary Kennedy, director of geriatric psychiatry at Montefiore Medical Center in New York.

Joint Disease

Although age is a risk factor for arthritis, the breakdown of cartilage in the joints is not inevitable. Minimizing weight gain goes a long way toward avoiding this problem, because every extra pound translates to 3 pounds of pressure on the knees while walking. It is also a good idea to limit foods that encourage inflammation in the body, particularly omega-6 fatty acids (found in corn and soybean oils and many snack and fried foods), the Arthritis Foundation says.

Cancer

Some 45 percent of colon cancers, 38 percent of breast cancers, and 69 percent of esophageal cancers would never occur if Americans ate better, weighed less, and exercised more, estimates the American Institute for Cancer Research. "It's not just cancers of the digestive tract. What you eat and what you weigh affect certain other cancer types as well," says Alice Bender, AICR's nutrition communications manager. The organization recommends limiting red meat to 18 (cooked) ounces per week and loading up on plant-based foods, which are high in the phytochemicals and antioxidants known to inhibit cancer cell growth in lab animals. Those with the deepest colors—like purple grapes, blueberries, and leafy green vegetables—tend to have the most beneficial compounds. One recent study, for example, showed that eating foods such as broccoli and kale that have lots of sulforaphane, an antioxidant, suppresses a bacterium linked to stomach cancer.

It looks as if food is the best source of healthful nutrients. "Numerous studies on supplements—of vitamin C, lycopene, beta carotene, and even fiber—have all proved disappointing," Bender says. Yet another reason to swap that cookie for a carrot.

Critical Thinking

1. Why is it more difficult for people over the age of 50 to lose or maintain their weight?

2. Which nutrients are needed in higher quantities by older adults?

3. What is the DASH diet? How many servings of fruits and vegetables and how much sodium is recommended per day on the DASH diet?

From *U.S. News & World Report,* February 2010, pp. 38, 41–43. Copyright © 2010 by U.S. News & World Report, LP. Reprinted by permission via Wright's Media.

Sugar Overload
Curbing America's Sweet Tooth

What led the American Heart Association to issue its new scientific statement on "Dietary Sugars Intake and Cardiovascular Health"?

The association cited the "worldwide pandemic of obesity and cardiovascular disease" in explaining its "heightened concerns about the adverse effects of excessive consumption of sugars."[1]

"Added sugars have become such a predominant feature of the American diet that we can't help but recognize their major contribution to excess calories," explains Van Horn. The average American swallows 350 to 475 calories' worth of added sugars each day (depending on the type of data used to estimate intakes).

Exactly what *are* added sugars? They include high-fructose corn syrup, ordinary table sugar, honey, agave syrup, and all other sweeteners with calories. (In this article, the word "sugars" refers to them all.)

To hear some critics talk, high-fructose corn syrup is the real villain. Table sugar gets a free pass. (See "Fear of Fructose".)

In fact, high-fructose corn syrup is roughly half fructose and half glucose, as is table sugar (sucrose) once it breaks down in the body. And although the fructose half may cause some problems, the glucose half causes others. So if there's a villain, it's *all* sugars.

"Added sugars are added sugars," says Rachel Johnson, a professor of nutrition at the University of Vermont who chaired the heart association panel that issued the new sugars advice.

Who can afford the roughly 400 calories' worth of added sugars that the typical American consumes each day?

"No adults, except those who are extremely physically active—we're talking about the Michael Phelpses of the world," says Linda Van Horn, a professor of preventive medicine at the Northwestern University Feinberg School of Medicine in Chicago. "The rest of us have no business consuming that many calories from sugars."

There's new evidence that added sugars—or sugar-sweetened beverages—may raise the risk of obesity, heart disease, diabetes, and gout.

What's wrong with sugars? For starters, they're not good for your teeth, especially if they come in sticky foods. Here are 10 reasons to cut back.

1. **You can't afford the empty calories.** The American Heart Association based its advice on what scientists call "discretionary calories"—that is, how much room you have for empty calories once you've eaten all the vegetables, fruit, lean protein, low-fat dairy, whole grains, and other foods you need to stay healthy. (It's like discretionary income that people can spend on luxuries once they've paid their bills.)

"There's no question that sugars are a major culprit in obesity, because they're a source of empty calories that most Americans don't need," says Van Horn. "They have no nutritional benefit whatsoever."

The fact is that most people simply can't afford a 500-calorie scone or a 600-calorie Venti White Chocolate Mocha when they stop at Starbucks.

"Added sugars either crowd out healthy foods, or they make you fat if you eat them in addition to healthy foods," explains Frank Sacks, a professor of cardiovascular disease prevention at the Harvard School of Public Health in Boston.

So the heart association turned to the discretionary calorie allowances calculated by the U.S. Department of Agriculture. (To find yours, go to mypyramid.gov.)

A typical woman, who should shoot for 1,800 calories a day, for example, would need about 1,600 calories a day from vegetables, fruits, lean protein, dairy foods, and whole grains to get the nutrients she needs.

That leaves about 200 calories to spend (like discretionary income) on whatever she wants. "We said, okay, half of that discretionary calorie allowance can come from solid fats and half can come from added sugars," explains Johnson. That's about 100 calories each.

A typical man should shoot for 2,200 calories a day. He gets about 150 calories to spend on each.

"Solid fats" include not just butter or margarine, but the extra fat you get if you choose dairy foods (milk, cheese, yogurt, ice cream) that aren't fat-free, poultry with skin, and cakes, cookies, pies, and other sweets that aren't fat-free. So unless you eat mostly fat-free foods, your 100-calorie solid-fat allowance is going to disappear quickly.

Sucrose

Sucrose (table sugar) is broken down—in the body and (to some extent) in foods—to half fructose and half glucose. At that point it is essentially identical to high-fructose corn syrup.

Sugar by Any Other Name

Here's the scoop on some popular sugars. Sucrose (table sugar) breaks down into 50% fructose, 50% glucose in the body.

Agave syrup or nectar *(84% fructose, 8% glucose, 8% sucrose).* From the Mexican Agave cactus.

Apple juice concentrate *(60% fructose, 27% glucose, 13% sucrose).* Made by cooking down apple juice.

Brown sugar *(97% sucrose, 1% fructose, 1% glucose).* Granulated white sugar mixed with a small amount of molasses.

Corn syrup *(8% to 96% glucose, 0% fructose, 0% sucrose).* A liquid made from cornstarch.

Evaporated cane juice *(100% sucrose).* Crystals made by evaporating liquid that has been pressed from sugarcane.

Fructose *(100% fructose).* Found naturally in fruits and vegetables. We get most of our fructose from high-fructose corn syrup.

Glucose or Dextrose *(100% glucose).* Small amounts are found naturally in fruit and vegetables, but most is made from cornstarch. It's also found in honey and most other sugars.

Grape juice concentrate *(52% fructose, 48% glucose).* Made by cooking down grape juice.

High-fructose corn syrup (HFCS) *(typically 55% fructose, 45% glucose or 58% glucose, 42% fructose).* Corn syrup with some of its glucose converted into fructose.

Honey *(50% fructose, 44% glucose, 1% sucrose).* Made by honeybees from plant nectar.

Maple syrup *(95% sucrose, 4% glucose, 1% fructose).* Boiled down tree sap from the sugar maple tree.

Molasses *(53% sucrose, 23% fructose, 21% glucose).* By-product of sugarcane refining. Blackstrap molasses is a good source of iron and calcium.

Orange juice concentrate *(46% sucrose, 28% fructose, 26% glucose).* Made by cooking down orange juice.

Raw sugar *(100% sucrose).* Partially refined sugar with some molasses left.

Table sugar, Confectioner's sugar, Baker's sugar, Powdered sugar *(100% sucrose).* Most is refined from sugarcane or beets.

Note: If percentages don't add up to 100, other sugars account for the difference.

Sources: USDA Nutrient Database and company information.

And guess what happens to your added sugars allowance if you want a glass of wine or beer.

"It's been shocking to some people when I've said that we've been fairly conservative, because if you're consuming alcohol regularly, you should be having even less added sugar," notes Johnson.

If you want more sugar, you can always burn more calories.

"What I tell people who can't live with the added-sugars recommendation is that they need to move more," says Johnson. "Then you can have more sugar."

2. **Sugar-sweetened beverages promote obesity.** We're eating 20 percent more added sugars now than we did in 1970. What's largely responsible for the leap in sugars intake?

"Soft drinks, soft drinks, soft drinks," says Johnson. In 1965, Americans got an average of 12 percent of their calories from beverages. In 2001, beverages accounted for 21 percent.[1]

"Soft drinks are the number-one source of added sugars in Americans' diets," says Johnson. And sugary liquids may make us fatter because they don't curb our appetite for more food.[2]

"When you give people liquid calories before a meal, they don't compensate by eating less at the meal or later, in the same way they do for calories from solid food," notes Johnson.

In a classic study at Purdue University, researchers gave 15 young adults 450 calories of sugars each day as either a liquid (a soft drink) or a solid (jelly beans).[3] After one month on the jelly beans, the volunteers compensated by eating less of other foods, so they gained no weight. But on the soft drinks, they actually ate slightly *more* food than before. That plus the calories in the soft drinks led them to gain weight.

Where's the Added Sugar?

Coke. Pepsi. Sprite. Regular sodas add the most sugar to a typical American's diet. But don't forget about coffee drinks, teas, sports drinks, and fruit drinks that have a health halo.

And in a recent trial that lasted 1½ years, people who cut back on liquid calories lost more weight than those who cut the same number of solid calories.[4]

"I keep telling people, 'If you're trying to cut back on added sugars, look at what you're drinking,' " says Johnson.

What's more, in a study of 51,000 women, those who went from drinking regular soda no more than once a week to at least once a day gained the most weight over four years.[5]

It's not just soda pop.

"If you look at consumption data, soft drinks are leveling off, but other sugar-sweetened beverages—sports drinks, energy drinks, sweetened teas—are taking off," Johnson notes.

"Just walk down the supermarket aisles. An entire one is filled with soft drinks and another is filled with other sugar-sweetened beverages that have a health halo."

3. **Sugar-sweetened drinks may raise the risk of heart disease.** "Sugars have for many years been considered neutral in their impact on cardiovascular disease," says Northwestern University's Linda Van Horn. "But in an obese environment like ours, we can't turn a blind eye to added sugars that contribute to excess calorie intake."

Fear of Fructose

"Made with no high-fructose corn syrup," brags the label of Thomas' Original English Muffins and dozens of other foods. What's wrong with high-fructose corn syrup (HFCS)?

Here's what the popular website run by Dr. Joseph Mercola (mercola.com) claims: "Part of what makes HFCS such an unhealthy product is that it is metabolized to fat in your body far more rapidly than any other sugar, and, because most fructose is consumed in liquid form (soda), its negative metabolic effects are significantly magnified."

"Among them: diabetes, obesity, metabolic syndrome, an increase in triglycerides and LDL (bad) cholesterol levels, liver disease."

There's some truth to some of those claims, but Mercola makes a common mistake: he seems to confuse high-fructose corn syrup with fructose, as though high-fructose corn syrup were mostly fructose. It's not.

"High-fructose corn syrup is typically 55 percent fructose, explains Kimber Stanhope, who conducts research on sugars at the University of California, Davis." "But sucrose, or table sugar, is 50 percent fructose."

Glucose makes up the rest of both HFCS and sucrose. So it's not surprising that researchers find few differences—in blood sugar, insulin, ghrelin (which stimulates appetite), or leptin (which curbs appetite)—when they pit high-fructose corn syrup against table sugar.[1]

"We still have no comparative data showing that HFCS or sucrose is better or worse than the other," says Stanhope.

What's the harm in minimizing high-fructose corn syrup? Nothing. "But people become so conscious of avoiding high-fructose corn syrup that they forget about avoiding other sweeteners," says University of Vermont researcher Rachel Johnson.

"I ate a granola bar the other day that listed brown rice syrup on the ingredient list. Doesn't that sound healthy? It's just a sweetener. Added sugars all add empty calories."

[1]*Am. J. Clin. Nutr.* 87: 1194, 2008.

Clearly, excess weight isn't good for the heart. A big belly is one part of the metabolic syndrome, which raises the risk of heart disease (and diabetes). But sugar-sweetened beverages may promote heart disease whether or not they make you gain weight.

When Harvard researchers tracked more than 88,000 women for 24 years, they found that—regardless of weight—those who drank at least two sugar-sweetened beverages a day had a 20 percent higher risk of heart disease than those who drank less than one sugar-sweetened beverage a month.[6]

"Our data suggest that soft drinks increase the risk above and beyond their impact on weight," notes study coauthor JoAnn Manson, a professor of medicine at Harvard Medical School.

And when scientists tracked 4,000 men and women in the Framingham Heart Study for four years, those who drank at least one soft drink a day had a 44 percent higher risk of being diagnosed with the metabolic syndrome than those who drank less than one soft drink a day, regardless of how much they weighed.[7]

Why else would sugar-sweetened drinks raise the risk of heart attacks? One possibility: the fructose in added sugars (like high-fructose corn syrup and table sugar) raises levels of fats called triglycerides. Higher-than-normal triglycerides are another sign of the metabolic syndrome.

4. **Fructose raises triglycerides.** Cholesterol isn't the only thing in blood that's linked to heart attacks. People with higher-than-normal triglycerides (at least 150) are also at risk, especially if their triglycerides soar after a meal.[8] And fructose raises triglycerides after meals.

For example, researchers at the University of Minnesota fed 24 men and women a diet that got 17 percent of its calories from either glucose or fructose.[9]

(That's a high dose, since Americans average 16 percent of their calories from added sugars, roughly half of it from fructose and half of it from glucose.)

After six weeks, triglyceride levels throughout the day were 32 percent higher when the men (but not the women) ate the high-fructose diet.

Peter Havel and colleagues at the University of California, Davis, got similar results when they studied 32 over-weight or obese men and women over 40. Participants got a hefty 25 percent of their calories from beverages sweetened with either fructose or glucose for 10 weeks.[10]

Once again, blood levels of triglycerides after a meal were higher on fructose than on glucose. "It's a strong and consistent effect," says researcher Kimber Stanhope, who works with Havel.

Triglycerides rose more in men, but they also rose in women, notes Stanhope, "possibly because the women in our study were older and heavier" than those in the earlier study.

Why would people on a high-fructose diet have higher triglycerides than people on a high-glucose diet?

When you consume a large dose of glucose, the liver doesn't pull much of it in if you don't need the calories. In contrast, fructose ends up in the liver whether you need the calories or not.

"The liver will take up nearly the entire amount of fructose," says Stanhope. "Very little of the fructose stays in the bloodstream."

What does the liver do with all that fructose? "It starts converting some of the fructose into fat," Stanhope explains. "Much of this fat gets sent into the bloodstream, resulting in higher levels of triglycerides."

That would explain why large doses of fructose boost triglyceride levels in the bloodstream and possibly in the liver. Would smaller doses do the same?

"We're testing lower doses right now," says Stanhope. "We're studying over 200 younger people, so it will take a while."

5. **Sugar-sweetened beverages may promote diabetes.** When researchers tracked roughly 91,000 women for eight years, those who drank at least one sugar-sweetened soft drink a day had an 83 percent higher risk of type 2 diabetes than those who drank less than one a month.[5]

When the scientists took weight out of the equation, soda drinkers had a 40 percent higher risk.

Tout de Sweet

A typical woman should get no more than 100 calories (about 6½ teaspoons) a day from added sugars, says the American Heart Association. A typical man should get no more than 150 calories (about 9½ teaspoons)—roughly what's in a 12 oz. can of Coke.

Here's how much added sugars you'd get in a sampling of popular foods. (The numbers don't include the naturally occurring sugars in fruit or milk.) To convert teaspoons to grams of sugar, multiply by 4. To convert teaspoons to calories from sugar, multiply by 16.

Food	**Added Sugars** *(teaspoons)*
Dairy	
Ice cream, vanilla *(½ cup)*	3
Chocolate milk, reduced fat 2% *(8 fl. oz.)*	3½
Yogurt, low-fat vanilla *(6 oz.)*	3½
Yogurt, low-fat fruit *(6 oz.)*	4½
Silk Chocolate Soymilk *(8 fl. oz.)*	5
TCBY Old Fashioned Vanilla Frozen Yogurt *(regular cup, 8.7 oz.)*	6*
Baskin-Robbins Vanilla Ice Cream Cone *(double scoop, 8.4 oz.)*	11½*
Chocolate shake, fast food *(16 fl. oz.)*	13
Dairy Queen Heath Blizzard *(medium, 14.5 oz.)*	26*
Baskin-Robbins Oreo Outrageous Sundae *(12.6 oz.)*	27*
Coldstone Creamery Founders Favorite *(Gotta Have It, 14.6 oz.)*	30½*
Beverages	
Propel Lemon *(24 fl. oz.)*	1½
Starbucks Caffè Mocha *(grande, 16 fl. oz.)*	3*
Starbucks Caramel Macchiato *(grande, 16 fl. oz.)*	4*
Starbucks Vanilla Latte *(grande, 16 fl. oz.)*	4*
Hawaiian Punch Fruit Juicy Red *(8 fl. oz.)*	4½*
SunnyD Tangy Original *(8 fl. oz.)*	4½*
Starbucks Cinnamon Dolce Latte *(grande, 16 fl. oz.)*	5*
Starbucks Tazo Shaken Iced Tea, any flavor *(grande, 16 fl. oz.)*	5
Gatorade Lemon-Lime *(20 fl. oz.)*	8½
Glacéau Vitamin Water Revive *(20 fl. oz.)*	8½
Starbucks Tazo Passion Shaken Iced Tea Lemonade *(grande, 16 fl. oz.)*	8½
Coca-Cola *(12 fl. oz. can)*	10
Snapple Lemon Tea *(16 fl. oz.)*	10½
Nestea Iced Tea Sweetened Lemon *(16.9 fl. oz.)*	12
Schweppes Tonic Water *(20 fl. oz.)*	14
SoBe Green Tea *(20 fl. oz.)*	15½
Sprite *(20 fl. oz.)*	16
Arizona Southern Style Sweet Tea *(23 fl. oz.)*	16½
Coca-Cola *(20 fl. oz.)*	16½
Minute Maid Lemonade *(20 fl. oz.)*	17
Pepsi *(20 fl. oz.)*	17½
Sunkist Orange Soda *(20 fl. oz.)*	21

Candy, Chocolate, etc.	**Added Sugars** *(teaspoons)*
Werther's Original Hard Candies *(3 pieces, 0.6 oz.)*	2½
Lindt Excellence 70% Cocoa Dark Chocolate *(4 squares, 1.4 oz.)*	3
Dove Dark Chocolate Promises *(5 pieces, 1.4 oz.)*	5
Hershey's Milk Chocolate Bar *(1.6 oz.)*	5½*
York Peppermint Patties *(1 patty, 1.4 oz.)*	6½
Jelly Belly Jelly Beans *(35 pieces, 1.4 oz.)*	7
M&M's Milk Chocolate *(56 pieces, 1.7 oz.)*	8
Maple syrup *(¼ cup, 2.9 oz.)*	12
Sweets *(1 item, unless otherwise noted)*	
Pepperidge Farm Milano, original *(3 cookies, 1.2 oz.)*	3
Entenmann's Crumb Coffee Cake *(1/10 cake, 2 oz.)*	3½
Mrs. Fields semi-sweet Chocolate Chip Cookie *(1.2 oz.)*	3½
Nabisco Oreo *(3 cookies, 1.2 oz.)*	3½
Pepperidge Farm Double Chocolate Milano *(3 cookies, 1.4 oz.)*	4
Entenmann's Rich Frosted Donut *(2.1 oz.)*	4½
Jell-O Strawberry *(1 snack cup, 3.5 oz.)*	4½
Sara Lee All Butter Pound Cake *(1 slice, 2.7 oz.)*	5
Entenmann's Glazed Buttermilk Donut *(2.1 oz.)*	5½
Krispy Kreme Chocolate Iced Kreme Filled Doughnut *(3.1 oz.)*	6
Entenmann's Chocolate Fudge Cake *(½ cake, 2.3 oz.)*	7
Krispy Kreme Glazed Chocolate Doughnut *(2.8 oz.)*	7
Starbucks Chocolate Chunk Cookie *(3 oz.)*	8
Starbucks Marble Loaf *(1 slice, 3.8 oz.)*	8
Panera Chocolate Chipper Cookie *(3.3 oz.)*	8½
Panera Chocolate Fudge Brownie *(3.5 oz.)*	8½
Starbucks Classic Coffee Cake *(4 oz.)*	8½
Hostess Twinkies *(2 cakes, 3 oz.)*	9
Starbucks Pumpkin Scone *(4.2 oz.)*	11
Entenmann's Super Cinnamon Buns *(6 oz.)*	11½
Hostess Sno Balls *(2 cakes, 3.5 oz.)*	11½
Panera Pecan Roll *(5.5 oz.)*	12
Panera Pumpkin Muffin *(6 oz.)*	12
Cinnabon Classic Cinnamon Roll *(7.8 oz.)*	14
Denny's Hershey's Chocolate Cake *(1 slice, 5 oz.)*	14
Dunkin' Donuts Coffee Cake Muffin *(5.8 oz.)*	14½
Uno Chicago Grill Chocolate Chocolate Malt Layer Cake *(1 slice, 9.5 oz.)*	25
Cereals & Cereal Bars	
Kashi TLC Trail Mix Chewy Granola Bar *(1 bar, 1.2 oz.)*	1½
General Mills Cinnamon Toast Crunch *(¾ cup, 1.1 oz.)*	2½
General Mills Honey Nut Cheerios *(¾ cup, 1 oz.)*	2½
Kellogg's Bite Size Frosted Mini-Wheats *(24 biscuits, 2.1 oz.)*	3
Kashi GoLean Crunch! Original *(1 cup, 1.9 oz.)*	3½
Kellogg's Cracklin' Oat Bran *(¾ cup, 1.8 oz.)*	4
Kashi GoLean Cookies 'N Cream Chewy Bar *(1 bar, 2.8 oz.)*	9
Miscellaneous	
Bush's Homestyle Baked Beans *(½ cup, 4.5 oz.)*	3
Cracker Jack *(½ cup, 1 oz.)*	4
Häagen-Dazs Chocolate Sorbet *(½ cup, 3.7 oz.)*	5

*CSPI estimate. Note: Added sugars are rounded to the nearest half teaspoon.

Sources: Company information and U.S. Department of Agriculture Nutrient Database. Chart compiled by Amy Ramsay.

Sweet Nothings

When researchers gave people either regular or diet soft drinks for several weeks, the participants gained weight only on the regular sodas.[1,2] But all non-caloric sweeteners are not created equal. Here's our take on their safety:

- **Acesulfame-potassium.** Tests conducted in the 1970s were of mediocre quality. One suggested an increased cancer risk in female rats.
- **Aspartame (NutraSweet, Equal).** Judging by two recent rat studies, it may slightly increase cancer risk. At the very least, new studies should be conducted.
- **Saccharin (Sweet'N Low).** In animal studies, it has caused cancer of the urinary bladder, uterus, ovaries, skin, blood vessels, and other organs.
- **Stevia.** Coke and Pepsi have started to use it to sweeten some beverages. It appears to be safe, though there should be more independent testing.
- **Sucralose (Splenda).** It appears to be safe, though there hasn't been much independent testing. (Sucralose isn't as natural as ads have implied. It's made by chlorinating sugar molecules.)

[1]*Am. J. Clin. Nutr.* 76: 721, 2002.

[2]*Am. J. Clin. Nutr.* 51: 963, 1990.

"Weight gain appears to account for half of the increased risk," says Manson.

What could explain the other half? "Sugar-sweetened soft drinks might also increase the risk of type 2 diabetes because they're high in rapidly absorbable carbohydrates," she suggests.

High-fructose corn syrup is roughly half fructose, which goes largely to the liver, so it doesn't raise blood sugar. But the glucose half of high-fructose corn syrup heads straight to the bloodstream.

"Consumption of sugar-sweetened soft drinks causes a fast and dramatic increase in blood sugar levels," says Manson. "In our studies, people who eat foods that raise blood sugar levels have a higher risk of diabetes."

6. Fructose may boost visceral fat. In the University of California, Davis, study, the 32 men and women gained about the same weight (roughly three pounds) after 10 weeks whether they drank beverages sweetened with fructose or glucose.[10] But there were differences.

The fructose eaters (especially the men) gained more deep abdominal—or visceral—fat than the glucose eaters. That's critical because visceral fat is linked to a higher risk of heart disease and diabetes.

In contrast, the glucose eaters gained more subcutaneous fat, which is just below the skin and is less likely to raise the risk of diabetes and heart disease.

Since this study was the first to see fructose's effect on visceral fat, Stanhope notes, "it would be good to see the result confirmed in other studies."

Another new finding: the fructose drinkers had a drop in insulin sensitivity. Reduced sensitivity to insulin is linked to a higher risk of heart disease and diabetes. But it's too early to know if Stanhope's results will hold up in future studies.

If fructose makes insulin less efficient, no one knows how. "It may be due to an increase in the amount of triglyceride stored in the liver," speculates Stanhope, "which could then lead to a chain of events that causes insulin receptors to perform less effectively."

7. Fructose may raise the risk of gout. Gout hurts. If your blood has too much uric acid, the excess ends up in joints (especially those of the big toe), where it can cause excruciating pain.

"Obesity is the major risk factor for gout because it's so common and it substantially increases the risk," says Gary Curhan, an associate professor of medicine at the Harvard Medical School.

But fructose is also a culprit. "We know that fructose increases uric acid, and that uric acid causes gout," says Curhan.

In a study of roughly 46,000 men, those who got at least 12 percent of their calories from fructose were nearly twice as likely to be diagnosed with gout over the next 12 years as those who got less than 7 percent of their calories from fructose.[11]

"After we adjusted for weight and all the other risk factors for gout that we know about, people with higher intakes of fructose had a substantially higher risk of gout," Curhan explains.

At least that's true in men, who are far more likely to get the disease. "We're just starting to look at women," says Curhan.

8. Fructose may promote over-eating. Leptin is a hormone made by fat cells. It's supposed to make you stop eating.

"Leptin tells your brain that you've got enough calories on board," says Robert Lustig, a professor of clinical pediatrics at the University of California, San Francisco, who served on the heart association sugar panel. "When you don't get that signal, you're still hungry."

When researchers fed rats a huge dose of fructose (60 percent of their diet) for six months, the animals became resistant to leptin—that is, leptin injections failed to curb their appetite.[12]

(Obese people can also be leptin-resistant. "They have lots of leptin, but it doesn't work," explains Lustig.)

Over time, a high-fructose diet blocks the leptin signal in the brain, notes Lustig. "So leptin can't extinguish hunger and can't extinguish reward." The result: you keep eating.

In fact, when the rats were allowed to eat as much palatable food as they wanted, they gained nearly twice as much weight as rats that got no fructose.

But so far, it's not clear what happens when people eat fructose in less-excessive amounts.

The Bottom Line

- Shoot for 100 calories (6½ teaspoons, or 25 grams) a day of added sugars if you're a woman and 150 calories (9½ teaspoons, or 38 grams) a day if you're a man. Even less may be better for your heart (see "What Should I Eat?" *Nutrition Action,* Oct. 2009).
- Don't drink sugar-sweetened beverages. Limit fruit juices to no more than 1 cup a day.
- Limit *all* added sugars, including high-fructose corn syrup, cane or beet sugar, evaporated cane juice, brown rice syrup, agave syrup, and honey.
- Don't worry about the naturally occurring sugar in fruit, milk, and plain yogurt.
- To estimate your calorie needs and get a more precise added-sugars limit, go to mypyramid.gov and click on "Get a personalized plan" in the "I Want To . . ." box.
- If a food contains little or no milk or fruit (which have natural sugars), the "Sugars" number on the package's Nutrition Facts panel will tell you how much added sugars are in each serving.

In two preliminary studies, 17 obese men and women and 12 normal-weight women had higher leptin levels over a 24-hour period when they consumed 30 percent of their calories from glucose-sweetened beverages with meals than when they consumed the same amount of fructose-sweetened beverages with meals.[13], [14] Few other studies have been done.

Does that mean we should be eating foods sweetened with glucose, which is what's in ordinary corn syrup?

"Why do we need corn syrup anyway?" asks Lustig. "We're better off getting carbs from foods that are packaged naturally with their own fiber. If we got carbs from whole grains, vegetables, fruit, and beans, we wouldn't overeat."

Fruit contains fructose (as well as sucrose and glucose). Do we need to limit apples and oranges? "I'm not concerned about fructose from fruit," says Lustig. "How many oranges can you eat in one sitting?"

9. **Minimizing added sugars keeps a lid on blood pressure.** "There's a possibility that sugar raises blood pressure," says Frank Sacks of the Harvard School of Public Health. "But it's far from definitive."

However, what *is* clear is that there's little place for sugar in a diet that's designed to lower blood pressure (see *Nutrition Action,* Oct. 2009, cover story).

The OmniHeart Study tested three diets on people with hypertension (blood pressure at least 140 over 90) or pre-hyper-tension (blood pressure at least 120 over 80).[15] Each diet was rich in fruits, vegetables, low-fat dairy foods, beans, nuts, and other foods that supply potassium, magnesium, and other key nutrients.

"The higher-carb OmniHeart diet did a great job of lowering blood pressure," says Sacks. It had just five teaspoons (80 calories) of added sugars a day. In people with hypertension, it trimmed systolic blood pressure (the top number) by an impressive 13 points.

But, adds Sacks, "the other two Omni-Heart diets—which were higher in either protein or unsaturated fat—did better." Those diets, which contained only two or three teaspoons (30 to 50 calories) of added sugars a day, cut systolic blood pressure by 16 points in people with hypertension.

"There's not much room for added sugars in most people's diets," concludes Sacks. "And certainly not if you're trying to optimize your diet to lower blood pressure."

His advice: "I never drink liquid calories, and I keep sweets and snacks out of the house. It's okay to indulge once in a while, but if I get hungry at night and there are no sweets around, I eat nuts or an apple."

10. **Most sugary foods are junk.** Coca-Cola, Pepsi, Cinnabon, Krispy Kreme, Dunkin' Donuts, Snapple, Entenmann's, Hostess, Sara Lee, Little Debbie.

Just about any sweets made by those and similar companies are high in sugars and low in nutrients. Many are also packed with virtually worthless white flour. And many are now supersized. Do you need a Cinnabon that's the size of a boxed lunch?

To stick to the heart association's new recommendations, you'll need to use your added sugars calorie allowance wisely. (To find out how much added sugar is in popular foods, see "Tout de Sweet").

"Be discriminating," suggests the University of Vermont's Rachel Johnson. "People enjoy sweet taste, and if you're discriminating, it has a role in a healthy diet. We're not all going to eat non-fat plain yogurt."

But "they're called discretionary calories for a reason," she adds. "Use them to enhance the palatability of already-nutritious foods."

"I'd rather see someone consume added sugars in a flavored yogurt or a whole-grain breakfast cereal or by putting maple syrup on oatmeal than consume them in a doughnut or soft drink."

Notes

1. *Circulation 120:* 1011, 2009.
2. *Physiol. Behav. 59:* 179, 1996.
3. *Int. J. Obesity 24:* 794, 2000.
4. *Am. J. Clin. Nutr. 89:* 1299, 2009.
5. *JAMA 292:* 927, 2004.
6. *Am. J. Clin. Nutr. 89:* 1037, 2009.
7. *Circulation 116:* 480, 2007.
8. *JAMA 298:* 309, 2007.
9. *Am. J. Clin. Nutr. 72:* 1128, 2000.
10. *J. Clin. Invest. 119:* 1322, 2009.
11. *BMJ 336:* 309, 2008.
12. *Am. J. Physiol. Regul. Integr. Comp. Physiol. 295:* 1370, 2008.
13. *J. Clin. Endocrinol. Metab. 89:* 2963, 2004.
14. *J. Clin. Endocrinol. Metab. 94:* 1562, 2009.
15. *JAMA 294:* 2455, 2005.

Critical Thinking

1. Describe the concept of discretionary calories. What is the recommended amount of discretionary calories for an average male and female?

2. Why does consuming high-fructose corn sweeteners increase the metabolic syndrome, type 2 diabetes, gout, and accumulation of visceral (abdominal) fat?

3. Why do fructose sweeteners promote overeating? Identify the hormone that is involved.

Fructose Sweeteners May Hike Blood Pressure

Human study confirms trend seen earlier in animals.

JANET RALOFF

The more fructose American adults add to their diets, the higher their blood pressure tends to be. The new finding adds fuel to a simmering controversy about whether this simple sugar—found in fruits, table sugar, soft drinks and many baked goods—poses a health hazard that goes beyond simply consuming too many empty calories.

If the new data are confirmed, they might go a long way toward explaining a more than tripling in hypertension rates over the past century—a period when "fructose consumption has increased dramatically in industrialized nations including the United States," the authors say.

The idea that fructose might play a role in hypertension is not new. In 2008, an international team of researchers found that among mice, "Fructose feeding decreased salt excretion by the kidney and resulted in hypertension." The scientists also homed in on a potential mechanism: the activity of a gene responsible for helping the small intestine absorb salt and secrete bicarbonate. When these researchers fed fructose to mice without the functioning gene or to animals eating a salt-free diet, the animals' blood pressure remained unaltered.

But that was in rodents.

Diana Jalal and fellow nephrologists at the University of Colorado Denver Health Sciences Center in Aurora decided to look for evidence that fructose might have a similar effect in people. So they pulled data collected from a representative cross-section of Americans as part of the National Health and Nutrition Examination Survey. Conducted every few years, the new study's data came from the 2003 to 2006 survey and included more than 4,500 adults with no prior diagnosis of hypertension.

Sure enough, when Jalal's group stratified the participants by blood pressure—and many had undiagnosed prehypertension or outright vascular disease characterized by significantly elevated blood pressure—mean intake of added dietary fructose climbed by group. Their findings appear in the *Journal of the American Society of Nephrology,* published online July 1 ahead of print.

Their focus was "added" fructose. The qualifier refers to fructose intake other than that occurring as a natural constituent of any fruits or other produce. And the reason: Americans are not renowned for downing even the recommended daily servings of fruits and vegetables, much less an excess.

So these nephrologists—kidney specialists—concentrated on the fructose present as a sweetener in processed foods and beverages. Although fructose constitutes half of table sugar, it's actually sweeter than the other constituent (glucose), so manufacturers have taken to sweetening most products with a high-fructose corn syrup. This somewhat increases the fructose content of the diet.

The new paper shows a barely significant trend toward increasing blood pressure with increasing fructose intake—until its authors applied a statistical technique (logistic regression analysis) to investigate the likelihood of blood pressure increasing as fructose consumption rises. Then they found a statistically significant link—but just for people with bonafide hypertension and only for systolic blood pressure (the higher of the two numbers in a blood-pressure reading).

Explains Jalal, her team's new data indicate that "High fructose intake is a strong predictor of a greater risk of hypertension." The average intake for people proved to be about 74 grams of added fructose per day, an amount equivalent to 2.5 soft drinks. People who ingest more than that "are at increased risk of high blood pressure when compared to the ones that ingest low fructose within each blood-pressure category," she says.

While the Denver group was working on this study, another came out last year focusing on "sugar-sweetened beverage consumption, a significant source of dietary fructose." It too focused on NHANES data—in this case, on almost 4,900 U.S. adolescents during the previous survey period: 1999 to 2004. And here, drinking sugary soda pop was again linked with elevated systolic blood pressure.

Of course, there are caveats. NHANES participants report their own dietary intake. The data are collected on diet the day before, not what each individual typically eats most days. And some people may be more sensitive to fructose impacts, whatever they might be.

Expect push back from the sweetener industry, especially the Washington, D.C.-based Corn Refiners Association, which has been defending high fructose corn syrup. Its website says: "Research confirms that high fructose corn syrup is safe and no different from other common sweeteners like table sugar and honey."

I asked Michel Conchol, another of the Denver authors, about what's next for his group: Will you conduct a feeding trial to control for differences in fructose contributions to the diet? Yes, he said: "We are already planning such a study."

Critical Thinking

1. The two studies cited in this article were analyses of National Health and Examination Survey (NHANES) data. What is NHANES?

2. What component of blood pressure (systolic or diastolic) is elevated in these two studies?

3. Do these two studies prove (show a cause and effect) that drinking added fructose sweeteners causes increased blood pressure? Explain your answer.

Food for Thought: Exploring the Potential of Mindful Eating

SHARON PALMER

Do you eat when you're not hungry? Do you find yourself wolfing down food without even remembering it? If you're like most people, the answer is yes. In today's world, people barely notice the act of eating, as they feed on demand from fast food drive-thrus, vending machines, and snack food cartons. The net result is that we've become increasingly out of touch with our body's sense of hunger and fullness, as well as the pleasures of eating. In a 2008 General Mills online hunger and eating survey that included 1,049 men and women aged 18 and over, only 6% indicated that they almost always notice physical hunger such as a growling stomach before they eat. When subjects were asked how often they multi-task (driving, walking, working, watching television, shopping online, etc.) while eating, a scant 3% reported never. Only 34% of participants indicated that they decide a meal or snack is over when they feel full.

Mindless Munching

It seems as if our society has refined the art of mindless eating as it grows ever busier and less connected to food and food preparation. "Mindless eating is when people are not paying attention when they are eating. They look down at their empty plate or bag of cookies and ask 'where did it go?' People are eating on the run without tasting food; without an awareness that they are putting it into their mouths. By buying prepared foods, people are putting less personal preparation into it. Even when you make a sandwich, there is a level of awareness and appreciation for the food," says Nancy Ostreicher, MS, health educator for the University of New Mexico Center for Life Mindful Eating and Living (MEAL) program, a mindfulness-based stress reduction program that incorporates eating exercises. What's the downside to a mindless eating habit? Experts believe that it may be contributing to our nation's obesity problem, which increases the risk for chronic disease.

A New Focus on Food

There is growing support for a new concept that is centered upon mindful eating. Mindful eating draws upon the recognized practice of mindfulness-based stress reduction, which helps people focus on the present moment rather than continuing habitual and unsatisfying behaviors. Mindfulness-based stress reduction has been shown to improve pain, anxiety, and depression. Building upon this strategy, mindful eating practices promote a satisfying relationship with food and eating on a deep emotional level and encourage a better sense of well-being.

"Mindful eating has to do with paying attention to your own personal experience with food. There is a physical awareness of the food; the taste, smell, texture, and how it feels traveling to your belly. There are all of the mental thoughts, including memories about food being pleasurable or displeasurable. Then you can expand that awareness to observations like who grew the food, how it was packaged, where it comes from, and who prepared it," explains Ostreicher.

Evidence supports the benefits of mindful eating in both mental and physical health. Researchers from the University of New Mexico recruited 25 participants for a mindfulness-based stress reduction course that included eating exercises. There was an observed decline in binge eating, as well as anxiety and depressive symptoms. This study was co-authored by Brian Shelley, MD, founder of the University of New Mexico Mindfulness-Based Stress Reduction Program.

On April 14, 2008, Shelley presented findings from a recent study on the effects of mindful eating at the 5th Annual Nutrition and Health Conference: State of the Science & Clinical Applications in Phoenix, Arizona, which was sponsored by the University of Arizona College of Medicine. When study subjects were provided with a MEAL curriculum that included mindfulness-based stress reduction and eating principles, there was an observed decrease in weight, improvements in markers of cardiovascular disease risk, and improvements in measures of mindfulness and binge eating. This study was followed up with a randomized control trial with a group of 20 mindfulness treatment subjects and a group of 20 support group control subjects. The overall weight loss between the groups was similar, but the effect size was slightly larger in the mindfulness group, and was accompanied with greater changes in waist-to-hip ratio and cardiovascular disease risk markers. At the 12-month mark, mindfulness participants maintained and continued to lose weight. Shelley believes that MEAL might be a viable option for treating obesity.

Practicing Mindful Eating

Mindful eating seems like a logical approach to managing your weight. The question is: Are you a mindful eater? Put yourself to the test. According to The Center for Mindful Eating, a mindful eater:

- Acknowledges that there is no right or wrong way to eat, but there are varying degrees of awareness surrounding the experience of food.
- Accepts that his/her eating experiences are unique.
- Is an individual who, by choice, directs his/her awareness to all aspects of food and eating on a moment-by-moment basis.
- Is an individual who looks at the immediate choices and direct experiences associated with food and eating, not to the distant health outcome of that choice.
- Is aware of and reflects on the effects caused by unmindful eating.
- Experiences insight about how he/she can act to achieve specific health goals as he/she becomes more attuned to the direct experience of eating and feelings of health.
- Becomes aware of the interconnection of earth, living beings, and cultural practices and the impact of his/her food choices on those systems.

Thinking Food Through, Step by Step

If you'd like to be more mindful in your eating approach, here are a few handy tips from mindful eating instructor Nancy Ostreicher when you sit down to your next meal:

1. Imagine that this is the first time you've ever seen this food.
2. Take one piece of the food and notice your impression of the food before you put it in your mouth: color, smell, texture, and how it feels in your hand.
3. Bring it to your nose and lips. Notice your feelings, thoughts, memories, expectations, and anticipation before you put it into your mouth.
4. Put it in your mouth. Without biting or swallowing it, notice the initial taste, texture, sensations, and activity inside your mouth.
5. Biting the food and chewing slowly, notice these same sensations and transformations of the food in your mouth.
6. Swallowing the food, notice the feeling of the food traveling to your stomach.
7. Think about what is going on in your mouth, throat, and stomach after swallowing.
8. Eat the second piece of food with awareness. Was your experience different than the first?
9. Consider how this experience with this food was different from how you usually eat this food. Think about your experience of feeling finished, satisfied or wanting more. What insights have you learned from this experience?

Mindful Eating at Your Fingertips

Looking for help on becoming a more mindful eater? Check out these resources:

- University of New Mexico Center for Life developed a Mindful Eating and Living (MEAL) six week training program to help guide participants through the practice of mindful eating (http://hsc.unm.edu/som/cfl/mindfulnessprog.shtml).
- The Center for Mindful Eating offers a wealth of information on mindful eating techniques, as well as links to articles, books, handouts, and workshops on mindful eating (www.tcme.org).

Critical Thinking

1. What is mindful eating? What diseases or medical conditions have been shown to improve with mindful eating practices?
2. What effect does eating convenience or already prepared food have on awareness and appreciation for food?
3. One aspect of mindful eating is increasing awareness of where food comes from and how many resources are involved in providing the food that is available to us. Using this concept, illustrate the number of people and resources involved in creating a pepperoni pizza.

From *Environmental Nutrition*, June 1, 2009. Copyright © 2009 by Belvoir Media Group LLC. Reprinted by permission. www.environmentalnutrition.com

The Best Diabetes Diet for Optimal Outcomes

Researchers have explored whether certain combinations of macronutrients more effectively manage the disease, but does a perfect eating plan exist?

Rita E. Carey, MS, RD, CDE

To say that dietary prescriptions for diabetes have varied over the last hundred years is an understatement. From the very-low-carbohydrate diets initiated before insulin was discovered and used therapeutically to the high-carbohydrate, high-fiber vegan diets endorsed today by some medical researchers, recommendations for optimal macronutrient intake for both type 1 and type 2 diabetes have covered nearly every conceivable option. Good scientific studies have identified a number of specific components in foods that may improve clinical diabetes outcomes and others that likely accelerate the pathogenesis of the disease. Yet, the optimal diet profile—the best balance of carbohydrate, protein, and fat—remains a topic of serious debate.

The following review will touch on the primary therapeutic diet patterns for diabetes considered today and some of the data that either support or refute their effectiveness in reducing hyperglycemia, promoting long-term weight loss, and reducing the risk of cardiovascular disease, the most common cause of death for individuals with diabetes.

Not One, but a Variety

The 2008 American Diabetes Association (ADA) position statement, as reported in *Diabetes Care,* notes that "although numerous studies have attempted to identify the optimal mix of macronutrients for the diabetic diet, it is unlikely that one such combination of macronutrients exists." Rather, the ADA indicates, the best mix of carbohydrate, fat, and protein varies depending on an individual's circumstances, caloric needs for weight control, and specific metabolic status (eg, lipid profile).

In other words, the ADA recognizes that a number of healthy diet patterns may be effective for maintaining good glycemic control and reducing the risk of comorbidities. The position statement also notes the important considerations of cultural and personal preferences, stages of change, and physical and social pleasures of eating in its dietary recommendations. Indeed, one of the goals of medical nutrition therapy for individuals with diabetes that's listed in the position statement is "to maintain the pleasure of eating by only limiting food choices when indicated by scientific evidence."

The ADA recognizes that a number of healthy diet patterns may be effective for maintaining good glycemic control and reducing the risk of comorbidities.

With the previous considerations in mind, the ADA does make some specific nutrition recommendations for weight loss, glycemic control, and the prevention of diabetic complications (see sidebar). Low-fat, calorie-restricted diets are traditionally recommended for weight loss. However, the ADA notes that low-carbohydrate diets (less than 130 g carbohydrate/day) may be effective for weight loss in the short term (ie, less than one year). Whether such diets sustain weight loss and support optimal lipid profiles over the long term remains to be determined. Evidence suggests that after one year, the difference in maintained weight loss between low-carbohydrate or low-fat diet patterns is insignificant.[1] In addition, a meta-analysis published in the *Archives of Internal Medicine* in 2006 found that some individuals had elevated LDL levels when following a low-carbohydrate diet.

Long-term effects of low-carbohydrate/high-protein diets on kidney function are also undetermined. Because very-low-carbohydrate diets can eliminate important nutrient- and energy-dense foods, the ADA maintains that the long-term benefits and metabolic effects of low-carbohydrate diets remain unclear.

Benefits of High-Fiber, Vegetarian Diets

The ADA position statement makes no mention of the effectiveness of high-fiber vegetarian or vegan diets for supporting good glycemic control or the overall health of individuals with diabetes. The ADA does, however, note that foods that make up the base of vegetarian and vegan diets (eg, grains, fruits, vegetables, legumes) offer considerable health benefits to people with diabetes, as does the reduction of saturated fat from animal products. The ADA recommends fiber intake of about 14 g/1,000 kcal/day, although data suggest that higher intake of fiber (about 50 g/day) improves glycemic control in people with type 1 and 2 diabetes, as well as lipid profiles in those with type 2.[2]

A study by Barnard et al published this year in *The American Journal of Clinical Nutrition* compared the effects of a low-fat vegan diet (less than 5% saturated fat, 10% total fat, 15% protein, and 75% carbohydrate) and a conventional diabetes diet following 2003 ADA guidelines (less than 7% saturated fat, 15% to 20% protein, 60% to 70% carbohydrate and monounsaturated fat, and less than 200 mg/day cholesterol) on glycemic control, weight loss, and plasma lipid levels. Individuals following the vegan diet ate an average of 22 g fiber/1,000 kcal/day, while those adhering to ADA guidelines consumed approximately 14 g/1,000 kcal/day. The actual trial lasted 52 weeks, but researchers followed the participants for 22 weeks afterward to assess long-term effectiveness of and adherence to the diets.

At the end of the extended observation period, researchers found that both diets were associated with modest sustained weight loss (–4.4 kg in the vegan group vs. –3 kg in the conventional group), as well as comparable reductions in hemoglobin A1c. However, more individuals in the vegan group were able to reduce medications. After controlling for these medication changes, significantly greater reductions were seen in A1c and total and LDL cholesterol concentrations in the vegan group.

A particularly interesting outcome was the greater reduction of triglycerides in the vegan group compared with the conventional group (–33.9 + 12.7 vs. –7.8 + 28.9). These results contrast with previous studies finding elevated triglycerides in high-carbohydrate diets.[3,4] Barnard et al argue that the participants in previous studies were not encouraged to consume most of their carbohydrates from high-fiber, low-glycemic index foods. Refined, carbohydrate-dense foods that are low in fiber are more likely to raise triglyceride levels. Weight loss was also cited as having an effect on lipid levels in this study, as was the ability of participants to self-regulate their caloric intake on either diet.

A Mediterranean Approach

Another macronutrient pattern considered for diabetes is the high-monounsaturated fatty acid (MUFA) or Mediterranean-style diet. The ADA recommends a diet that provides 60% to 70% of calories from a mix of carbohydrate and monounsaturated fat.

ADA Recommendations

- Either low-carbohydrate or low-fat, calorie-restricted diets may be effective strategies for weight loss in the short term.
- Monitor renal function, lipid profiles, and protein intake (in patients with nephropathy) and adjust hypoglycemic therapy as necessary for those following a low-carbohydrate diet.
- Monitoring carbohydrate is a key strategy for achieving glycemic control.
- Patients with diabetes should consume an assortment of fiber-containing foods and attain the USDA dietary fiber recommendation (14 g/1,000 kcal).
- There is not enough consistent, sufficient evidence to prove that low-glycemic load diets reduce diabetes risk. For diabetes management, the use of the glycemic load/index may provide an added, though modest, benefit over that observed when only total carbohydrate is considered.
- Limit saturated fat to less than 7% of total calories and minimize trans fat intake.
- For good health, include carbohydrate from fruits, vegetables, whole grains, legumes, and low-fat milk in the diet.

—Adapted from the American Diabetes Association. Nutrition Recommendations and Interventions for Diabetes. *Diabetes Care.* 2008:31(Suppl 1):S61–S78.

Gerhard et al attempted to determine the optimal energy distribution from MUFA and carbohydrate in the diabetic diet in a study published in *The American Journal of Clinical Nutrition* in 2004. This study was very small (only 11 subjects) but yielded interesting results.

Researchers found that a low-fat (20% of calories from fat) vs. a high-MUFA diet (40% of calories from total fat, 26% MUFA) resulted in more weight loss and improved triglyceride levels. Glycemic control did not differ significantly between the two groups. The low-fat diet was higher in fiber and contained foods with a lower caloric density than those in the high-MUFA diet. Subjects in this study were also allowed to self-regulate their intake. The authors suggest that when individuals are allowed to regulate their intake according to satiety, a low-fat, high-fiber, high-volume diet may have advantages for weight loss (but not necessarily glycemic control) over a high-MUFA diet.

A more recent study published this year in *Diabetes Care* found no significant difference in outcomes (weight, lipid levels, and glycemic control) between two groups consuming either a high-MUFA or high-carbohydrate diet over one year. Both groups had modest weight reductions over 52 weeks (approximately 4 kg) along with improved lipid, blood pressure, A1c, and fasting glucose levels. No detail was offered regarding the fiber content or glycemic index of the carbohydrate-dense foods that participants consumed. The authors of this study concluded that both low-fat and high-MUFA diets provide clinical benefits to individuals with type 2 diabetes.

Some researchers have expressed concern over the effects of a high-fat diet on pancreatic beta-cell health and insulin resistance. However, most of the deleterious effects of a high-fat diet seem to be attributable to saturated fatty acids, not MUFAs. A study published in *Diabetes* in 2003 concluded that the fatty acids in monounsaturated oils mitigate the negative effects of saturated palmitic acid on beta-cell death. In addition, circulating saturated fatty acids appear to cause pronounced insulin resistance, whereas MUFA apparently does not.[5]

Low Carb and Beyond

The ADA position statement names low-carbohydrate diets as a viable alternative for weight loss in the short term. Low-carbohydrate diets have been defined as providing anywhere from 50 to 150 g carbohydrate/day.[6] Weight loss is believed to occur not when individuals replace carbohydrate with fat or protein but when deficits in appetite cause a drastic reduction in caloric intake from high-carbohydrate foods. Still, questions about the sustainability of the diet and long-term effects on lipid profiles, glycemic control, cardiovascular disease, and kidney function remain.

Some scientists are now considering diet/genome interactions to explain differences between individual glycemic responses to food. Apparently, a number of genetic factors may influence how an individual reacts physiologically to his or her dietary pattern. For example, a gene implicated in diet/genome interactions is Rad.[7] In experiments with mice, Rad overexpression caused mice eating a high-fat diet to become more insulin resistant and glucose intolerant than normal mice eating the same diet. Rad overexpression has been identified in humans, and this finding suggests that a high-fat diet may have a more profound impact on glucose homeostasis in some individuals.[7] Genetic studies may eventually provide a way to fine-tune individual diets for optimal glycemic control and improved clinical diabetes outcomes.

Best Advice

So what is the optimal macronutrient balance in a diet for someone with diabetes? It appears that low-fat, high-fiber diets may be more effective than low-carbohydrate diets over the long term for sustaining weight loss and improving clinical diabetes outcomes (eg, lipid profile, glycemia). This may also be true of low-fat vs. high-MUFA diets.

The bottom line is that no one can truly say which diet is best. One of the biggest barriers to determining the ultimate diet profile for individuals with diabetes is likely the lack of consistency in study design and size. Not all studies encourage the intake of unrefined, carbohydrate-dense foods that are high in fiber or rate low on the glycemic index scale.

Cohort sizes are often very small. Observation time can range from three to 72 months or more. Most studies also rely on the diet recall of free-living subjects to determine compliance with dietary prescriptions or establish intake patterns. Feeding subjects a controlled diet in a controlled environment would yield more accurate results, but this is usually not feasible or affordable in a study lasting several months or years.

Considering the circumstances and metabolic profile of each individual before suggesting a dietary pattern for diabetes is likely still the best practice.

Notes

1. Gardner CD, Kiazand A, Alhassan S, et al. Comparison of the Atkins, Zone, Ornish and LEARN diets for change in weight and related risk factors among overweight premenopausal women: The A to Z weight loss study: A randomized trial. *JAMA.* 2007;297(9):969–977.
2. Franz MJ, Bantle JP, Beebe CA, et al. Evidence-based nutrition principles and recommendations for the treatment and prevention of diabetes and related complications. *Diabetes Care.* 2003;26 (Suppl 1):S51–S61.
3. Barnard ND, Scialli AR, Turner-McGrievy G, Lanou AJ, Glass J. The effects of a low-fat, plant-based dietary intervention on body weight, metabolism, and insulin sensitivity. *Am J Med.* 2005;118(9):991–997.
4. Nordmann AJ, Nordmann A, Briel M, et al. Effects of low-carbohydrate vs low-fat diets on weight loss and cardiovascular risk factors: A meta-analysis of randomized controlled trials. *Arch Intern Med.* 2006;166(3):285–293.
5. Chavez JA, Summers SA. Characterizing the effects of saturated fatty acids on insulin signaling and ceramide and diacylglycerol accumulation in 3T3-L1 adipocytes and C2C12 myotubes. *Arch Biochem Biophys.* 2003;419(2):101–109.
6. Westman EC, Feinman RD, Mavropoulos JC, et al. Low-carbohydrate nutrition and metabolism. *Am J Clin Nutr.* 2007;86(2):276–284.
7. Dedoussis GV, Kaliora AC, Panagiotakos DB. Genes, diet and type 2 diabetes mellitus: A review. *Rev Diabet Stud.* 2007;4(1):13–24.

Critical Thinking

1. Why is a high fiber, low fat (where most fats are from monounsaturated and omega-3 fats) diet the best overall long-term diet advice for a person with type 2 diabetes?

2. What type of fat has a negative impact on pancreatic beta cells and insulin resistance? How do monounsaturated fats interfere with this process?

3. When considering carbohydrate intake in research studies, what is the most important factor to consider regarding the carbohydrates?

RITA E. CAREY, MS, RD, CDE, is a clinical dietitian and diabetes educator at Yavapai Regional Medical Center and the Pendleton Wellness Center in Prescott, Ariz.

UNIT 4

Obesity and Weight Control

Unit Selections

Learning Outcomes

After reading this unit, you should be able to

- Summarize the "food environment" in the United States. Explain why many health professionals refer to our food environment as toxic.

- Develop recommendations of how families can effectively impact the nutrition and health of their children.

- List the diseases or medical conditions that are linked to increased weight gain during pregnancy.

- Discuss how excessive maternal weight gain during pregnancy can impact the health of the fetus.

- Identify the primary factors that have contributed to the obesity epidemic in the world.

- Describe how the Federal Trade Commission, The Centers for Disease Control and Prevention, the Food and Drug Administration, and the Department of Agriculture together are tackling the way food is marketed to children.

- Discuss the health consequences associated with children being overweight or obese.

Student Website

www.mhhe.com/cls

Internet References

American Society of Exercise Physiologists (ASEP)
   www.asep.org
Calorie Control Council
   www.caloriecontrol.org
Centers for Disease Control and Prevention: Overweight & Obesity
   www.cdc.gov/obesity
Shape Up America!
   www.shapeup.org

Overweight and obesity have become epidemic in the United States during the last century and are rising at a dangerous rate worldwide. Approximately 5 million adults are overweight or obese according to the standards set by the U.S. government using a body mass index (BMI) range of 30 to 39.9. Reports suggest that by the year 2050, half of the U.S. population will be considered obese if current trends continue; however, recent analysis indicates that the rate of increase in overweight and obesity in the United States is nearing a plateau rather than the upward slope.

Overweight and obesity is prevalent in males and females of all ages, races, and ethnic groups. Approximately 15 percent of children in the United States between the ages of 6–19 are obese, and 30 percent are overweight. Because of this, childhood obesity has gained much needed attention in the media and health arenas. Considering the prevalence of U.S. children and adolescents who are overweight or at risk, the appropriate method of action is prevention. Prevention efforts are geared toward curtailing obese children from maturing into obese adults who burden our current healthcare system and government supported healthcare reimbursement programs with exorbitant costs of obesity-related chronic diseases. The major health consequences of obesity are heart disease, diabetes, gallbladder disease, osteoarthritis, and some cancers. The cost for treating the degenerative diseases secondary to obesity is approximately $100 billion per year in the United States.

Even though health and nutrition professionals have tried to prevent and combat obesity with behavior modification, a healthy diet, and exercise, it seems that these traditional ways have not proven effective. Fast-food restaurants are the mainstay for many Americans because they offer quick, inexpensive food. Supersizing has become the norm because, in many instances, it's cheaper to order a biggie combo than smaller items individually. Americans are so accustomed to our fast food nation that many people become infuriated when asked to pull up and wait an extra minute for a 2,400 calorie meal. The problem is exacerbated by the food industry's historical plight to earn profit and market share by providing U.S. consumers with the fatty, sugary, and salty foods that we demand. Considering all of these challenges, we should not be surprised that obesity has become an epidemic. Food companies spend millions of dollars in advertising foods loaded with simple sugars, fat, and salt. Their aggressive advertising, coupled with food accessibility and large portion sizes, has created the current obesity pandemic. Other obstacles to maintaining a healthy diet are low accessibility and the high cost of eating a healthy diet.

More recently, scientists have reported that fat is a dynamically active endocrine organ that releases hormones and inflammatory proteins that may predispose a person to chronic diseases such as heart disease. In addition, research has discovered the role of the "hunger hormone" and how individual differences affect our ability to lose weight. A positive association was recently found between obesity, especially central obesity, and different types of cancer. Thus, there is a great need for a multifaceted public health approach that would involve mobilization of private and public sectors and focus on building better coping skills and increasing activity.

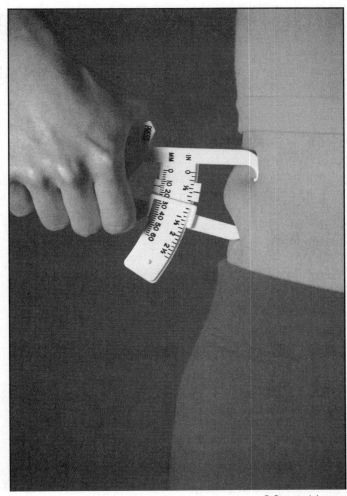

© Comstock Images

Globalization is causing the rest of the world and especially developing third world countries to mimic the unhealthy Western diet that contributes to obesity. Obesity and its health consequences are now becoming a global epidemic. Sweetened beverages and the sedentary Western way of life that has been adopted by many developing countries are some of the major contributors of this epidemic.

Intervention should be the top priority of policymakers. At the public sector, inclusion of health officials, researchers, educators, legislators, transportation experts, urban planners, and businesses would cooperate in formulating ways to combat obesity is crucial. A sound public health policy would require that weight-loss therapies have long-term maintenance and relapse-prevention measures built into them. Healthy People 2010 is the U.S. government's prevention agenda designed to ensure high quality of life and reduce health risks. One of the 28 areas it focuses on is overweight and obesity. Its main objectives are to reduce the proportion of overweight and obese children, teens, and adults by half and to increase the proportion of adults who are at a healthy weight.

Underage, Overweight

The federal government needs to halt the marketing of unhealthy foods to kids.

SCIENTIFIC AMERICAN

The statistic is hard to swallow: in the U.S., nearly one in three children under the age of 18 is overweight or obese, making being over-weight the most common childhood medical condition. These youngsters are likely to become heavy adults, putting them at increased risk of developing cardiovascular disease, type 2 diabetes and other chronic ailments. In February First Lady Michelle Obama announced a campaign to fight childhood obesity. Helping parents and schools to instill healthier habits in kids is an important strategy in this battle. But the government must take further steps to solve the problem.

In an ideal world, adults would teach children how to eat healthily and would lead by example. But in reality, two thirds of U.S. adults are themselves overweight or obese. Moreover, the food and beverage industry markets sugar- and fat-laden goods to kids directly—through commercials on television, product placement in movies and video games, and other media. Its considerable efforts—nearly $1.7 billion worth in 2007—have met with sickening success: a recent study conducted by researchers at the University of California, Los Angeles, found that children who see more television ads tend to become fatter. You might expect that watching TV, being a sedentary activity is responsible for obesity but the study found that obesity is correlated not with television per se but with advertising. The more commercial programming children watched, the fatter they got compared with those who watched a comparable amount of public television or DVDs. The majority of products marketed during children's programming are foods.

As nutritionist Marion Nestle of New York University has written, society needs to "create a food environment that makes it easier for parents and everyone else to make better food choices." Protecting children from junk-food marketing would help create conditions conducive to achieving a healthy weight.

Unfortunately like the tobacco industry before it, the food industry cannot be trusted to self-regulate in this regard. In a study published in the March *Pediatrics,* investigators looked at the prevalence of food and beverage brands in movies released between 1996 and 2005. They noted, for instance, that although Coca-Cola and PepsiCo have pledged to not advertise during children's television programming, their products routinely appear in movies aimed at kids.

Likewise, in the March *Public Health Nutrition,* researchers reported a 78 percent increase from 2006 to 2008 in the use of cartoon characters, toys and other child-oriented cross promotions on food packaging—much of it for nutritionally bereft foods. A whopping 55 percent of these cross promotions came from food manufacturers that have opted into the Children's Food and Beverage Advertising Initiative, sponsored by the Council of Better Business Bureaus, which promises to limit advertising to kids but allows participants to decide for themselves whether to restrict in-store marketing. Such examples of ineffectual commitments on the part of the food industry abound.

In December a group of U.S. agencies—the Federal Trade Commission, the Centers for Disease Control and Prevention the Food and Drug Administration, and the Department of Agriculture—proposed standards for foods and beverages that are marketed to children between the ages of two and 17. The agencies sensibly recommended that such foods must provide a meaningful contribution to a healthy diet by meeting specified requirements; that the amounts of saturated fat, trans fat, sugar and salt in these foods must not exceed limits set by the group; and that certain clearly healthy foods-such as those that are 100 percent fruits, vegetables or whole grains—may be marketed to kids without meeting the other two standards.

The interagency working group is due to submit a report containing its final recommendations to Congress by July 15. The standards are worthy but have one problem: as they stand, they would be voluntary. They should be mandatory, not optional, and the FDA should implement and enforce them.

The estimated cost of treating obesity-related ailments in adults was $147 billion for 2009. With the health care system already faltering, allowing companies to decide for themselves whether to peddle junk food to kids is a fox-and-henhouse policy this country simply cannot afford any longer.

Critical Thinking

1. Which nutrients are being targeted by the Federal Trade Commission, the Centers for Disease Control, and Food and Drug Administration as being unhealthy for children and, thus, should not be marketed to kids between the ages of 2 to 17?

2. From 2006 to 2008, what percentage increase was observed in the use of cartoon characters, toys, and kid-oriented promotion on food packaging?

3. How have Coca-Cola and PepsiCo addressed the popular opinion to decrease marketing of unhealthy products to kids?

Engaging Families in the Fight against the Overweight Epidemic among Children

Mick Coleman, Charlotte Wallinga, and Diane Bales

"Epidemic!" "Alarming!" "A threatening storm!" These powerful descriptors have been used by the Centers for Disease Control and Prevention (CDC) (Polhamus et al., 2004), the American Academy of Pediatrics (Committee on Nutrition, 2003; Council on Sports Medicine and Fitness and Council on School Health, 2006), and other medical professionals (Olshansky et al., 2005) to describe the increase in the number of U.S. children who are overweight. Indeed, data compiled from the National Health and Nutrition Examination Survey by the CDC (2007) show that the prevalence of overweight preschool-age children, 2 to 5 years old, increased from 5% in the period 1971–74 to 13.9% in the period 2003–04. During the same time periods, the prevalence of overweight 6- to 11-year-olds increased from 4% to 18.8% and the prevalence of overweight 12- to 19-year-olds increased from 6.1% to 17.4%. Across age groups, the prevalence of overweight children remains higher among low-income and minority groups than among children as a whole (Anderson & Butcher, 2006).

In this article, we provide an update on the overweight epidemic with early childhood educators in mind. We begin with information about the consequences of being overweight for children's health. We then examine the multiple factors that contribute to the overweight epidemic. Next, we look at the case for involving families in the fight against the overweight epidemic among children. Finally, we share three principles and associated strategies that early childhood educators can use to help families guide their children toward a healthy lifestyle.

Consequences Associated with Children Being Overweight

Cardiovascular Disease. It is estimated that a majority (61%) of overweight children from 5 to 10 years old have one or more cardiovascular risk factors (Freedman, Dietz, Srinivasan, & Berenson, 1999), such as high blood pressure, high cholesterol, and hardening of the arteries (Daniels, 2006; Freedman et al., 1999). While these biological processes can take decades to progress to a stroke or heart attack, it is feared that becoming overweight during childhood may accelerate their impact and lead to an early death (Daniels, 2006).

Diabetes
Diabetes in children also is attributed to the increased incidence of children being overweight (Daniels, 2006; Ludwig & Ebbeling, 2001). Diabetes, in turn, can lead to blindness, heart disease, kidney disease, and loss of limbs (The Center for Health and Health Care in Schools, 2005).

Asthma
The risk of asthma is higher among children who are overweight (Gilliland et al., 2003). In addition, overweight children with asthma have been found to use more medicine, make more visits to the emergency room, and spend more days wheezing than non-overweight children with asthma (Belamarich et al., 2000).

Sleep Apnea
Being overweight carries a higher risk of sleep apnea, an abnormal collapse of the airway during sleep, both in adults and children (Daniels, 2006). As a result, overweight children may exhibit daytime sleepiness, which, in turn, can lead to a decrease in physical activity and further heighten the risk for being overweight (Daniels, 2006). In addition, daytime sleepiness can negatively impact children's classroom performance. Over the long term, sleep apnea also can increase blood pressure, further raising the risk of heart disease.

Quality and Length of Life
Overweight children and their parents report significantly lower quality of life scores for physical, emotional, social, and

school functioning than do families with children diagnosed as "healthy" (Schwimmer, Burwinkle, & Varni, 2003). Perhaps more alarming, because of the increased incidence of childhood overweight, young children today may live less healthy and shorter lives than their parents (Olshansky et al., 2005). Should this occur, being overweight would indeed prove to be the "threatening storm" that reverses the steady rise in life expectancy observed during previous centuries.

Factors Contributing to the Overweight Epidemic among Children

Children become overweight when they eat too many calories and do not get enough physical activity to burn off those calories (Anderson & Butcher, 2006; U.S. Department of Health and Human Services, 2001). Although genetics and body metabolism both contribute to this imbalance, certain lifestyle factors also must be considered (Anderson & Butcher, 2006; Council on Sports Medicine and Fitness and Council on School Health, 2006).

The Food Environment

Children in the United States have an overwhelming abundance of food choices. Unfortunately, not all foods found in grocery stores are healthy, few fast food meals are healthy, and pre-packaged foods and soft drinks are often high in fat, sugar, and calories. Advertisements also can be confusing and sometimes misleading. For example, although many prepackaged foods are advertised as healthy (e.g., "reduced fat"), they may contain as many or more calories than the foods they are designed to replace (CDC, 2005a). We only need to look at the vending machines at our work sites to realize that milk, juices, and healthy snacks are far less available than their less healthy counterparts. Unfortunately, vending machines and food advertising through television programming remain a fact of life in too many elementary and middle schools, perhaps, in part, because of the added income they bring to schools (Anderson & Butcher, 2006; Cawley, 2006).

Portion Sizes

Yet another factor contributing to the confusing food environment is portion size (Cawley, 2006). Food manufacturers began producing larger portion sizes in the 1970s and continued to do so at an increasing rate through the 1980s and 1990s, leading children and adults to eat more and take in more calories during meals and snacks (CDC, 2005a; Young & Nestle, 2002). It easy to understand why children have difficulty establishing healthy eating patterns.

Schedules

Skipping breakfast and eating fast food are characteristics of a national mindset in which food quantity and convenience override considerations of food quality and health. Even though many ready-to-eat healthy foods are available (e.g., fruits), families often prefer prepackaged foods because they have longer shelf lives, do not require cleaning, and appeal to the tastes of children. Nevertheless, results from research suggest that eating food away from home, especially at fast food establishments, contributes to children becoming overweight (Davis et al., 2007). Likewise, skipping breakfast is a risk factor for becoming overweight (Davis et al., 2007).

Technological Advances and Urban Design

While technology has contributed to the quality of our lives, it also has reduced our level of physical activity. For example, as children spend more time watching television, they spend less time engaged in outdoor physical activities. Likewise, many families live in communities designed more for vehicles than for walking and biking (Fierro, 2002). Urban sprawl, combined with inadequate sidewalks and heavy traffic, prevents children from walking or riding bikes to school and parks (Anderson & Butcher, 2006).

Play and Physical Education

Recess and time for free play have been eliminated or shortened in many school systems (U.S. Department of Health and Human Services, 2004). In addition, rules regarding physical education for elementary school children vary widely (National Conference of State Legislatures, 2005). These changes have come about at least in part due to the increased concern over preparing children to meet mandated test scores (Anderson & Butcher, 2006). In response, such groups as the American Association for the Child's Right to Play (www.ipausa.org) are advocating for the 60 minutes of daily physical activities often recommended by the medical profession (Council on Sports Medicine and Fitness and Council on School Health, 2006; Davis et al., 2007).

The Case for Engaging Families as Health Educators

Increasingly, families are being viewed as essential in the fight against the overweight epidemic among children. Families, more than any other social institution, serve as both mediators and monitors of children's health behaviors.

Families as Mediators

Families mediate their children's eating behaviors through their choice and preparation of snacks and meals, as well as through their decisions of where to eat when outside the home. Families serve as mediators of children's physical activities through the rules they set regarding the amount of time children spend watching television and playing computer games. Likewise, families determine the degree to which children are involved in such physical activities as games, recreational pursuits, home chores, and yardwork.

Families as Monitors

Families also serve as monitors of their children's eating and physical activity patterns. Although some families appear to

Table 1   Families as Health Educators: Guides for Developing Healthy Lifestyle Activities for Families

Family-based Activities. In order to make healthy living truly a family affair, strive to develop activities that involve all family members in a household and not just a child or a parent-child dyad. Otherwise, efforts to fight family overeating and inactivity may not be successful.

Time Efficiency. Because families lead busy lives, develop family involvement activities that can be incorporated into their usual routines (e.g., dinner, bedtime, housework). Families are more likely to try healthy lifestyle activities if they fit into their daily schedules.

Simplicity. The fewer materials and directions needed to complete an activity, the better. Families may not bother to attempt a healthy lifestyle activity if that activity involves numerous materials and directions.

Clarity. Check all printed materials for clarity. If doubt remains about certain words or phrases, ask a few families to read the materials and provide you with feedback. Identify volunteers to translate printed materials into the languages represented in your classroom.

Fun. No one wants to eat bland food or engage in boring or unpleasant physical activities. Use your creativity and consult with community nutritionists and recreation specialists to develop fun and creative activities that reinforce healthy eating and exercise.

Encourage Rather Than Preach. Avoid a "preaching" stance by acknowledging that we all have a right to watch television, play video games, and eat a piece of cake. Disallowing these things altogether will only serve to sabotage families' efforts. Note the importance of moderation, not total elimination, when suggesting activities that help move families toward a more active and healthy lifestyle.

have difficulty recognizing the potential health risks associated with being overweight (Young-Hyman, Herman, Scott, & Schlundt, 2000), a number of family-based intervention programs have achieved success in lowering the weight of overweight children (see Epstein, Valoski, Wing, & McCurley, 1994; Golan & Crow, 2004; Golan, Weizman, Apter, & Fainaru, 1998; Harvey-Berino & Rourke, 2003; Lindsay, Sussner, Kim, & Gortmaker, 2006). Indeed, one of the most basic ways that parents can monitor and contribute to their children's development of healthy eating patterns is by establishing a family rule about eating dinner together (Lindsay et al., 2006).

The importance of a family-based approach to addressing the overweight epidemic becomes even clearer when we consider how families must juggle multiple schedules and unique demands, which can interfere with their ability to serve as effective monitors of their children's eating patterns and exercise activities. As a result, consideration must be given to respecting the realities of family life when planning family activities to promote healthy eating and exercise. Table 1 presents guides that we have followed in carrying out training related to healthy living. These guides also were the foundation for our development of the activity ideas found in Table 2 and Figure 1.

Involving Families in the Fight against the Overweight Epidemic

Early childhood educators have the expertise to bridge the gap between factual health information and the application of family involvement practices to promote family-oriented healthy eating and exercise. Three recommendations from the CDC (2005b) for involving families in promoting a healthy approach to eating and physical activity are especially relevant to early childhood teachers' work with families.

Guide 1. Encourage Families to Serve as Role Models

A family-based approach to fighting against the factors contributing to children being overweight is in keeping with current recommendations that recognize the importance of parents as children's most important role models in adapting a healthy lifestyle (Council on Sports Medicine and Fitness and Council on School Health, 2006; Davis et al., 2007; Lindsay et al., 2006). Families that model healthy eating patterns, regularly participate in physical activities, and talk about the benefits associated with a healthy lifestyle set an example for children to follow. Younger children, in particular, are more likely to mimic the behavior of important adults like parents and guardians. Some ideas to share with families to help them model healthy living habits can be found in Table 2.

Guide 2. Encourage Families to Engage in Healthy Activities in Different Settings

Help families discover practical ways to eat healthy meals and exercise throughout the week. Family activity calendars, like the one presented in Figure 1 for families of preschool and kindergarten children, can provide the encouragement families need to work toward a healthy lifestyle within and outside the home.

Guide 3. Advocate for Quality School and Community Physical Activity Programs

Families may not always see themselves as having the knowledge or skills needed to serve as health advocates for their children. Help promote families' knowledge, confidence, and skills in the following ways:

Figure 1   Themes and Ideas for an Activity Calendar

Theme	Mon	Tue	Wed	Thu	Fri
Practice Fundamental Motor Skills	*Trapping.* Sit on the floor and roll a large ball back and forth. Roll it to one side, then the other side. Roll it slowly, then quickly.	*Catching.* Help your child practice catching a large ball by rolling it down a slide or chute. Then, toss the ball back and forth to each other.	*Hopping.* Hop like a rabbit or grasshopper. See how long you can hop on one foot.	*Weaving.* Weave through an obstacle course of chairs or sheets hung over an outdoor line.	*Throwing.* Practice throwing a ball through a hula hoop from different distances and angles.
Encourage Creative Movement	Attach a large scarf to your child's pants or around her waist. Do the same for yourself. Pretend you have been swept up by the wind and are floating in the sky. What do you see below?	Observe how bugs move on the ground. Take turns making up your own creative bug movements.	Use ribbons attached to your wrists as butterfly wings. Fly around and visit your favorite flowers and plants.	Some communities have free introductory dance classes. Take your family to different classes. Which ones do family members enjoy the most?	Put on a fast song. Everyone make up a silly dance, the sillier the better.
Family Relaxation and Recreation	As a family, take a stroll around the neighborhood after dinner. Using hints, play a game of "guess what I see."	As a family, color and decorate heavy paper plates. Use them as frisbees. Aim for a tree or play toss and catch.	Read a book with or to your child. Make up a story together. Be sure to write it down and draw pictures so you can enjoy it again later.	Use the Internet or library to look up dances from different cultures. Try a new dance each week.	As a family, bowl, play a round of miniature golf, ride bikes, dance, etc. Don't make it competitive. Just have fun.
Movement Games	Try walking in a straight line while balancing a balloon or foam ball in your hand. Repeat, this time walking in a circle or along a winding path.	Play "Simon Says" by directing your child to move in different ways. Repeat, with your preschooler giving you directions.	Make up your own family movement game. Remember to keep it simple so everyone can play and have fun.	Divide into pairs and play a game of opposites. If your partner hops forward, you hop backward. If you partner crouches on her knees, you jump up in the air.	As a family, form a line and play a movement game of follow the leader. Take turns being the leader.

Table 2   Ideas for Helping Families Become Healthy Role Models

Incorporate the following ideas into classroom newsletters, family workshops, and parent-teacher conferences to help families become healthy role models for their children.

Starting Smart: Teaching Young Children About Healthy Foods While Grocery Shopping

1. Help your child name the different types of vegetables and fruits on display in the produce section. Note that these foods are good for our bodies. When passing by the cookie and candy aisles, note that we should eat only a little of these items, and only occasionally. Help reinforce this message by "skipping" past these aisles with your child as you move on to more healthy foods.

2. Make a shopping list using pictures of healthy foods. Help your child cut out and paste the pictures onto sheets of paper. As your child decorates each page, note that the foods in the pictures are good for our bodies because they give us energy and help our bodies stay strong and healthy. Arrange the pictures in an order that reflects the layout of your grocery store. Hand your child a few pictures of the healthy food you are shopping for before entering each aisle. Your child can use the pictures to help you look for the healthy food. This game will also help distract him from looking for less healthy foods.

3. Point out the different colors, shapes, and textures associated with such foods as bell peppers, apples, onions, grapes, tomatoes, nuts, and lettuces. Help your child pick foods with the colors, shapes, or textures she would like to try in a snack or meal.

Eating In, Eating Out: Managing the Food Environment

1. Make sure that fresh and dried fruit, juice, milk, and water are readily available and easily accessible to everyone in the family. Putting juice and water in colorful pitchers will help catch your child's attention. Ask your child to draw pictures of his favorite fruits. Paste the pictures onto serving bowls to encourage him to go to those bowls for his snacks.

2. Ask your child to name her favorite healthy foods and write these on a large sheet of paper. Work with your child to write her own recipe, using some of the foods from her list. Use the recipe when preparing a family snack or meal.

3. When eating out, help your child find and make healthy choices by limiting your and his choices to only healthy items. Share the healthy choice you have made and repeat the healthy choices available to your child.

Serve as an Exercise Role Model

1. Take your child shopping for your exercise clothing and equipment. Talk about why you wear these clothes and how you use the equipment.

2. When dressing for exercise, talk to your child about why you are stretching, drinking water, and dressing in certain types of clothes. After exercising, talk to your child about how you feel.

3. Allow your child to play with your exercise equipment in a supervised and safe environment. Do not try to teach athletic skills. Instead, let her experiment with different movements.

Exceptions to the Rule

1. Practice moderation, not elimination. Allow your child to eat sweets now and then, explaining the importance of not making them a part of our daily diet. Repeating this message will help your child develop the mindset needed to follow a balanced diet.

2. At the end of holiday celebrations, help your child divide the candy he received into small portions and put them into individual sandwich bags. Give him two bags each week. One can serve as a special snack for the week. Encourage him to share the other bag with a family member. Serve something healthy (milk, water, or an apple) to drink or eat with the candy.

Practices to Avoid

1. Avoid the mindset of "Do as I say, not as I do," as it strikes children as being unfair. When they see adults eating candy or fast food, they have a difficult time understanding why they cannot do the same. Eating healthy is a family affair. Everyone should follow the same rules.

2. Avoid forcing your child to eat foods she does not like. Instead, use a "try me" approach to encourage your child to try new foods. Visit the following United States Department of Agriculture website to learn about the variety of foods you can serve that have similar nutritional qualities: www.mypyramid.gov/pyramid/index.html

3. Avoid using food as a reward. Such rewards often consist of unhealthy sweets, and this can promote unhealthy food choices and eating patterns.

4. Avoid placing your child on a strict diet. This will only interfere with her ability to develop the knowledge, skills, and motivation needed to follow a balanced diet. If you believe your child is overweight, consult with a nutritionist or your family physician to develop a plan of action that addresses both eating and physical activity patterns of behavior.

Television and Electronic Games

1. Follow the recommendation of the Council on Sports Medicine and Fitness and the Council on School Health (2006) of limiting your child's television viewing to no more than 2 hours per day. Help remind your child of this family rule by monitoring his television viewing and using the hands of a clock to show how much time he has left to watch television before it is turned off for the day.

(continued)

Table 2   Ideas for Helping Families Become Healthy Role Models *(continued)*

2. Take inventory of the number of electronic games in your home versus games and materials that promote physical activity, such as bikes, badminton sets, jump ropes, balls, and rackets and bats. Are your purchases more heavily weighted toward sedentary electronic games? If so, make a concentrated effort to balance out your purchases when selecting gifts for your child during the holidays and on her birthday.

3. Take television shows and electronic games outside. Work with your child to plan a version of her favorite television show or an electronic game that can be played outside. Follow two rules. First, the game must be safe and nonviolent. Second, it must involve movement. For example, you may plan a game called the human pinball machine. Friends and family members can take turns serving as stationary "bumpers" located at arm's length from each other (the bumpers cannot move from their spot) and "balls." Each "ball" attempts to run through the pinball machine without being touched by the stationary "bumpers."

- *Note how your center or school promotes healthy eating and physical activity.* Point out classroom menus and outdoor play equipment to families when conducting registration and orientations. Explain how menus and physical activities are developed. Encourage dialogue by asking families about their children's favorite foods and physical activities.

- *Make health part of parent-teacher conferences.* Address children's nutritional habits and physical activities that you have observed in the classroom. Compare your observations to those made by families in the home environment. Provide families with a list of community youth groups that offer free or inexpensive age-appropriate activities, like dance and swimming. Visit with a local school nutritionist or your local cooperative extension agent to gather ideas for quick and healthy snacks for families to try at home. Invite these experts to conduct family night workshops on such topics as childhood nutrition, reading and understanding food labels, using the food pyramid, and identifying misleading food advertisements. Invite professionals from your local department of recreation to demonstrate noncompetitive games that families can play at home, as well as fun activities that promote children's fundamental motor skills, like those presented in Figure 1.

- *Encourage families to share.* Inviting family members to the classroom to share their recreational hobbies is an inexpensive way to introduce children to a variety of physical activities. If children do engage in the activity being demonstrated, pair the visiting parent with an early childhood physical education teacher to ensure that developmentally appropriate practices are followed.

- *Engage families in the learning process.* Recruit families to work with children in growing a garden of herbs and vegetables in pots or raised beds. Families that are unable to come to the classroom can be provided with tip sheets on how to grow herbs and vegetables at home. Invite families to help children prepare healthy salads and other dishes using the herbs and vegetables they harvest.

Conclusion

There are no easy solutions to addressing the epidemic of children who are overweight. The authors hope that the information and ideas presented in this article will help early childhood educators play an active role in working with families to help children develop the eating and activity patterns needed for a healthy lifestyle.

References

Anderson, P. M., & Butcher, K. F. (2006). Childhood obesity: Trends and potential causes. *The Future of Children: Childhood Obesity, 16*(1), 19–45.

Belamarich, P. F., Luder, E., Kattan, M., Mitchell, H., Islam, S., Lynn, H., & Crain, E. F. (2000). Do obese inner-city children with asthma have more symptoms than nonobese children with asthma? *Pediatrics, 106*(6), 1436–1441.

Cawley, J. (2006). Markets and childhood obesity policy. *The Future of Children: Childhood Obesity, 16*(1), 69–88.

Center for Health and Health Care in Schools. (2005). *Childhood overweight: What the research tells us.* School of Public Health and Health Services, The Georgia Washington University Medical Center. Retrieved June 29, 2008, from www .healthinschools.org/~/media/Files/obesityfs.ashx

Centers for Disease Control and Prevention. (2005a). *Overweight and obesity: Contributing factors.* Retrieved June 29, 2008, from cdc.gov/nccdphp/dnpa/obesity/contributing_factors.htm.

Centers for Disease Control and Prevention. (2005b). *Healthy youth! Promoting better health strategies.* Retrieved June 29, 2008, from www.cdc.gov/HealthyYouth/physicalactivity/promoting_ health/strategies/families.htm

Centers for Disease Control and Prevention. (2007, May 22). *Overweight prevalence.* Retrieved June 29, 2008, from www.cdc.gov/print.do?url=http%3A%2F%2Fwww.cdc. gov%2Fnccdphp%2Fdnpa%.

Committee on Nutrition. (2003). Prevention of pediatric overweight and obesity. *Pediatrics, 112*(2), 424–430.

Council on Sports Medicine and Fitness and Council on School Health. (2006). Active healthy living: Prevention of childhood obesity through increased physical activity. *Pediatrics, 117*(5), 1834–1842.

Daniels, S. R. (2006). The consequences of childhood overweight and obesity. *The Future of Children: Childhood Obesity, 16*(1), 47–67.

Davis, M. M., Gance-Cleveland, B., Hassink, S., Johnson, R., Paradis, G., & Resnicow, K. (2007). Recommendations for prevention of childhood obesity. *Pediatrics, 120* (Supplement 4), S229–S253.

Epstein, L. H., Valoski, A., Wing, R. R., & McCurley, J. (1994). Ten-year outcomes of behavioral family-based treatment for childhood obesity. *Health Psychology, 13*(5), 373–383.

Fierro, M. P. (2002). *The obesity epidemic—How states can trim the fat. Issue Brief.* National Governors Association Center for Best Practices. Online: www.nga.org/portal/site/nga

Freedman, D. S., Dietz, W. H., Srinivasan, S. R., & Berenson, G. S. (1999). The relation of overweight to cardiovascular risk factors among children and adolescents: The Bogalusa heart study. *Pediatrics, 103*(6), 1175–1182.

Gilliland, F. D., Berhane, K., Islam, T., McConnell, R., Gauderman, W. J., Gilliland, S., Avol, E., & Peters, J. M. (2003). Obesity and the risk of newly diagnosed asthma in school-age children. *American Journal of Epidemiology, 158*(5), 406–415.

Golan, M., & Crow, S. (2004). Targeting parents exclusively in the treatment of childhood obesity: Long-term results. *Obesity Research, 12*(2), 357–361.

Golan, M. A., Weizman, A., Apter, A., & Fainaru, M. (1998). Parents as the exclusive agents of change in the treatment of childhood obesity. *American Journal of Clinical Nutrition, 67*(6), 1130–1135.

Harvey-Berino, J., & Rourke, J. (2003). Obesity prevention in preschool Native-American children: A pilot study using home visiting. *Obesity Research, 11*(5), 606–611.

Lindsay, A. C., Sussner, K. M., Kim, J., & Gortmaker, S. (2006). The role of parents in preventing childhood obesity. *The Future of Children: Childhood Obesity, 16*(1), 169–186.

Ludwig, D. S., & Ebbeling, T. B. (2001). Type 2 diabetes mellitus in children: Primary care and public health considerations. *Journal of the American Medical Association, 286*(12), 1427–1430.

National Conference of State Legislatures. (2005). *Childhood obesity: An overview of policy options in legislation for 2003–2004.* Online: www.ncsl.org/programs/health/childhoodobesity.htm.

Olshansky, S. J., Passaro, D. J., Hershow, J. L., Carnes, B. A., Brody, J., Hayflick, L., Butler, R. N., Allision, D. B., & Ludwig. D. S. (2005). A potential decline in life expectancy in the United States in the 21st century. *New England Journal of Medicine, 253*(11), 1138–1145.

Polhamus, B., Dalenius, K., Thompson, D., Scanlon, K., Borland, E., Smith, B., & Grummer-Strawn, L. (2004). *Pediatric nutrition surveillance 2002 report.* Atlanta, GA: U.S. Department of Health and Human Services, Centers for Disease Control and Prevention.

Schwimmer, J. B., Burwinkle, T. M., & Varni, J. W. (2003). Health-related quality of life of severely obese children and adolescents. *Journal of the American Medical Association, 289*(14), 1813–1819.

U.S. Department of Health and Human Services. (2001). *The surgeon general's call to action to prevent and decrease overweight and obesity.* Rockville, MD: Public Health Service, Office of the Surgeon General.

U.S. Department of Health and Human Services. (2004). *Healthy People 2010 Progress Review: Nutrition and overweight.* Online: www.healthypeople.gov/data/2010prog/focus19/default.htm.

Young, L. R., & Nestle, M. (2002). The contribution of expanding portion sizes to the U.S. obesity epidemic. *American Journal of Public Health, 92*(2), 246–249.

Young-Hyman, D., Herman, L., Scott, D. L., & Schlundt, D. G. (2000). Care giver perception of children's obesity-related health risk: A study of African-American families. *Obesity Research, 8*(3), 241–248.

Critical Thinking

1. What percentage of overweight children, 5–10 years old, have high blood pressure, high cholesterol, and/or hardening of the arteries?

2. What are the six health-related consequences associated with children being overweight?

3. What are three examples of how families can serve as positive role models for overweight kids?

MICK COLEMAN is Professor, **CHARLOTTE WALLINGA** is Associate Professor, and **DIANE BALES** is Associate Professor, Department of Child and Family Development, University of Georgia, Athens.

From *Childhood Education,* Spring 2010, pp. 150–156. Copyright © 2010 by the Association for Childhood Education International. Reprinted by permission of the authors and the Association for Childhood Education International, 17904 Georgia Avenue, Suite 215, Olney, MD 20832.

Birth Weight Strongly Linked to Obesity

New evidence suggests gain during pregnancy is key.

NANCI HELLMICH

Women who gain a lot of weight during pregnancy are more likely to have high-birth-weight babies, which may increase the children's risk of becoming obese later in life, a new study suggests.

The findings add to growing evidence of the importance of appropriate weight gain during pregnancy.

For several decades, researchers have observed that a high birth weight increases the risk that a child will gain too much weight later in life. Some studies of animals suggest excess calories affect the fetus, including the fat tissue and the organs that regulate body weight.

Now researchers at Children's Hospital in Boston and Columbia University in New York have studied the medical records of more than 500,000 women who had two or more pregnancies, a total of more than 1 million babies. A newborn who weighed more than 8 1/2 pounds at birth was considered at a high birth weight.

By comparing siblings, researchers for the first time were able to control for mothers' genetic influences on birth weight.

The findings, reported online in The Lancet: The women gained an average of 30 pounds during pregnancy; those who gained 50 pounds were twice as likely to have a high-birth-weight baby than those who gained 20.

"Although birth weight is not the only determinant of adult weight, these findings suggest that an optimal time to begin obesity prevention efforts is before birth," says pediatric endocrinologist David Ludwig of Children's Hospital, lead author of the study.

Matthew Gillman of Harvard Medical School, who is also researching pregnancy and weight gain, says follow-up studies are needed to establish the link between gestational weight gain and childhood obesity.

In the meantime, there are other reasons to be concerned, Ludwig says. Pregnant women who are overweight or obese are at greater risk of problems such as complications during labor and delivery (including C-sections), gestational diabetes and high blood pressure.

How much should you gain?

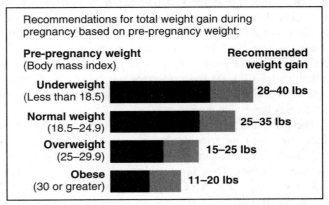

Recommendations for total weight gain during pregnancy based on pre-pregnancy weight:

Pre-pregnancy weight (Body mass index)	Recommended weight gain
Underweight (Less than 18.5)	28–40 lbs
Normal weight (18.5–24.9)	25–35 lbs
Overweight (25–29.9)	15–25 lbs
Obese (30 or greater)	11–20 lbs

Source: Institute of Medicine   By Frank Pompa, USA TODAY

A word of caution: "Being severely underweight during pregnancy, as well as severely limiting food intake, can also be problematic to fetal growth and development," says Alan Fleischman, medical director for the March of Dimes, which works to improve babies' health. Too little weight gain increases the risk of having a low-birth-weight baby of less than 5 1/2 pounds.

Critical Thinking

1. Pregnant women who are overweight or obese are at greater risk for developing certain medical conditions. What are three of these medical conditions?

2. How does excessive maternal weight gain during pregnancy impact the health of the fetus?

3. What is the recommended weight gain for a normal weight pregnant woman? How does this recommendation differ from the recommended weight gain for an obese pregnant woman?

The Fat Plateau

Americans are no longer getting fatter, it appears.

THE ECONOMIST

A few years ago, Burger King, a fast-food chain, conducted a study of the eating habits of some of its most frequent customers. A few dozen "SuperFans", as the firm calls them, recorded and photographed everything they ate for two weeks. The results were collected in a book called "Food for Thought". Unsurprisingly, this book is not publicly available: amateur photos of heaps of junk food are hardly an enticing advertisement for a firm that supplies the stuff. Nonetheless, "Food for Thought" gives an insight into why some Americans have such poor diets.

The fast-food fans in the book typically lead chaotic lives. They often toil long, irregular hours for not much money. They grab food when they can, skipping many meals and gorging at unorthodox times. They favour whatever is quick, convenient and comforting. ("I selected the pie because it was easy to grab out of the fridge," says one.) They often have an imperfect grasp of nutritional science. ("I am eating chocolate muffins at work because they are not too heavy," says another.) Oddly for a piece of corporate research, the book contains passages that are quite moving. One single dad's diary shows him eating nothing but junk for days on end. Then, one evening, he visits his aunt's house and she cooks him a feast of real food: pork, okra stew, collard greens and corn bread.

At 33.8%, America's obesity rate is ten times higher than Japan's. In all, 68% of Americans are either obese or overweight. (Some studies yield lower numbers, but since they typically ask people how much they weigh, rather than weighing them, scepticism is in order.) Few problems, besides death, afflict more people. Americans are more likely to be overweight than to pay federal income tax.

But the good news is that the nation may have stopped getting fatter. A study published this month in the *Journal of the American Medical Association (JAMA)* found that American women were no more likely to be obese in 2008 than they were nearly a decade before. For men, there was a small rise in obesity over the same period, but no change in the past three years. Among children, too, there was no change in obesity rates except among the very heaviest boys, whose numbers increased slightly. Could it be that the American obesity epidemic has reached a plateau?

If the national girth really has stopped expanding, that would be a blessing, though of course it is a big fall in obesity that is really required. Although a little extra heft is no big deal, many Americans are so ample that it ruins their health. That places a burden on the health-care system: each obese American racks up medical bills 42% higher than an American of normal weight, according to Eric Finkelstein and Justin Trogdon, writing in *Health Affairs*. Add to that the indirect costs of obesity, such as lost productivity due to sickness or premature death.

The startling Republican victory in Massachusetts this week throws Barack Obama's health reforms up in the air. But the issue will not go away. And a plateau in the obesity rate would make some kind of reform a bit less expensive. It will not lead to a sudden dip in health-care costs, predicts Mr Trogdon. But it could substantially slow the rate at which they are rising. Previous projections typically assumed that Americans would keep on ballooning. As a thought experiment in 2008, Youfa Wang of the Johns Hopkins Centre for Global Health drew a line from recent trends and projected that 100% of Americans would be over-weight by 2048. By 2030, his model showed health-care costs attributable to excess weight approaching a trillion dollars a year.

The latest numbers remind us how little is known about public health. Of course, people put on weight when they consume more calories than they burn off. But no one knows for sure why America's obesity has trebled since 1960. Plausible theories abound. As people grow richer food becomes relatively cheaper. Time grows more precious: hence the lure of fast food. Desk work burns fewer calories than spadework. And labour-saving devices do just that if we still washed dishes and clothes by hand, we would burn off five pounds of flesh each year, reckons Barry Popkin, the author of a book called "The World is Fat". All this is no doubt true, but it does not explain why Americans are fatter than people in other rich countries, nor why they appear to have stopped getting fatter.

No to Nannies

Kathleen Sebelius, the health secretary, says that "fighting obesity is at the heart" of health reform. But telling people to eat more healthily is like telling them not to have risky sex. Americans are suspicious of the nanny state at the best of times, let alone when it nags them to curb their most basic instincts. Some regulations help: forcing restaurants to post calorie counts on dishes, for example, prompts diners to pick less calorific treats. But politicians are reluctant to attack voters' favourite vices too vigorously. A recent proposal to tax sugary drinks, for example, went nowhere. Opponents argued that it would disproportionately affect the poor. True enough, but the poor are disproportionately likely to be overweight.

The constant barrage of pro-vegetable propaganda in schools may have raised awareness of the need for a balanced diet, reckons Mr Trogdon. And popular pressure has prompted many fast-food outlets to offer salads and other wholesome fare. But even if good food were freely available, losing weight is hard. Every year, 25% of American men and 43% of American women attempt it. "[F]ailure rates are exceedingly high," notes a *JAMA* editorial. But there is hope. Eating is social. Studies suggest that people guzzle more if they have overweight friends and relatives, and less if they don't. So if Americans have stopped getting fatter, their children have a better shot at staying trim.

Critical Thinking

1. What are the primary factors that have contributed to the obesity epidemic in the United States?

2. What is the latest percentage of obese or overweight Americans? How does this percentage differ from the obesity rate percentage?

3. Describe the typical fast food fan depicted in the book, *Food for Thought*.

In Your Face
How the Food Industry Drives Us to Eat

BONNIE LIEBMAN AND KELLY BROWNELL

Excess pounds raise the risk of diabetes, heart disease, stroke, cancer (of the breast, colon, esophagus, kidney, and uterus), gallbladder disease, arthritis, and more. And once people gain weight, the odds of losing it and keeping it off are slim.

"Estimates are that this generation of children may be the first to live fewer years than their parents," says Kelly Brownell. "Health care costs for obesity are now $147 billion annually."

What are we doing about it? Not enough.

"The conditions that are driving the obesity epidemic need to change," says Brownell. Here's why and how.

Q: Why do you call our food environment toxic?
A: Because people who are exposed to it get sick. They develop chronic diseases like diabetes and obesity in record numbers.

Q: How does the environment influence what we eat?
A: When I was a boy, there weren't aisles of food in the drugstore, and gas stations weren't places where you could eat lunch. Vending machines in workplaces were few and far between, and schools didn't have junk food. Fast food restaurants didn't serve breakfast or stay open 24 hours. Today, access to unhealthy choices is nearly ubiquitous.

Burgers, fries, pizza, soda, candy, and chips are everywhere. Apples and bananas aren't. And we have large portion sizes—bigger bagels, burgers, steaks, muffins, cookies, popcorn, and sodas. We have the relentless marketing of unhealthy food, and too little access to healthy foods.

Q: Does the price structure of food push us to buy more?
A: Yes. People buy a Value Meal partly because that large burger, fries, and soft drink cost less than a salad and bottle of water. A large popcorn doesn't cost much more than a small. A Cinnabon doesn't cost much more than a Minibon.

Q: And most stores are pushing junk food, not fresh fruit?
A: Yes. There's a Dunkin' Donuts at our Stop 'n Shop supermarket and at the Wal-Mart near us. And if you look at retail stores, they're set up in ways that maximize the likelihood of impulse purchases.

For example, the candy is on display at the checkout line at the supermarket. And when you go to a modern drugstore, the things you usually go to a drugstore to buy—like bandages, cough medicine, pain reliever, your prescriptions—are all at the back. People typically have to walk by the soda, chips, and other junk food to navigate their way there and back.

Old Genes, New World

Q: You've said that our biology is mismatched with the modern world, How?
A: Thousands of years ago, our ancestors faced unpredictable food supplies and looming starvation. Those who adapted ate voraciously when food was available and stored body fat so they could survive times of scarcity.

Our bodies were programmed to seek calorie-dense foods. They were exquisitely efficient calorie-conservation machines, which matched nicely with a scarce food supply.

But now we have abundance. And there's no need for the extreme physical exertion that our ancestors needed to hunt and gather food. It's a mismatch.

Q: How do ads encourage overeating?
A: Overeating is written into the language that companies use—names like Big Gulp, Super Gulp, Extreme Gulp. At one point, Frito-Lay sold dollar bags of snack foods called the Big Grab. The burger companies describe their biggest burgers with words like the Monster Burger, the Whopper, the Big Mac. The industry capitalizes on our belief that bigger is better and promotes large amounts of their least healthy foods.

Q: Why do we want a good deal on a bad food?
A: Everybody likes value. Getting more of something for your money isn't a bad idea. You like to do that when you buy an automobile or clothing or laundry detergent or anything.

But when the incentives are set up in a way that offers value for unhealthy food, it's a problem. If you buy the big bag of Cheetos, you get a better deal than if you buy the little bag. A big Coke is a better deal than a little Coke. But if you buy six apples, you don't always get a better deal than if you buy three.

Q: Is indulgence a code word for overeating?
A: Right. You deserve a reward and we're here to offer it to you. And ads describe foods as sinful. Or we make light of eating too much, like the ad that said "I can't believe I ate the whole thing."

Are We Irresponsible?

Q: *How does the food industry blame people for the obesity epidemic?*

A: The two words it uses most frequently are personal responsibility. It plays well in America because of this idea that people should take charge of their own lives and because some people have the biological fortune to be able to resist our risky environment.

But it also serves to shift blame from the industry and government to the individuals with a weight problem. It's right out of the tobacco-industry playbook.

Q: *What else is in the food industry's playbook?*

A: Industry spokespeople raise fears that government action usurps personal freedom. Or they vilify critics with totalitarian language, characterizing them as the food police, leaders of a nanny state, and even food fascists, and accuse them of trying to strip people of their civil liberties.

They also criticize studies that hurt the food industry as "junk science." And they argue that there are no good or bad foods—only good or bad diets. That way, soft drinks, fast foods, and other foods can't be targeted for change.

Q: *So people think it's their fault?*

A: Many people who struggle with weight problems believe it's their own fault anyway. So exacerbating that is not helpful. But removing the mandate for business and government to take action has been very harmful.

For example, if you look at funding to reduce obesity, it has lagged far behind the extent of the problem. It's because of this idea that people are responsible for the way they are, so why should government do anything about it?

Q: *Are people irresponsible?*

A: There's been increasing obesity for years in the United States. It's hard to believe that people in 2010 are less responsible than they were 10 or 20 years ago. You have increasing obesity in literally every country in the world. Are people in every country becoming less responsible?

We looked into the literature to find data on other health behaviors like mammograms, seat belt use, heavy drinking, and smoking. All those other behaviors have remained constant or have improved in the U.S. population.

If irresponsibility is the cause of obesity, one might expect evidence that people are becoming less responsible overall. But studies suggest the opposite.

So if people are having trouble acting responsibly in the food arena, the question is why? There must be enormous pressure bearing down on them to override their otherwise responsible behavior.

Q: *It's not as though society rewards obesity.*

A: No. Obesity is stigmatized. Overweight people, especially children, are teased and victimized by discrimination. Obese children have lower self-esteem and a higher risk of depression. They're less likely to be admitted to college. And obese adults are less likely to be hired, have lower salaries, and are often viewed as lazy and less competent. So the pressure to overeat must be overwhelming.

Q: *Are the pressures worse for children?*

A: Yes. Kids don't have the natural cognitive defenses against marketing. And they're developing brand loyalty and food preferences that can last a lifetime.

To allow the food industry to have free range with our children has come at a tremendous cost. A third of kids are now overweight or obese. And when you project ahead to the adult diseases that will cause, it's incredible. Someday, our children may wonder why we didn't protect them from the food companies.

Q: *Do we do anything to protect kids?*

A: We do some nutrition education in schools, but it's a drop against the tidal wave of what the food industry is doing to educate those children.

The Robert Wood Johnson Foundation is by far the biggest funder of work on childhood obesity, and it's now spending $100 million a year on the problem. The food industry spends that much every year by January 4th to market unhealthy food to children. There's no way the government can compete with that just through education.

If parents ate every meal with their children, that would amount to 1,000 teaching opportunities per year. Yet the average child sees 10,000 food ads each year. And parents don't have Beyoncé, LeBron, and Kobe on their side.

Q: *So if irresponsibility isn't to blame, what is?*

A: When you give lab animals access to the diets that are marketed so aggressively in the United States, they become obese. We have abundant science that the environment is the causative agent here. So the environment needs to be changed.

That's what public policy is all about. We require that children get vaccinated and ride in child safety seats. We have high taxes on cigarettes. Your car has an air bag. The government could educate us to be safe drivers and hope for the best. Or it could just put an air bag in every car. Those are examples of government taking action to create better defaults.

Keeping It off

Q: *Why is it so important to prevent obesity?*

A: Because it's so difficult to fix. The results of studies on treating obesity are very discouraging, especially if one looks at long-term results. The exception is surgery, but that's expensive and can't be used on a broad scale. So this is a problem that screams out to be prevented.

Q: *Why is it so hard to keep weight off?*

A: There's good research, much of it done by Rudolph Leibel and colleagues at Columbia University, that shows that when people are overweight and lose weight, their biology changes in a way that makes it hard to keep the weight off.

Take two women who weigh 150 pounds. One has always weighed 150 and the other was at 170 and reduced down to 150. Metabolically, they look very different. To maintain her 150-pound weight, the woman who has dropped from 170 is going to have to exist on about 15 percent fewer calories than the woman who was always at 150.

Q: Why?

A: It's as if the body senses that it's in starvation mode so it becomes more metabolically efficient. People who have lost weight burn fewer calories than those who haven't, so they have to keep taking in fewer calories to keep the weight off. That's tough to do day after day, especially when the environment is pushing us to eat more, not less.

And Leibel and others have shown that there are changes in hormones, including leptin, that explain why people who lose weight are hungry much of the time.

Q: Are you saying that our bodies think we're starving when we lose just 10 percent of our body weight?

A: Right. It's not hopeless, but the data can be discouraging. The results of weight-loss studies are clear. Not many people lose a significant amount of weight and keep it off. All these environmental cues force people to eat, and then this biology makes it hard to lose weight and keep it off.

Q: Does genetics play a role in obesity?

A: Yes. Genetics can help explain why some people are prone to gain weight and some are not. But genetics can't explain why there are so many overweight people. The reason we have more obesity than Somalia, let's say, is not because we're genetically different. The fact that so many people are overweight is all environment.

Addictive Foods

Q: Are some foods addictive?

A: My prediction is that the issue of food and addiction will explode onto the scene relatively soon, because the science is building almost by the day and it's very compelling. I think it's important to put the focus on the food, rather than the person. There are people who consider themselves food addicts, and they might be, but the more important question is whether there's enough addictive properties in some foods to keep people coming back for more and more. That's where the public health problem resides.

Q: What are those properties?

A: What's been studied most so far is sugar. There are brain-imaging studies in humans and a variety of animal studies showing that sugar acts on the brain very much like morphine, alcohol, and nicotine. It doesn't have as strong an effect, but it has a similar effect on reward pathways in the brain. So when kids get out of school and they feel like having a sugared beverage, how much of that is their brain calling out for this addictive substance? Are we consuming so many foods of poor nutrient quality partly because of the addictive properties of the food itself?

Q: What do you mean by reward pathways?

A: There are pathways in the brain that get activated when we experience pleasure, and drugs of abuse like heroin hijack that system. The drugs take over the system to make those substances extremely reinforcing and to make us want those things when we don't have them.

The drugs do that by setting up withdrawal symptoms when we don't have them. The drugs set up the addiction by creating tolerance, so you need more over time to produce the same effect. The drugs set us up to have cravings. The same reward system is activated by foods, especially foods high in sugar.

Q: Do we need more research in people?

A: Yes, but we already have animal and human studies, some done by highly distinguished researchers. I think this is a top priority because if we get to the point where we say that food can be addictive, the whole landscape can change.

Think of the morality or legality of marketing these foods to children. Could the industry ever be held accountable for the intentional manipulation of ingredients that activate the brain in that way? The stakes are very high.

Q: How much does exercise matter to losing weight?

A: Exercise has so many health benefits that it's hard to count them. It lowers the risk for cancer, heart disease, and cognitive impairment as people age. There's a very long list of reasons to be physically active, but weight control may not be one of them. Recent studies have suggested that the food part of the equation is much more important than the activity part.

Q: Because you can undo an hour of exercise with one muffin?

A: Yes. The food industry has been front and center in promoting exercise as the way to address the nation's obesity problem. The industry talks about the importance of physical activity continuously, and they've been quite involved in funding programs that emphasize physical activity. The skeptics claim that that's the way to divert attention away from food.

Answers

Q: So what's the answer to the obesity epidemic?

A: The broad answer is to change the environmental conditions that are driving obesity. Some of the most powerful drivers are food marketing and the economics of food, so I would start there. I don't think we have much chance of succeeding with the obesity problem unless the marketing of unhealthy foods is curtailed.

Q: Not just to kids?

A: No, but children would be a great place to start. Second would be to change the economics so that healthy food costs less and unhealthy food costs more. So a small tax on sugar-sweetened beverages—say, one penny per ounce—would be part of that effort.

Ideally, the tax revenues would be used to subsidize the cost of fruits and vegetables. That creates a better set of economic defaults. Now, especially if you're poor, all the incentives are pushing you toward unhealthy foods.

Q: Like zip codes where there are no grocery stores?

A: That's a great example of a bad default. Another, which applies not just to the poor, would be what children have available in schools. You can sell a lot of junk in schools and then try to educate your way out of it. Or you can just get rid of the junk food and kids will have healthier defaults. They'll eat healthier food if that's what's available. You can inspire that just by changing the default.

Imagine the optimal environment to combat obesity. We would have affordable and healthful food, especially fresh fruits and vegetables, easily accessible to people in low-income neighborhoods. TV commercials for children would encourage them to eat fresh fruits and vegetables rather than pushing processed snacks that are associated with TV and movie characters. And every community would have safe sidewalks and walking trails to encourage physical activity.

Q: *So people wouldn't have to struggle to avoid eating junk?*
A: Right. We have a terrible set of defaults with food: big portions, bad marketing, bad food in schools. These conditions produce incentives for the wrong behaviors. So the question is: can we create an environment that supports healthy eating, rather than undermines it?

If you count the number of places where you can buy sugared beverages and salty snack foods and candy, it's enormous. If you count the number of places where you can buy baby carrots and oranges, it's a fraction of that.

So if you were creating an environment from scratch, you would do the opposite of what we have. The population deserves a better set of defaults.

Critical Thinking

1. What is meant by the quote, "our biology is mismatched with the modern world."

2. What types of foods are considered addictive?

3. The author talks about the U.S. food defaults. What are the U.S. food defaults that are causative factors in our toxic food environment?

KELLY BROWNELL is a professor in the Department of Psychology at Yale University. He is also a professor of epidemiology and public health. Brownell co-founded and directs Yale's Rudd Center for Food Policy and Obesity, which works to improve the world's diet, prevent obesity, and reduce weight stigma. Brownell, who is a member of *Nutrition Action*'s scientific advisory board, has published more than 300 scientific articles and chapters and 14 books including *Food Fight: The Inside Story of the Food Industry, America's Obesity Crisis, and What We Can Do About It* (McGraw-Hill). He spoke to *Nutrition Action*'s Bonnie Liebman from New Haven.

From *Nutrition Action HealthLetter,* May 2010, pp. 3–6. Copyright © 2010 by Center for Science in the Public Interest. Reprinted by permission.

Why We Overeat

DAVID A. KESSLER AND BONNIE LIEBMAN

"In 1960, when weight was relatively stable in America, women ages 20 to 29 averaged about 128 pounds," writes David Kessler in *The End of Overeating.* "By 2000, the average weight of women in that age group had reached 157." Among women 40 to 49, the trend was similar. "The average weight had jumped from 140 pounds in 1960 to 169 in 2000."

Two out of three American adults are now either overweight or obese. One in six children aged 2 to 19 is obese. Excess weight increases the risk of diabetes, heart disease, cancer (of the breast, colon, esophagus, kidney, and uterus), stroke, gallbladder disease, arthritis, and more.

Americans spend billions on weight-loss schemes, yet most diets fail over the long term. "That is because we have not understood why eating certain foods only makes us want to eat more of them," says Kessler. "No one has recognized what's really happening."

Here's how the food industry leads us to overeat . . . and how to fight back.

Q: *Why did you write* The End of Overeating?

A: There was a fundamental mystery that I wanted to understand. Why is it so hard for so many of us to resist eating even if we're not hungry? Why does that chocolate chip cookie have so much power over me? Why do we engage in behavior we don't want to engage in?

I started listening to people say, "I eat when I'm hungry, I eat when I'm not hungry, I eat when I'm happy, I eat when I'm sad." And I'd ask, "Do you understand why?" And they'd say "No."

Q: *Do people blame themselves?*

A: Yes. The result is a lot of misinformation and myths or people feeling bad about themselves or just throwing in the towel and saying, "There's nothing I can do."

I wanted to help people understand why it's so hard to resist food. And for the first time, we now have the science to say to people, "It's not your fault, and there are things you can do to control it."

Q: *What does the science say?*

A: First, we know what drives overeating. We published a paper called "Deconstructing the Vanilla Milkshake." We asked: Is it sugar or fat or the flavor that drives intake?

Chocolate Chip Cookie Molten Cake. Cake (fat, sugar), chocolate filling (fat, sugar), ice cream (fat, sugar), chocolate shell (fat, sugar).

Cheese Dip. Heavy cream (fat), cheese (fat), tortilla chips (fat, salt).

Southwestern Eggrolls. Fried tortilla (fat), chicken (salt), cheese (fat), ranch dressing (fat, salt).

Bacon Cheeseburger. Ground beef (fat), bacon (fat, salt), cheese (fat), sauce (fat, salt).

Buffalo Chicken Wings. Fried wings (fat), hot sauce (salt), butter (fat), dressing (fat, salt).

Cheese Fries. Fried potatoes (fat), beef chili (fat, salt), cheese (fat), dressing (fat, salt).

Java Chip Frappuccino. Coffee mix (sugar), whipped cream (fat, sugar), chocolate chips (fat, sugar), chocolate drizzle (sugar).

We gave rats a series of solutions containing combinations of sugar, corn oil, and vanilla, and found that sugar was the prime driver. But when you add fat to sugar, you increase the drive synergistically.

Q: *The rats pressed a lever more times to get it?*

A: Yes. If you combine sugar and fat, animals will work harder to get it. They'll want it more. If you give sugar alone, you'll get some dopamine spike, but if you put sugar and fat together, you stimulate more brain activation. And we know that humans prefer sugar mixed with cream more than the same amount of sugar mixed with skim milk.

Q: *How is dopamine—a neurotransmitter that conveys messages from one nerve cell to another—part of overeating?*

A: Dopamine focuses your attention. As human beings, we are wired to focus on the most important stimuli in our environment. If a bear walked into your office right now, your dopamine would spike. If your child is sick today, that's what you're thinking about. That's what captures your attention.

For some, alcohol can be a salient stimulus. Or illegal drugs, gambling, sex, smoking. But for many of us, it's food.

Of all the cues in this room right now, of all the things I could be thinking about, those little chocolate chip cookies over there are capturing my attention. Why? Because of my past experience, chocolate chip cookies will activate my brain.

Q: *Before you take the first bite?*

A: Yes. I'm not tasting them. It's not genuine hunger, but the anticipation, that makes us eat long after our calorie needs are satisfied.

Q: *And the sight of the cookies is the cue?*

A: Yes, but I could also be cued by the location, the time of day, or just getting in my car because it anticipates the consumption.

I could be walking down Powell Street in San Francisco and I start thinking about chocolate-covered pretzels because six months earlier I went into a store on Powell Street that had chocolate-covered pretzels. I didn't even remember that, but the street itself was a cue. And we're such effective learners.

The street cue stimulates brain activation. It causes arousal. And then it becomes part of working memory. You're thinking about it. You want it.

Food or Drug?

Q: *Do some foods keep the brain activated more than others?*

A: Yes. We've known that dopamine would spike—and stay elevated—in response to drugs like cocaine or amphetamines. But with food, we thought you would get a little dopamine elevation and then we would habituate—that is, the food would lose its capacity to activate our brains.

But if you combine sugar and fat, that brain activation doesn't always habituate. And as you make food more multisensory, some people don't get habituation. Their dopamine stays elevated.

Q: *What do you mean by multisensory?*

A: I mean that the food is more complex. For example, ice cream combines sugar and fat and cold. But if you add Heath bars, Reese's Peanut Butter Cups, crumbled cookies, and hot fudge, that adds more texture and aroma and temperature. The more multisensory you make food, the more reinforcing it becomes. The more people come back for more.

Q: *So it gets harder to resist over time?*

A: For some people, yes. I was talking to an individual who works in publishing. Big guy. The hardest thing for him to do every day, he says, is to get past the newsstand on the way to the train because the newsstand sells KitKat candy bars. For each of us, it's something different. But at its core, fat, sugar, and salt are highly salient stimuli.

Q: *How does salt make us want to eat more?*

A: A food industry executive told me that the industry creates dishes to hit what he called the three points of the compass. Sugar, fat, and salt are what make food compelling and indulgent. The most palatable foods have two or three

of them. [See boxes.] They lead to a roller coaster in the mouth—the total orosensory experience. We get captured.

Q: *What's the roller coaster?*

A: It's the cycle of cue-activation-arousal-release. We get cued—by sights, sounds, smells, time of day, location. The brain circuits get activated. There's arousal. And then you either distract yourself with something that's more important or you consume it and there's a release.

Q: *So eating is a thrill ride?*

A: Yes. If I gave you a pack of sugar and said, "Go have a good time," you'd look at me and say, "What are you talking about?"

Now I add to that sugar some fat, I add texture, color, temperature, mouthfeel, the outward appearance, the smell, and I put it on every corner, make it available 24/7.

Then I add the emotional gloss of advertising. I say you can eat it with your friends. Have a good time. I make it into a food carnival, and what do you expect to happen?

Q: *It's hard to resist.*

A: Right. Let me give you another example. Nicotine alone is a moderate reinforcing substance in animals. I add to that nicotine the smoke, the cellophane crinkling of the pack, the color of the pack, the image of the cowboy, the sexiness, the glamour that the industry created 50 years ago, the emotional gloss of advertising.

And what did I do? I took a moderately reinforcing substance and made it into an addictive product. So sugar alone is not enough.

Q: *Is everyone equally vulnerable to these foods?*

A: No. You can ask people if they have these three characteristics:

One: Do you lose control in the face of highly palatable foods? Is it very hard to resist them?

Two: Do you feel a lack of satiation—a lack of feeling full—when you're eating?

Three: Do you have a preoccupation? Do you think about foods in between meals? Or as you're eating something, are you thinking about what you'll be eating next?

When you ask these questions, some people have no idea what you're talking about. But about 50 percent of obese, 30 percent of overweight, and 20 percent of healthy-weight individuals score very high on those three characteristics.

Q: *Are these normal people?*

A: Yes. We're not talking about eating disorders. This is in the normal spectrum. There's no psychopathology. So when you add them up, it's some 70 million Americans who have this constellation of characteristics. It's not a disease. It's a syndrome that I call conditioned hyper-eating.

Q: *Is there evidence of what's going on in their brains?*

A: Yes. If you expose these people to the cues—a picture of chocolate, say—and you scan their brains, you see elevated activation in a part of the brain called the amygdala.

Q: *What does the amygdala do?*

A: That's where we process and store memories of emotions. When individuals who aren't conditioned hypereaters start to consume chocolate, for example, the activation shuts off. But in conditioned hypereaters, the activation remains elevated and it doesn't stop until they stop consuming the chocolate.

So the reason some foods are so hard for conditioned hypereaters to resist is that the reward circuits of the brain are in overdrive, and they're overriding the body's homeostatic mechanisms.

Q: *Those mechanisms should have made them stop eating?*

A: Yes. If you look at children at the age of two or three, they compensate. If you give them more calories in one meal, they'll eat less later in the day. But if they get exposed to sugar, fat, and salt all day for a few years, they lose the ability to compensate. By age four or five, they're eating all the time.

Q: *So eating these foods changes your brain?*

A: Yes. Every time you get cued and consume the stimulus, you strengthen the neural circuits, so the next time you're more likely to do it again. Strengthening those circuits is what we define as learning, even though it's not the kind of conscious learning we think about.

Q: *Does that explain why it's tough to keep weight off?*

A: Yes. Why don't diets work? Sure, I can deprive someone by cutting their calories for 30, 60, or 90 days. And they'll lose weight.

But, first of all, deprivation increases the reward value of food unless you substitute something you want more. And after you lose the weight, the old circuitry is still there.

Unless you've replaced it with new circuitry—new learning—if you're put back in your old environment, you continue to get bombarded by the old cues, so of course you'll gain the weight back.

Q: *Because the old circuitry remains?*

A: Yes. And if I become stressed, fatigued, hungry, if I'm trying to catch a plane and there's nothing else around, I will still grab those chocolate-covered pretzels. For most of us, the trick is to learn new circuitry. (See "Food Rehab," box)

The Food Industry

Q: *How does the food industry take advantage of conditioned hypereating?*

A: They understand that sugar, fat, and salt drive consumption. They've layered and loaded it into foods. They understand the combinations that will drive intake by giving you the greatest neural activation.

Industry also knows the bliss points—how much sugar, fat, and salt is just enough and not too much. And they understand the outputs—that people keep coming back for more.

Food Rehab

Here's some of the advice David Kessler gives in *The End of Overeating* (Rodale, $25.95) to help you resist the pull of unhealthy foods.

1. **Replace chaos with structure.** Determine ahead of time what you'll eat for meals and snacks. Block out everything else.
2. **Practice just-right eating.** Figure out how much food you need. (Odds are, it's less than you think.) Put it on your plate and don't go back for more.
3. **Pick foods that will satisfy, not stimulate, you.** What satisfies you is personal, but try foods that occur in nature, like whole grains, beans, non-starchy vegetables, and fruit, combined with lean protein and a small amount of fat.
4. **Rehearse.** Anticipate your moves like an elite athlete before a competition. For example, tell yourself, "If I encounter chocolate-covered pretzels, I'll keep walking."
5. **Seize control.** Stay alert to emotional stressors or other stimuli that trigger automatic behavior. Recognize emotions (like sadness, fatigue, or anxiety) that might lead you to overeat.
6. **Stop that thought.** Change the channel. Turn off the image of the trigger food before you start to debate whether to eat it.
7. **Think negative.** Pair the unhealthy food with a stream of (unappealing) images. "That's the flip side of what advertising agencies do when they link an Olympic athlete to a pair of sneakers or an attractive woman to a new piece of technology," says Kessler.

They haven't necessarily understood the black box in between—the neuroscience. Industry would say that it's just giving consumers what they want. But what they're giving consumers is food that excessively activates the brains of millions.

Q: *So we get a fatty, salty food like french fries smothered in cheese and bacon, which adds even more fat and salt?*

A: Right. They've optimized those ingredients to maximize the drive for food. We used to eat for nutrition—to satisfy ourselves. Now we eat for stimulation.

We're getting cued. We get that arousal. That attention. That release. The food isn't satisfying us. It's taking us on a roller coaster ride.

Q: *It's food as entertainment?*

A: Yes. If you go at 5 P.M. to a food court like the one at Washington D.C.'s Union Station, it's a food carnival. You optimize sugar, fat, and salt to drive consumption and add the emotional gloss, which amplifies the reinforcing value.

You'll want it. You'll love it. You'll have a good time. They make it into a carnival. Who doesn't want to get on the rides?

Q: *How can people fight back?*

A: How do you cool down the stimulus? The same way we did it with tobacco. We used to look at tobacco as something we wanted, something that would make us feel better, that would make us cool, sexy.

The real success was that we changed how people viewed the stimulus. We changed from seeing tobacco as glamour to perceiving it as a deadly, disgusting product.

When you're dealing with a reinforcing stimulus, that's important. If you view it as something that you want, something that's going to comfort you, you'll approach it. If you view it as something you don't want, that's your enemy, you're going to avoid it. So social norms and attitudes do affect us and affect brain impulses.

Q: *Did it help to tell teens that the tobacco industry was trying to hook them?*

A: Yes. And if our behavior is becoming conditioned and driven, that has immense policy implications. Then you start seeing advertising not just as information protected under the First Amendment, but as a cue that stimulates and drives consumption.

Once our kids become conditioned and their behavior is driven by sugar, fat, and salt, then that vending machine in the hallway and that fast food restaurant are cues.

Q: *Don't we want the food industry to make good-tasting food?*

A: Yes. We need foods that are rewarding. Food has to be pleasurable. But we've taken highly reinforcing substances and made them more reinforcing. And we've taken down the barriers by putting fat, sugar, and salt on every corner, making it socially acceptable and available 24/7.

Q: *What policies could help people?*

A: First, restaurants should list calories on the menu. We also need well-funded campaigns to let people know that big food—food that's layered and loaded with fat, salt, and sugar—is unhealthy. And we need to rethink advertising for highly palatable foods.

Q: *How?*

A: Advertising is not just neutral information. It's a cue that amplifies the reward value of highly stimulating foods. It affects how the brain responds. Once you understand that, then I think that's a legitimate reason to limit advertising of foods that have excess fat, sugar, and salt. And we need to go to the next step on food labeling.

Q: *Beyond Nutrition Facts?*

A: Yes. I was recently in the cafeteria at Google's headquarters. It was striking. They have red, yellow, or green in front of each lunch item. Green means have as much as you want. Yellow means have a moderate amount. Red means taste it but be careful how much you eat. It had a real effect on me.

We need something like that on the front of food packages. It's not just about individual ingredients any more.

Also, the industry needs to set responsible portion sizes. The reality is that we're going to finish the package because once our brains are activated, it's virtually impossible to stop.

Q: *How have people responded to the book?*

A: It takes courage for people who weigh 300 pounds to come to these book events. But to see them shake their heads and say, "Finally, someone is explaining to me why I do this," that's why I wrote the book.

Critical Thinking

1. Why is a food that contains fat and sugar more addictive than a food that is high in sugar?

2. What area of the brain is activated by anticipation of consuming an addictive food?

3. Name the three components of a food that make it compelling and indulgent.

4. What causes a "hypereater" to eat in excess?

DAVID A. KESSLER was commissioner of the U.S. Food and Drug Administration from 1990 to 1997, during which the agency overhauled and redesigned the Nutrition Facts labels that are on most foods. His first book, *A Question of Intent: A Great American Battle with a Deadly Industry,* describes the FDA's attempt to regulate cigarettes as nicotine-delivery devices. In 2000, the Supreme Court ruled that the FDA did not have the power to regulate tobacco. In June, Congress passed legislation to give the FDA that authority. Kessler spoke to *Nutrition Action*'s Bonnie Liebman by phone from San Francisco.

UNIT 5

Health Claims

Unit Selections

Learning Outcomes

After reading this unit, you should be able to

- Contrast the types of health claims that can be published on product labels: nutrient content claims and structure/function claims.
- List the nutrients that are required to be included on the Nutrition Facts panel.
- Criticize the current format of the Nutrition Facts label.
- Create recommendations for improvements in the type of information provided and how this information should be presented.
- Identify the form of omega-3 fatty acid found in flax.
- Explain why fish oil is considered the more potent source omega-3 fatty acids compared to flax oil.
- List the beneficial characteristics of flax, other than containing omega-3 fatty acids.
- Compare the effects of phytosterols and lipid-lowering medications on heart disease.
- Describe how consumers can protect themselves from misleading nutrition-related information.
- Identify reputable sources for nutrition-related information written in a clear, easily understood manner.

Student Website
www.mhhe.com/cls

Internet References

Federal Trade Commission (FTC): Diet, Health & Fitness
www.ftc.gov/bcp/menus/consumer/health.shtm
Food and Drug Administration (FDA)
www.fda.gov/default.htm
National Council against Health Fraud (NCAHF)
www.ncahf.org
Office of Dietary Supplements: Health Information
http://ods.od.nih.gov/Health_Information/Health_Information.aspx
QuackWatch
www.quackwatch.com

Technological advances in the 21st century have resulted in high-speed communication of scientific results and the possibility for miscommunication. Even if the scientific protocol, study, design, data collection, and analysis are impeccable, it is still possible to report the findings in a confusing and biased manner. According to an American Dietetic Association (ADA) survey, 90 percent of consumers polled get their nutrition information from television, magazines, and newspapers.

Some Americans are so confused and overwhelmed by the controversies surrounding food and health that they have stopped paying attention to the contradictory claims reported by news media. The media very frequently misinterprets results, simplifies the message, and does not provide the proper context to accurately interpret the information. In addition, the media is eager to publish sensational information and not solid science.

The dietary supplement industry is experiencing a huge transformation. Americans spend approximately $25 billion on alternative treatments. Antioxidant supplements are very popular among Americans, and even though they are available in our diet, many choose not to obtain them from food. Consumers, especially baby boomers, are opting for combination or condition-specific supplements. One of the articles in this unit reveals why the baby boomer generation is quickly buying up supplements for specific conditions and why members of generation Y are going for the nutrition and sports-performance type supplements. Additionally, there has been a recent interest in brain health due to the growing incidence of Alzheimer's and cognitive decline in old age. Because of this, there are several new products related to cognitive function on the market. One of the articles in this unit provides information on foods, food components, and other products that are thought to improve mental health.

Functional foods—foods that may provide a health benefit beyond basic nutrition—constitute one of the fastest growing segments of the food industry, especially among the affluent aforementioned baby boomers. The U.S government has no regulatory category of functional foods, but has set prerequisites as to what may qualify as a health and structure–function claim. Phytosterols have been documented to lower low-density

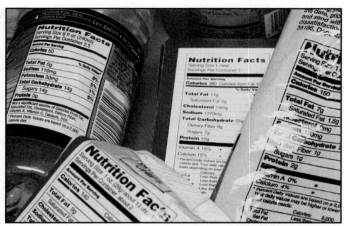

© C. Sherburne/PhotoLink/Getty Images

lipoprotein cholesterol and are as effective, safer, and cheaper than medications to lower blood lipids. New food products with added phytosterols are revolutionizing the market and our outlook for disease treatment. Flax meal, flax seeds, and flax oil are all products derived from flax, which has been reported to lower heart disease risk, reduce inflammation, diabetes, depression, and anxiety among other health benefits. Consumers are increasingly interested in purchasing and using flax for its health-promoting properties.

A topic of current interest with many touted health claims is omega-3 fatty acids and the best source for these beneficial fats. Demand for supplements and fortified foods containing omega-3s has culminated in a vast number of products on the market. Since the metabolic pathways of these PUFAs are complex, there is a great deal of confusion when it comes to information presented on the label and in the media. "Brain Food," by Linda Milo Ohr provides advice on how to intelligently interpret the claims about omega-3 fatty acids. "The Benefits of Flax" from *Consumer Reports on Health* discusses the difference between omega-3s from flax seed oil versus fish oil.

Influencing Food Choices
Nutrition Labeling, Health Claims, and Front-of-the-Package Labeling

For nearly 2 decades, nutrition labeling and health claims found on food packaged in the United States have supplied consumers with information based on a food's nutritional content and the potential health benefits from consuming the food. To further assist consumers in making food choices based on nutrient content, a number of organizations—professional and trade associations, grocery chains, and food manufacturers—have developed a variety of tools and labeling programs to supplement the Food and Drug Administration–regulated nutritional labeling effort. This article highlights Web resources that address nutritional labeling, health claims, in-store nutrition navigation, and several front-of-the-pack labeling programs.

KATHLEEN L. CAPPELLANO, MS, RD, LDN

Nutrition Labeling

The United States is one of 7 nations that require nutrition labeling on food packaging. The Nutrition Labeling and Education Act, signed into law in 1990, authorized the Food and Drug Administration (FDA) to require food manufacturers to include nutrition labeling in the form of a Nutrition Facts label on the packaging of most domestic and imported prepared foods. The law also requires that all nutrient content and health claims meet FDA regulations. Foods exempt from this requirement include meat, poultry, and eggs, which are regulated by the US Department of Agriculture, and alcoholic beverages containing more than 7% alcohol. The Nutrition Facts panel discloses the caloric, total fat, saturated and unsaturated fat, cholesterol, sodium, sugar, fiber, and carbohydrate content of the food. As of January 1, 2006, manufacturers are required to include the *trans*-fatty acid content per serving on the Nutrition Facts label.[1]

Food and Drug Administration

The FDA's website furnishes information about food labeling regulations, label claims, food allergens, and links to food labeling and packaging survey reports and to print resources such as its comprehensive Food Labeling Guide (www.fda.gov/Food/GuidanceComplianceRegulatory Information/GuidanceDocuments/FoodLabelingNutrition/ FoodLabelingGuide/default.htm).[2] By following the FDA's Nutrition Labeling Consumer Information link: www .fda.gov/Food/LabelingNutrition/ConsumerInformation/ default.htm, one can access pages that describe how to use the Nutrition Facts label (www.fda.gov/Food/Labeling Nutrition/ConsumerInformation/ucm078889.htm) and a description of *trans*-fat labeling in English (www.fda .gov/Food/LabelingNutrition/ConsumerInformation/ ucm109832.htm) and Spanish (www.fda.gov/Food/ LabelingNutrition/ConsumerInformation/ucm110019 .htm).[3–6] Another page, www.fda.gov/Food/Labeling Nutrition/ConsumerInformation/ucm121642.htm, leads to food labeling and nutrition education tools.[7] Colorful posters containing nutrition information for the 20 most frequently consumed fresh fruits, vegetables, and fish in the United States are available in multiple-size PDF format. These materials can be displayed or distributed by retailers participating in the voluntary point-of-purchase program.[8]

Make Your Calories Count

A user-friendly interactive program for learning about the Nutrition Facts label includes an overview and diagram of a sample label and explanations on how to interpret information pertaining to serving size; calorie and protein content; nutrients to limit such as fat, saturated and *trans* fat, cholesterol, sugar, and sodium; and guidance to purchase foods containing nutrients that are typically lacking in American diets such as vitamins A and C, calcium, iron, and fiber (www. fda.gov/Food/LabelingNutrition/ConsumerInformation/ ucm114022.htm).[9]

Health Claims

Explanation of the 3 types—health, nutrient content, and structure/function claims allowed on packaging of food and dietary supplements—can be found at www.fda.gov/ Food/LabelingNutrition/LabelClaims/ucm111447.htm.[10] A summary of health claims approved for use on food and dietary supplement labels is accessible in Appendix C of the Food Labeling Guide at www.fda.gov/Food/Guidance ComplianceRegulatoryInformation/GuidanceDocuments/ FoodLabelingNutrition/FoodLabelingGuide/ucm064919 .htm.[11]

Nutrient Content Claims

The Nutrition Labeling and Education Act allows the use of nutrient content claims that describe nutrient levels by using terms such as *free, high,* and *low* and/or *lite* on food packaging. Most nutrient content claim regulations pertain to nutrients for which there is an established daily value—reference points for intakes based on a 2,000-calorie diet. Appendix A: Definitions of Nutrition Content Claims,[12] www.fda .gov/Food/GuidanceComplianceRegulatoryInformation/ GuidanceDocuments/FoodLabelingNutrition/Food LabelingGuide/ucm064916.htm, and Appendix B: Additional Requirements for Nutrient Content Claims to the Food Labeling Guide,[13] www.fda.gov/ Food/GuidanceComplianceRegulatoryInformation/ GuidanceDocuments/FoodLabelingNutrition/Food LabelingGuide/ucm064916.htm, provide examples of nutrient content claims.[12,13] The FDA Modernization Act of 1997 permits manufacturers to submit notification of a nutrient content claim based on scientific evidence typically supported by the Food and Nutrition Board of the Institute of Medicine at the National Academy of Sciences to the FDA. Health claims may be used on product packaging 120 days after receipt of notification if the FDA takes no action to modify or prohibit the claim.[14]

Structure/Function Claims

Structure/function claims on packaged foods, dietary supplements, and pharmaceuticals describe how a nutrient or ingredient may benefit normal function in humans.

Guidance regarding compliance to the regulations on structure/function claims can be accessed at www.fda .gov/Food/GuidanceComplianceRegulatoryInformation/ GuidanceDocuments/DietarySupplements/ucm103340 .htm.[15]

Nutrition Labeling—Too Much or Too Little?

There has been much debate about the shortcomings of FDA's nutrition labeling program. Critics believe that the Nutrition Facts panel is too confusing—shoppers are rushed or distracted with little time to decipher the label and ingredients list. Calorie and total fat information reportedly is most useful to consumers in selecting food. However, the nutritional information appearing on labels varies across product categories given the differences in nutrient content among foods and is often inconsistent, particularly with respect to portion sizes even within the same product category. The percentage of daily value is a difficult concept for some to comprehend. Furthermore, the small font size used on the packaging is hard to read for some people. Nutrition labeling may be of limited use to the increasing number of Americans for which English is not the primary language.

Voluntary Labeling Programs— Stars, Stamps, and Checkmarks

Hannaford Guiding Stars

The Hannaford Guiding Stars program (www.hannaford .com/Contents/Healthy_Living/Guiding_Stars/index .shtml) is the first storewide navigation system to offer at-a-glance nutrition information for more than 25,000 foods including fresh produce, meat, seafood, deli items, and packaged foods. Bottled waters and foods with less than 5 calories per serving are not rated.[16]

The Guiding Stars scoring system, which is based on a "good, better, and best" approach was developed by nutrition scientists and an advisory panel of nutrition and medical experts. The nutrient data are analyzed from the information on the Nutrition Facts label and the US Department of Agriculture's nutrient database. A food with a poor nutritional score is given a "no star" ranking; a product with a 3-star score contains more micronutrients and/or whole grains and less *trans* and saturated fats, cholesterol, added sugars, and/or sodium. The scoring does not distinguish between foods that are organically or conventionally produced. The stars are placed on the unit price tags on grocery shelves, on produce signs, and those appearing on meat, poultry, and seafood cases.[17]

Front-of-Pack Nutrition Labeling

Professional and trade associations, grocers, and food manufacturers have developed a number of nutrition labeling tools to educate consumers and influence food purchasing. Nutrition scientists and food industry representatives hypothesize that a single, credible front-of-the pack labeling system that is recognizable and uniform across categories will benefit consumers greatly. They welcome a quick and easy means to bring attention to the caloric content of foods and to identify those rich in certain nutrients and/or food groups.

Nutrition scientists and food industry representatives hypothesize that a single, credible front-of-the pack labeling system that is recognizable and uniform across categories will benefit consumer greatly.

American Heart Association

The American Heart Association's (AHA's) food certification program, established in 1995, is designed to provide guidance for healthy people older than 2 years (www.americanheart.org/presenter.jhtml?identifier=2115).[18]

The heart-check program has 3 levels of certification: standard, for those products meeting the criteria for saturated fat and cholesterol; whole-grains certification, for foods meeting saturated fat, cholesterol, and whole-grains criteria; and whole-oat soluble fiber certification, for foods that meet the saturated fat and cholesterol criteria and contain 0.75 g of β-glucan per serving. A list of approximately 800 AHA-certified foods arranged by food category and manufacturer can be accessed at http://checkmark.heart.org. Foods ineligible for heart-check certification include bottled water, alcoholic beverages, meal replacements, certain beef cuts, nuts, products containing stanol-sterols, foods manufactured by tobacco companies, and those that do not align with AHA science.[19]

Whole Grains Council

The Whole Grains Council (www.wholegrainscouncil.org/find-whole-grains) is a nonprofit consumer advocacy group that works to increase consumption of whole grains for better health by encouraging manufacturers to create products using whole grains; help consumers find whole-grain foods and understand their health benefits; and ensure accurate reporting about whole grains among the media. In 2002, food manufacturers, scientists, and chefs convened at a Whole Grains Summit to outline a number of goals, one being the development of a packaging symbol—the Whole Grain Stamp—to help American shoppers easily select and purchase whole products as a means to reach the goal of consuming the recommended 3 daily servings of whole grains.[20]

The Whole Grain Stamp program participants must file information about each qualifying product and be a member of the Whole Grains Council. Manufacturers are bound by a legal agreement to abide by all the rules and guidelines of the program, thus providing a safeguard to consumers. The Whole Grain Stamps first appeared on grocery shelves in 2005 when stamps displayed on packaging described a food as a "good source" with a minimum of 8 g per serving; an "excellent source" containing 16 g of fiber; or "100% excellent" for products that contained all whole grains and at least 16 g of fiber for serving. The phase 2 program launched in June 2006 uses the Basic Stamp on the packaging for foods that contain at least 8 g of whole grain but may also contain refined grains, extra bran, germ, or refined flour. A product bearing the 100% Stamp must contain all whole grains as grain ingredients and 16 g of whole grain per serving. The stamps also include a number indicating the number of whole grains per serving.[21]

With recent expansion to Canada, Mexico, the Dominican Republic, and the United Kingdom, more than 2,100 products have used the Whole Grain Stamps on their packaging as of September 2008. A list of these products searchable by country and/or category, that is, granola and snack bars, beverages, breads and cereals, pasta, pizzas, entrees, and side dishes, is accessible at www.wholegrainscouncil.org/find-whole-grains/stamped-products.[22]Frequently-asked-questions pages for consumers and manufacturers can be found at www.wholegrainscouncil.org/whole-grain-stamp/stamp-faq-consumers and www.wholegrainscouncil.org/whole-grain-stamp/stamp-faq-manufacturers.[23,24]

Smart Spot

Pepsico's Smart Start program (www.pepsico.com/Purpose/Health-and-Wellness/Smart-Spot.html), launched in 2004, marks products with the Smart Spot symbol that are nutritious and contribute fiber and at least 10% of the daily value for nutrients such as protein, calcium, and vitamins A and C; meet limits for fat, saturated and *trans* fat, cholesterol, sodium, and added sugar; or are reduced in calories, fat, saturated or total fat, sodium, and sugar.[25]

Smart Choices Program

Led by the nonprofit Keystone Center, a partnership of scientists, university faculty, and representatives from the food and beverage industry and health and research organizations convened in 2007 to establish a comprehensive voluntary front-of-the pack labeling initiative to help consumers make smart food selections. This effort they hoped would improve shoppers' nutrition knowledge and encourage selection of healthful foods and would subsequently positively impact the health of the U.S. public.

The Smart Choices program (http://smartchoices program.com) launched in August 2009 marked products in 19 food product categories with a symbol displayed on the front of the package to guide shoppers in making quick and smarter food and beverage selections within a product category.[26] To help consumers make fast calorie comparisons, Smart Choices products also included calorie information on the front of the package indicating the number of calories per serving and servings per container.

The Smart Choices program was voluntarily suspended in late October pending an FDA ruling on package-front nutrition labeling.[27]

References

1. American Heart Association nutrition labeling. www .americanheart.org/presenter.jhtml?identifier=4631. Accessed June 16, 2009.

2. Food labeling guide guidance for industry. April 2008. www .fda.gov/Food/GuidanceComplianceRegulatoryInformation/ GuidanceDocuments/FoodLabelingNutrition/ FoodLabelingGuide/default.htm. Accessed July 2, 2009.

3. FDA nutrition labeling consumer information. www.fda.gov/ Food/LabelingNutrition/ConsumerInformation/default.htm. Accessed July 2, 2009.

4. How to understand and use the nutrition facts label. www .fda.gov/Food/LabelingNutrition/ConsumerInformation/ ucm078889.htm. Accessed July 2, 2009.

5. *Trans* fat now listed with saturated fat and cholesterol on the nutrition facts label. www.fda.gov/Food/ LabelingNutrition/ConsumerInformation/ucm109832.htm. Accessed July 2, 2009.

6. Los Ácidos Grasos Trans Ahora Serán Listados Junto con las Grasas Saturadas y el Colesterol en la Etiqueta de Información Nutricional. www.fda.gov/Food/LabelingNutrition/ ConsumerInformation/ucm110019.htm. Accessed July 2, 2009.

7. Label Education Tools. Food labeling and nutrition education tools. www.fda.gov/Food/LabelingNutrition/ ConsumerInformation/ucm121642.htm. Accessed July 2, 2009.

8. Nutrition Information for Raw Fruits, Vegetables and Fish www.fda.gov/Food/LabelingNutrition/ FoodLabelingGuidanceRegulatoryInformation/ InformationforRestaurantsRetailEstablishments/ucm063367 .htm. Accessed July 3, 2009.

9. Make Your Calories Count. www.fda.gov/Food/ LabelingNutrition/ConsumerInformation/ucm114022.htm. Accessed July 3, 2009.

10. Claims that can be made for conventional foods and dietary supplements. www.fda.gov/Food/LabelingNutrition/ LabelClaims/ucm111447.htm. Accessed July 3, 2009.

11. Appendix C: Health claims April 2008 guidance for industry. A food labeling guide. www.fda.gov/ Food/GuidanceComplianceRegulatoryInformation/ GuidanceDocuments/FoodLabelingNutrition/ FoodLabelingGuide/ucm064919.htm. Accessed July 3, 2009.

12. Appendix A: Definitions of nutrition content claims April 2008. Guidance for industry, a food labeling guide. www.fda.gov/Food/ GuidanceComplianceRegulatoryInformation/GuidanceDocuments/ FoodLabelingNutrition/FoodLabelingGuide/ucm064911.htm. Accessed July 3, 2009.

13. Appendix B: Additional requirements for nutrient content claims guidance for industry, a food labeling guide. www.fda.gov/Food/ GuidanceComplianceRegulatoryInformation/GuidanceDocuments/ FoodLabelingNutrition/FoodLabelingGuide/ucm064916.htm. Accessed July 3, 2009.

14. Nutrient content claims notification for choline containing foods. www.fda.gov/Food/LabelingNutrition/LabelClaims/ FDAModernizationActFDAMAClaims/ucm073599.htm. Accessed July 3, 2009.

15. Guidance for industry: structure/function claims, small entity compliance. www.fda.gov/Food/ GuidanceComplianceRegulatoryInformation/ GuidanceDocuments/DietarySupplements/ucm103340.htm. Accessed July 3, 2009.

16. Hannaford Guiding Stars. www.hannaford.com/Contents/ Healthy_Living/Guiding_Stars/index.shtml. Accessed June 16, 2009.

17. Hannaford Guiding Stars frequently asked questions. www. hannaford.com/Contents/Healthy_Living/Guiding_Stars/faqs. shtml. Accessed June 16, 2009.

18. American Heart Association. www.americanheart.org/presenter. jhtml?identifier=2115. Accessed June 16, 2009.

19. American Heart Association food certification program list of foods. http://checkmark.heart.org. Accessed June 16, 2009.

20. WholeGrains Council.org. www.wholegrainscouncil.org/ find-whole-grains. Accessed June 16, 2009.

21. Whole Grains Stamp program. www.wholegrainscouncil.org/ whole-grain-stamp. Accessed June 16, 2009.

22. Whole Grains Stamp Products. www.wholegrainscouncil.org/ find-whole-grains/stamped-products. Accessed June 16, 2009.

23. Whole Grains Council consumer FAQs. www .wholegrainscouncil.org/whole-grain-stamp/stamp- faq-consumers. Accessed June 16, 2009.

24. Whole Grains Council FAQ manufacturers. www. wholegrainscouncil.org/whole-grain-stamp/stamp- faq-manufacturers. Accessed June 16, 2009.

25. Smart Spot. www.pepsico.com/Purpose/Health-and-Wellness/ Smart-Spot.html. Accessed October 28, 2009.

26. Smart Choices Program™. http://smartchoicesprogram.com. Accessed October 28, 2009.

27. Food label program to suspend operations. The New York Times business section, October 24, 2009. www.nytimes .com/2009/10/24/business/24food.html?_r=2. Accessed October 26, 2009.

Critical Thinking

1. What is the Food and Nutrition Labeling Act of 1990?
2. Which nutrients are required to be included on the nutrition facts panel?
3. What is the difference between health claims, nutrient content claims, and structure/function claims on product labels?

KATHLEEN L. CAPPELLANO, MS, RD, LDN, is an instructor at the Friedman School of Nutrition Science and Policy, Tufts University, Boston, Massachusetts, and former Nutrition Information Manager at the Jean Mayer United States Department of Agriculture Human Nutrition Research Center on Aging at Tufts University. A member of the American Dietetic Association and Dietitians in Business and Communications practice group, Cappellano has over a decade of experience in evaluating and writing about medical, health, and food and nutrition websites. KATHLEEN L. CAPPELLANO, MS, RD, LDN, Friedman School of Nutrition Science and Policy. Tufts University, 150 Harrison Ave, Boston, MA 02111 (kathleen.cappellano@tufts.edu).

The Benefits of Flax

Flax products have been popping up all over grocery-store shelves lately, with claims such as "special protection for women's health" and "fights the blues." Here's our take on the seed's potential benefits, as well as some advice on how to incorporate it into your diet.

As Good as Fish Oil?

Flax products come in three forms: supplements, oil, and the seed itself. All of those, like fish oil, contain omega-3 fatty acids. In fish oil, those substances protect the heart in several ways, notably thinning the blood and lowering levels of LDL (bad) cholesterol and triglycerides. Moreover, those fatty acids might offer other health benefits, including protection against mild depression, Alzheimer's disease, and macular degeneration.

But it's unclear if the fatty acids in flax, which come in the form of alpha-linolenic acid (ALA), provide the same benefits. That's because the body has to convert ALA into the two fatty acids, eicosapentaenoic acid (EPA) and docosahexaenoic acid (DHA), found in fish oil. And to get meaningful amounts of those compounds you may have to consume lots of flax, according to a September 2008 study in the American Journal of Clinical Nutrition. It found that even large doses of flax oil—four to six 600-milligram capsules—boosted blood levels of EPA by only about 35 percent and had no effect on DHA.

Benefits Beyond the Heart

Still, flax oil might provide at least some coronary protection. And flaxseeds, especially crushed or ground, may offer certain benefits that fish oil does not. For example, they are rich sources of lignans, compounds that alter the way the body handles estrogen. That may explain why preliminary research hints that flaxseed can lower the risk of breast cancer. And one small study of women with mild menopausal symptoms found that about 3 tablespoons of flaxseed a day eased their hot flashes and night sweats as effectively as supplemental estrogen. Finally, the seeds contain lots of fiber, protein, magnesium, and thiamin.

How to Get more into Your Diet

- Add a tablespoon of crushed or ground flaxseed to your hot or cold breakfast cereal or yogurt.
- Add a teaspoon of crushed or ground flaxseed to mayonnaise or mustard when making a sandwich.
- Use crushed or ground flaxseed in place of eggs in baking. Mix 1 tablespoon with 3 tablespoons of water as a substitute for 1 large egg, and let it sit for a few minutes. Note that this will change the texture of the food.
- Look for products that contain flax, including cereals, granola bars, and breads.

Recommendation

Flax-oil supplements might be worth a try for people who want some of the benefits of fish oil but don't like the taste of fish or fish-oil pills, or avoid fish because they're vegetarians. But the supplements aren't good for people who can't take fish oil for safety reasons, because they may interact with the same blood-thinning drugs. And women with a history of breast, ovarian, or uterine cancers, as well as endometriosis or fibroids, should talk with their doctor before consuming flaxseeds because of their possible effect on estrogen. But most other people can safely add flaxseed to their diet.

Critical Thinking

1. Define alpha-linolenic acid (ALA), eicospentaenoic acid (EPA), and docosahexaenoic acid (DHA).

2. Why is fish oil considered the more potent source of omega-3 fatty acids as compared to flax oil?

3. What are the beneficial characteristics of flax in addition to containing omega-3 fatty acids?

Brain Food

Linda Milo Ohr

Cognitive health is a growing concern for consumers of all ages. Parents are continually learning about the importance of omega-3 fatty acids for their babies, toddlers, and adolescents. Teenagers and adults need to stay mentally sharp and focused for school and work. And baby boomers and seniors face conditions such as Alzheimer's and cognitive decline as they age.

This increased interest in brain health is evident in the growing number of brain-related products and brain-healthy ingredients that are available in the market. For example, *Minute Maid® Enhanced Pomegranate Blueberry Juice Blend* from Coca-Cola Co., Atlanta, Ga. (www.thecoca-colacompany.com, www.minutemaid.com), contains omega-3/DHA—50 mg/8 oz. It also contains choline and vitamin B-12, which "play a role in brain and nervous system signaling"; vitamin E to "help shield the omega-3s in the brain from free radicals"; and vitamin C, which is "highly concentrated in brain nerve endings."

In addition to these ingredients, other brain boosters include fruits, botanicals, walnuts, and more. Here is information on some of these "foods for thought."

Omega-3 Fatty Acids

A proven ingredient for brain health for all ages, omega-3 fatty acids such as docosahexaenoic acid (DHA), arachidonic acid, and eicosapentaenoic acid aid in development as well as benefit certain mental conditions. Most recently, Ryan and Nelson (2008) indicated that higher DHA levels are associated with improved listening comprehension and vocabulary skills in preschool children. They gave 400 mg/day of DHA (n = 85) or matching placebo (n = 90) to 4-year-old children for 4 mo. A preplanned regression analysis yielded a statistically significant positive association between a higher DHA level in the blood and higher scores on the Peabody Picture Vocabulary Test, a cognitive test designed to measure listening comprehension and vocabulary skills.

Omega-3 fatty acids have also been linked to improving various clinical and behavioral conditions involving mental function, including depression, bipolar disorder, schizophrenia, aggression, attention deficit hyperactivity disorder, Alzheimer's, and Parkinson's disease. Ma et al. (2007) showed that DHA decreased an important risk factor for late-onset Alzheimer's disease. Using a mouse model, a diabetic rat model, and cultured human cells, the study found that DHA increased the production of LR11, a protein vital to clearing the brain of the enzymes that make amyloid beta plaques often associated with Alzheimer's disease.

Currently, a National Institutes of Health-funded study is studying the effects of DHA in slowing the progression of Alzheimer's disease. Patients with mild-to-moderate Alzheimer's disease will be treated for 18 mo, taking either 2 g/day of DHA or a placebo. The results are anticipated by December 2009. The DHA is produced by Martek Biosciences Corp., Columbia, Mo. (phone 410-740-0081, www.martek.com).

Blueberries

High in antioxidants, blueberries are gaining recognition as brain-healthy foods. U.S. Dept. of Agriculture Agricultural Research Service scientists studied the effect of a blueberry extract on mice that carried a genetic mutation for promoting increased amounts of amyloid beta plaque in the brain (Bliss, 2007). They found increased activity of a family of enzymes, called kinases, in the brains of amyloid-plaqued mice that were fed blueberry extract. Two of the kinases found are important in mediating cognitive function.

Other research has shown that Alaskan wild-bog blueberries contain compounds that can reduce inflammation in the central nervous system that is associated with the progression of neurodegeneration (Society for Neuroscience, 2007). Another study at the Center for Aging and Brain Repair at the University of South Florida College of Medicine, Tampa, Fla., showed that supplementing the diet of old rats with blueberries for 8 weeks resulted in maintenance and rejuvenation of brain circuitry.

Grapes

Wang et al. (2008) found that grape-seed-derived polyphenolics, *MegaNatural®-AZ* from Polyphenolics, Madera, Calif. (phone 559-661-5556, www.polyphenolics.com), significantly reduced Alzheimer's disease-type cognitive deterioration. They gave mice with Alzheimer's disease either water containing grape seed extract or plain water for 5 mo and found that the mice treated with grape seed extract had significantly reduced Alzheimer's disease-type cognitive deterioration compared to the mice in the control group. This was due to the prevention of amyloid beta plaque forming in the brain.

Another study suggested that Concord grape juice in the diet may provide benefits for older adults with early memory decline (Welch, 2008). Subjects drank a total of 15–21 oz of either Concord grape juice or a placebo for 12 weeks. Those who drank the grape juice showed significant improvement in list learning, and trends suggested improved short-term retention and spatial memory.

Walnuts

Walnuts, already associated with a reduced risk of coronary heart disease, contain alpha-linolenic acid, an essential omega-3 fatty acid, and other polyphenols. Researchers at the USDA Human Nutrition Research Center at Tufts University, Boston, Mass., showed that diets containing 2%, 6%, or 9% walnuts were found to reverse several parameters of brain aging, as well as age-related motor and cognitive deficits in old mice (Society for Neuroscience, 2007).

Walnuts, already associated with a reduced risk of coronary heart disease, contain alpha-linolenic acid, an essential omega-3 fatty acid, and other polyphenols.

Researchers from Baldwin-Wallace College, Berea, Ohio, showed that walnut extracts may play a role in developing novel treatments for Alzheimer's disease. The enzyme acetylcholinesterase has been shown to induce amyloid beta plaque formation. Using chemical techniques in the absence of living cells, the researchers showed that walnut extract and two of its major components, gallic and ellagic acids, not only inhibit the site of acetylcholinesterase associated with amyloid beta protein aggregation, but also inhibit the site of acetylcholinesterase responsible for the breakdown of acetylcholine.

Botanicals and Botanical Blends

Ginseng is one of the most widely used medicinal herbs in the world. According to the National Center for Complementary and Alternative Medicine, Bethesda, Md. (www.nccam.nih.gov), traditional and modern uses of ginseng include increasing a sense of well-being and stamina, as well as improving both mental and physical performance.

In February 2008, Naturex, South Hackensack, N.J. (phone 201-440-5000, www.naturex.com), announced that it would be participating in "New Technologies for Ginseng Agriculture and Product Development," a program oriented to validating

several health claims on North American ginseng. Research will focus on various medical and health areas, including metabolic syndrome, stress, physical endurance, cardiovascular diseases, immuno-modulation, reproductive health, and neuroprotective and psychiatric disorders.

A novel dietary supplement, *Think Gum*™, from Think Gum LLC, Los Angeles, Calif. (www.thinkgum.com), includes a blend of botanicals touted to enhance mental performance. The chewing gum contains peppermint, rosemary, ginkgo biloba, vinpocetine from periwinkle plants, and the Indian herb bacopa. The company's website cites studies backing each herb's mental benefit, like improving mental clarity and protecting brain cells.

A wild green-oat extract, *Neuravena®*, from Frutarom USA Inc., North Bergen, N.J. (phone 201-861-9500, www.frutarom.com), has been shown to enhance stress-coping abilities as well as learning performance. The extract's phytonutrients are thought to affect the activity of cerebral enzymes closely related to mental health and cognitive function.

Phospholipids

Phospholipids are building blocks in the brain and are often linked to improving memory and mental health. Phosphatidylcholine is a major source of choline, which is used to produce the neurotransmitter acetylcholine, a chemical messenger molecule that seems to be involved in neuron networks.

A Food and Drug Administration-approved qualified health claim for dietary supplements states that soy-derived phosphatidylserine (PS), another phospholipid, may reduce the risk of cognitive dysfunction in the elderly. Earlier this year, a commercial form of PS, *Sharp-PS*™, from Enzymotec, Israel (phone +972-4-654-5112, www.enzymotec.com), received "No Questions" from FDA for its GRAS notification. The company also offers *Sharp-PS*™ *Silver*, a blend of PS and DHA for improving mental and cognitive ability, and *Sharp-PS*™ *Gold*, a PS and DHA conjugate for better memory and mental performance.

L-Carnitine

L-carnitine is essential for transporting long-chain fatty acids across the mitochondrial membrane for subsequent fat breakdown and energy production. Known to benefit exercise and weight management, L-carnitine has also been shown to aid in mental function in the elderly.

Malaguarnera et al. (2007) reported that L-carnitine lessened fatigue and boosted mental function. They gave 66 males and females age 100 years and older either 2 g of L-carnitine or a placebo once daily. After 6 mo, researchers concluded that oral administration of L-carnitine facilitated an increased capacity for physical and cognitive activity by reducing fatigue and improving cognitive functions.

The acetyl derivative of L-carnitine, acetyl L-carnitine (ALC), is found throughout the central nervous system. According to information from Lonza Inc., Allendale, N.J. (phone 201-316-9200, www.lonza.com, www.carnipure.com), ALC plays a broad role in central nervous system metabolism as a source of acetyl groups both for the synthesis of acetylcholine and for energy-producing reactions.

Citicoline

Citicoline is a naturally occurring, water-soluble molecule that is used by the brain to make phospholipids. Information from Kyowa Hakko, New York (phone 212-319-5353, www.kyowa-usa.com), explains that one way citicoline supports brain health is by increasing the activity of the mitochondria in neurons to produce energy, particularly high-energy ATP.

Silveri et al. (2007) recently confirmed the ability of *Cognizin®* citicoline to improve brain energy by increasing levels of specific markers for ATP and increasing activity in the frontal-lobe region of the brain. The frontal lobe directs complex thought, decision-making, and attention. Age-related declines in cognitive abilities are also related to deteriorating frontal-lobe function.

Critical Thinking

1. Which form of omega-3 fatty acids is found to be most beneficial to preserving cognitive health?

2. Which two types of fruit are recommended for cognitive function?

3. What are the health benefits of consuming walnuts?

From *Food Technology,* September 2008, pp. 65–68. Copyright © 2008 by Institute of Food Technologists. Reprinted by permission.

"Fountain of Youth" Fact and Fantasy

What you really need to know about antioxidants and your health.

Are antioxidants the new "fountain of youth"? Media reports and nutritional products promote the idea that these vitamins and nutrients can reduce or even reverse the damage caused to the body by "free radicals," combating chronic disease and the ravages of aging. In a new book, *Understanding the Antioxidant Controversy: Scrutinizing the Fountain of Youth* (Praeger, $49.95), Tufts scientist Paul E. Milbury, PhD, and co-author Alice C. Richer, RD, explore what science really does—and doesn't—know about the benefits of antioxidants. Milbury is a scientist at Tufts' Jean Mayer USDA Human Nutrition Research Center on Aging and an assistant professor at the Friedman School. Richer is a Registered/Licensed Dietitian in private practice at Spaulding Rehabilitation Hospital outpatient centers and a medical writer.

In this excerpt from their book, Milbury and Richer look at the bottom line on antioxidants and what the latest research findings mean to you and your health.

Research studies to date in vitro and in animals show consistent evidence supporting antioxidant health benefits, yet human trials have been disappointing. There is also recent evidence that suggests, under certain circumstances, supplementation may actually do more harm than good. Individual antioxidants in the form of dietary supplements are more potent and bioavailable than they are in foods, and they do not exhibit the **synergistic effects** with other compounds found within natural food sources. Therefore, supplements most likely do not possess all the physiologically active components needed to be truly effective in preventing disease incidence and progression. In addition, individual genetics and/or physical status may have as significant an effect on health as antioxidant nutrients do.

We saw in the early years of America that poor diets caused many nutrition-related, life-threatening and debilitating diseases. Food fortification programs, such as vitamin D and iodine, proved to be beneficial and improved public health by eradicating or preventing most associated illnesses. Today nutrition deficiencies are rare in America. Poor diet is usually the result of individual choice, lack of knowledge, extreme poverty, or illness. The average American has the opportunity to obtain his or her **daily nutrient needs from diet alone.** Nevertheless, many Americans do not achieve optimal levels of vitamin C and E and perhaps the flavonoids (see box, next page).

Possible decreased nutrient value of crops and an aging population that is living longer, has more disposable income, believes supplements to be safe and effective, and is willing to self-medicate in an effort to feel better and decrease health care costs has driven the popularity

and increased use of antioxidant supplement sales. Almost daily media reports extolling the virtues of antioxidants for increased longevity and improved health have steadily increased this trend in use of **antioxidant dietary supplements** and functional foods/nutraceuticals.

Deflating the Hype

Years of self-promoting lobbying efforts by the dietary supplement industry urged Congress to preserve consumer freedom of choice and Congress, believing that all supplements were safe, allowed passage of the **Dietary Supplement Health and Education Act** (DSHEA) in 1994. DSHEA effectively deregulated supplements and weakened the FDA's ability to safeguard the public by allowing harm to occur before action can be taken to protect the public. As to the safety of these products "caveat emptor" is the rule of the day—the exact opposite of what the consumers assume is the case. Surveys of older Americans find that approximately 75% want the government to review and approve supplements for safety and verify all marketing claims *before* they are sold in the market. In many ways we have returned to pre-1906 legislation days when unproven and harmful patent medicines and cures were rampant.

Consumers are beginning to realize that many claims made about supplements and functional foods are marketing "hype" designed to increase product sales and manufacturer bottom lines, not necessarily to improve the health and safety of the consumer. Judy Foreman, a writer for the *Boston Globe,* sums up this growing disenchantment with supplements in her May 14, 2007, "Health Sense" column. She writes her "love affair with vitamins and supplements is over: with a few exceptions . . . I'm tossing them out." She further explains that reports about vitamins and minerals influenced her to take specific supplements, mostly antioxidants. But as scientific studies began to accumulate disputing previous claims of improved health or showed they could be dangerous, she stopped taking most of them. She does admit that multivitamins will remain a part of her daily regime for now because she fails to eat enough fruits and vegetables. But even this has her concerned after reading the recent ConsumerLab .com analysis that revealed many multivitamins are either contaminated with lead, do not dissolve properly, or do not contain the ingredients or amounts listed on the label. She notes one benefit of not taking these supplements is "the handful of twenties I'm not spending on supplements!"

As food manufacturers enhance foods to enter the **functional foods/nutraceuticals** market, concerns about "**hypersupplementation**" will rise. The majority of supplement users are better educated, have higher incomes, are older, and take an active and preventive approach toward their health. However, antioxidant vitamin and mineral intakes from the available American diet provide sufficient, and at times more than, Dietary Reference Intakes (DRI) levels of these essential micronutrients. In addition, dietary supplements and functional foods/nutraceuticals support the concept that food is medicine and may sway individuals from eating a balanced diet from natural food sources, believing that they can acquire the same or superior benefits from supplementation at a lower overall cost. Instead of improving eating patterns to include more fruits, vegetables and whole grains, people tend to eat the same foods they have always eaten (often processed and high in sugars and fats) with the "insurance" of a supplement to "fix" all that is wrong with their diet. Aging Americans, who also tend to have an increased use of pharmaceutical medications, have a tendency to incorporate supplements and functional foods/nutraceuticals into what may already be a nutritionally adequate diet. Nutrient and drug interactions, toxicities, and overdoses may contribute to a potential public safety disaster.

Antioxidant Guidelines

The antioxidant nutrients—**vitamins C** and **E, carotenoids, selenium** and **polyphenols**—do appear to have a positive correlation in chronic disease reduction and better overall health. But lifestyle factors (exercise, tobacco and alcohol use, and diet choices key among them) and genetic factors also factor heavily into disease incidence. Scientific evidence is insufficient to prove that antioxidant nutrients are the exclusive reason for benefits observed from high phytochemical intake of fruits and vegetables. Antioxidants also do not appear to be a quick fix in prevention or treatment of chronic health problems that may have taken decades to develop, despite the hopes of so many Americans.

Finding Flavonoids

Most people are familiar with the antioxidant vitamins and minerals—vitamin C, E, the carotenoids like beta-carotene, selenium—and have some idea how to obtain them from food. If not, you can always check Nutrition Facts labels. But what about the antioxidants collectively known as flavonoids, which have been associated with a wide variety of possible health benefits?

Flavonoids are a subclass of plant polyphenols that represent over 6,000 compounds identified to date. Flavonoids are compounds that plants have conserved and diversified over a billion years of evolution. These polyphenolic compounds fulfill many different functions for plants, including protecting the plant from predators and environmental stresses. Plants also use flavonoids as both deterrents and attractants for insects and fruit-eating animals. During pollination, plants attract insects and birds to their flowers by using the anthocyanin flavonoids. When seeds need protection, bitter-tasting flavonoids in seed husks deter fruit-eating animals and insects. When seeds are ready for dispersal, plants add sugar to mask the bitter flavonoids and again add anthocyanins to signal birds and animals that the fruits are ripe.

But it is not just fruits that contain flavonoids. Flavonoids are ubiquitous, although in differing forms and concentrations, throughout all plant parts. So it is not unexpected that catechins, well-known flavonoids, are found in both the tender leaves of the tea plant, the fruits of the apple tree and the root bulbs of the onion.

Despite the ubiquitous presence of flavonoids in our plant-based foods, the determination of flavonoid intakes has only recently been undertaken. The task of analyzing the great variety of flavonoids present in foods is challenging, and existing food databases are incomplete.

But you can start finding foods rich in flavonoids with this quick guide to common dietary sources:

Anthocyanidins—Berries (red, blue, purple), cherries, grapes (red, purple), plums, red wine, rhubarb

Flavanols—Apples, berries, chocolate, grapes (green, red), red wine, teas (green, white, black, oolong)

Flavanones—Citrus fruits and juice (orange, grapefruit, lemon)

Flavonols—Apples, berries, broccoli, kale, scallions, teas, yellow onions

Flavones—Celery, hot peppers, parsley, thyme

Isoflavones—Legumes, soy foods, soybeans

Catechin, Epicatechin—Apples and cider, apricots, beans, blackberries, cherries, grapes, peaches, red wine, teas (black, green)

Hydroxybenzoic acids—Black currants, blackberries, raspberries, strawberries

Proanthocyanidins—Apples, apricots, avocados, bananas, beans (red kidney, pinto, black), beer, berries, cherries, chocolate, cinnamon, curry, grapes (green, grape seed), Indian squash, juices (cranberry, apple, grape), kiwis, mangos, nectarines, nuts, peaches, pears, plums, red wine

The leading causes of death in the United States—coronary heart disease, cancer, stroke, and diabetes—have been associated with poor diet choices. Many positive health outcomes have been associated with increasing dietary intake of fruits, vegetables, legumes and whole grains—all high in naturally occurring antioxidant nutrients. Combining different fruits and vegetables has also been discovered to have an even greater disease-fighting potential (for example, mixing tomatoes with broccoli instead of consuming separately has been shown to provide a much more potent combination in prostate cancer reduction).

In 1991, the National Cancer Institute and the Produce for Better Health Foundation partnered to create the **5 A Day For Better Health Program.** The 5 A Day Program focuses on increasing public awareness about eating a diet high in fruits and vegetables for better health and reduction of stroke, high blood pressure, diabetes and cancer risks. Despite this national marketing effort, fruit and vegetable consumption appears to have remained below recommended levels. The **Healthy People 2010** objectives for our nation recommended increasing fruit and vegetable consumption of at least two daily servings of fruit to 75% of the population, and at least three daily servings of vegetables to 50% of the population. But "The State of Aging and Health in America 2007 Report," which is submitted by the CDC, stated that approximately 29.8% of all Americans are currently meeting these goals. However, a *Journal of the American Dietetic Association* study, using data from the NHANES 1999–2000 and 1994–1996 CSFII, reported 40% of Americans ate the recommended amount of at least five servings of fruits and vegetables daily between 1999 and 2000. Despite these discrepancies in study results, which highlight just how difficult it is to really accurately assess food and nutrient intakes, the bottom line still reveals that Americans continue to eat below optimal levels of fruits and vegetables (although consumption was estimated to have increased by 3% between 1990 and 2000). Cultural food preferences, environmental barriers, cost, convenience, advertising and lack of education are just some of the barriers affecting fruit and vegetable consumption in the United States.

The clearest answer about what to do when advising others about antioxidants appears to be what mothers and home-economic teachers have recommended for years: eat a healthy and well-balanced diet with an emphasis on intake of fruits, vegetables, legumes and whole grains. Obviously, exercise and lifestyle habits (avoiding tobacco, alcohol and drug abuse) and genetic legacy factor into our prospective overall health. But controlling what we eat and making healthy, nutrient-dense food choices (not gulping down a dietary supplement pill in place of them) appear to be the best choice when trying to prevent or delay chronic illnesses and improve quality of life as we age.

It should be kept in mind, however, that there is a function and role for dietary supplements. Specific at-risk populations—such as those who live in poverty, the elderly who have changing gastric secretions that may affect how much of a nutrient is absorbed, those consuming below 1,600 calories per day, and those who suffer from diseases that affect nutrient absorption—benefit from supervised dietary supplementation. Supplements are a relatively inexpensive form of nutrients that can be administered, if taken consistently, in a more precise and reliable dose than through fruits and vegetables. As such, they may be beneficial for certain life stage groups, such as during pregnancy and the elderly years when appetite and nutrient intake or absorption are diminished.

Two Smart Eating Plans

Based on the growing body of evidence that using foods to meet nutrient needs is safer and more beneficial to our health, the Department of Health and Human Services (HHS) and the USDA published dietary guidelines that promote health and reduce risk for chronic disease. These guidelines, reviewed every five years, take into account current research and the state of health in America, seeking to provide an overall pattern of eating that will improve health and that the general public can easily follow. The **Dietary Guidelines for Americans 2005** promotes the need for all healthy Americans to choose meals and snacks high in variety and that are nutrient-dense but low in excess calories, saturated and trans fat, added sugars, and alcohol.

At-risk populations have specific nutrition risks. People over age 50 are often low in vitamin B12, pregnant women are often low in iron, women of childbearing age need to fortify their daily diet with folic acid (from functional foods or supplements) to prevent birth defects, and older adults or people who are dark-skinned (or get very little exposure to sunlight) are often deficient in vitamin D.

HHS and USDA recommend two food guides for better health: the **USDA Food Guide** and the **DASH Eating Plan.** These guides allow individuals to meet their daily DRIs without the need of additional supplementation. But if a person's diet is not varied, doesn't include enough fruits, vegetables and whole grains, or is below 1,600 calories, then functional foods or multivitamins may be of benefit.

In general, it appears that most American adults consume less than recommended amounts of calcium, potassium, fiber, magnesium and vitamins A (carotenoids), C and E, even though the Institute of Medicine draws different conclusions. Children and adolescents consume less than recommended amounts of calcium, potassium, fiber, magnesium and vitamin E. At-risk populations tend to consume less of vitamin B12, iron, folic acid and vitamins E and D. Americans generally consume too many calories and too much saturated fat, cholesterol, added sugars and salt.

The first key point the USDA Food Guide and the DASH Eating Plans stress is the inclusion of more dark green and orange vegetables, fruits, legumes, whole grains and low-fat milk and milk products and less refined grains, total fats, added sugars and calories in the daily diet. The second point they stress is picking foods that are nutrient-dense. Nutrient-dense foods provide substantial amounts of vitamins and minerals in few calories. For example, fruits and vegetables are nutrient-dense foods because they contain antioxidants (vitamins, minerals and phytochemicals) and fiber at low calorie levels. In comparison, processed foods often high in sugar, fat and salt—such as cookies and potato chips—are poor nutrient-dense food choices because they contain very little (and sometimes no) nutrient values at a high calorie level.

In addition to the HHS and USDA dietary guidelines, the CDC partners with other government agencies and not-for-profit and industry groups to increase public awareness about the benefits of fruits and vegetables and increasing their consumption through the **National Fruit & Vegetable Program** (formerly the 5 A Day For Better Health Program). They support the HHS and USDA dietary guidelines and provide a website <www.fruitsandveggiesmorematters.org> that helps people learn about the benefits of eating these natural antioxidants and also gives tips, ideas and recipes to assist people to increase them in their diet.

Individuals may also want to incorporate more organic produce into their diets as well. Although organic produce is more expensive, one study indicates their value may be worth the extra expense. Studies are still ongoing to determine whether there is a significant difference between organic and conventional produce. Nevertheless, organic products are becoming more popular and available. As demand continues to increase, more suppliers will enter the market and prices should come down.

What about Supplements and Nutraceuticals?

In general, all vitamin and mineral needs should be consumed via natural food sources. But because most Americans do not eat the recommended amounts of fruits and vegetables, eat on the run (therefore eating at fast food restaurants or not balancing meals), and/or follow weight-reducing diets, taking a multivitamin/multimineral is an appropriate choice to compensate for possible nutrient deficits in the diet. To date the evidence neither supports nor opposes taking a daily multivitamin as "insurance." Even if a healthy diet is eaten, which follows all recommendations, taking an additional multivitamin/multimineral supplement as an inexpensive "insurance" is unlikely to exceed the ULs for nutrients. Natural or synthetic brands make no difference in absorption of most nutrients and it is best to purchase the least-expensive brand that is free of fillers and other additives (such as sugar, yeast or artificial colorings) that conform to **US Pharmacopeia** (USP) guidelines. Multivitamin/multimineral supplements should be taken within 30 minutes before or after meals.

Concerns about quality of multivitamins on the market surfaced when a recent **ConsumerLab.com** analysis found some products were contaminated with lead, did not have the correct amounts of listed nutrients, and/or did not dissolve properly. (Both ConsumerLab.com and the USP are independent agencies that test health products and pharmaceuticals, including supplements.) This study supports the concept that ingesting daily nutrients from foods is the best option. However, adding functional foods/nutraceuticals and multivitamins/multiminerals to adequate diets may become problematic and may lead to hypersupplementation. With a nutraceutical that provides 100% of most daily nutrients—such as Kellogg's SmartStart Antioxidant Cereal—including this cereal every day along with a balanced and adequate diet plus a multivitamin/multimineral can quite possibly lead to taking in excess recommended nutrient intakes.

When considering functional foods/nutraceuticals, the following questions should be asked before consuming them:

- **Should I be eating this?** Don't add this food just for its medicinal value.
- **How meaningful is the claim?** When a product claims that it affects the body, that is, "supports the immune system" or "enhances mood," what scientific evidence backs up the claim? Beware ORAC (oxygen radical absorbance capacity) claims. Marketers often suggest a high ORAC value "proves" superior antioxidant value. The ORAC assay, however, is only one of many assays that measure the capability of a product or food to "quench radicals" and are useful in the lab setting and in vitro only. All these assays, including the ORAC, are limited and none truly measure "radical quenching" of all radicals. They do not predict health effects of antioxidants in humans. Marketing claims about product antioxidant capacity are often overstated, unscientific and written out of context.
- **Do I need this(these) nutrient(s)?** Healthy people who eat well-balanced diets do not need to add these products to their diet. If an individual is in an at-risk category or has diseases that may affect nutrient absorption, then their diet must be carefully evaluated before adding them into a daily diet.
- **Am I overdosing?** Be sure to know what the maximum amount of any nutrient is safe to take and the sources of the nutrient to avoid toxicities.

(Healthletter *editor's note: Consult with your physician before beginning any supplement regimen.*)

There is some evidence that free radicals can cause oxidative damage to cells. Antioxidants appear to reduce this damage and are worth incorporating into our daily diets, although supporting evidence has been conflicting. But the source of antioxidants should come from a balanced diet that includes a variety of fruits, vegetables, legumes and whole grains. Much more research needs to be done and the media and the average American need to take a wait-and-see approach, rather than jump on the latest fad, which could endanger their health. The media should also give more publicity to the government programs that have been already been put into place to help Americans improve their health. Lastly, health-care professionals need to be better informed about current self-care trends that Americans are embracing and actively query their patients about what they are doing, educating them on the benefits and dangers.

Hippocrates seems to have summed it up best: "Let food be thy medicine, thy medicine shall be thy food."

To Learn More

US Pharmacopeia, www.usp.org.
Consumer Lab, www.consumerlab.com.

HHS & USDA Dietary Guidelines, www.health.gov/dietaryguidelines.
Fruit & Veggies Matter, www.fruitsandveggiesmorematters.org.
DASH eating plan, www.nhlbi.nih.gov/health/public/heart/hbp/dash.

Critical Thinking

1. Why are phytochemicals in supplement form potentially more harmful than those in food?

2. What impact did the Dietary Supplement Health and Education Act of 1994 have on the supplement industry, the FDA, and consumer safety?

3. Describe the history of the five fruits and vegetable campaign. Has this campaign been successful?

As seen in *Tufts University Health & Nutrition Letter,* May 2008; excerpted from *Understanding the Antioxidant Controversy: Scrutinizing the Fountain of Youth, 1st ed.,* by Paul E. Milbury and Alice C. Richer, (Praeger, 2007). Copyright © 2007 by Paul E. Milbury and Alice C. Richer. Reprinted by permission of Greenwood/ABC-CLIO, LLC.

Miscommunicating Science

This article explores the rapidly evolving nature of communications from the perspective of the food or nutrition scientist who wishes not to miscommunicate; tongue-in-cheek tips are offered to scientists who are not afraid to mislead or misinform the public and hinder public understanding of their work. Analysis is offered of the chief causes of miscommunication and public misunderstanding of science.

SYLVIA ROWE, MA AND NICK ALEXANDER, BA

What follows can be considered a kind of primer on how to tell it wrong—how to take a scientific project, worthy or not worthy, and communicate it so that (1) few people can be expected to understand the project, (2) few people can be expected to care about the project, or (3) best yet, different people will draw entirely different conclusions from the project, and (4) in any event, most people will fail to understand the truth that the science has revealed. That would be called *miscommunication,* and if you wish to be sure that you know how to communicate, you must also know how to miscommunicate and understand the potential for misunderstanding.

If you wish to be sure that you know how to communicate, you must also know how to miscommunicate.

A Brief History

In the beginning, there was the spoken word. Presumably, communication was first conducted through grunts and other noises, then later, through symbolic sounds, sounds that stood for concepts and objects. Not all of this, of course, was science communication—much of it was gossip, threats, warnings, emotional utterances, and the like. However, those early human noises devoted to information gathering and the quest for new ideas were certainly the first efforts at science communication. In those prehistoric times, there must have been a great deal of misunderstanding, of miscommunication.

The evolution of transmitting science information, new discoveries, new thoughts about the world, and the nature of things can be looked at as a kind of refining process toward common understanding. Western science is a process of group think, a communal effort at discovering physical truth, and, clearly, that process is enhanced through clear communication. Therefore,

scientists developed a specialized language to express precision and reduce the chances for misunderstanding and miscommunication.

There must have been all sorts of barriers to communication in the beginning: language difficulties (amplified enormously with the multitude of spoken dialects around the world) and time and space difficulties (messengers and minstrels had to carry information from place to place and formal meetings had to be scheduled months and years in advance to allow for travel time). For formal disciplines such as science, protocols had yet to be developed to specify the ground rules for transparency, experimental design, replicability, and the other requisites of scientific process.

Then came the written word, far more permanent than the spoken word and susceptible to scientific dispute resolution—papers could be drafted and circulated, albeit inefficiently, through crude and uncertain delivery systems. Then came the journals—the earliest journal in English was published by The Royal Society of London in the mid 17th century, a good 250 years after Gutenberg's famous improvement of mechanical publishing.[1] Newspapers and a formalized journalistic structure helped to disseminate scientific discoveries and theories and popularize them.

Subsequent 19th-century revolutions in transportation, communication, and electronics technology have expanded science and other forms of communication exponentially. However, the explosion of technological innovation in the 20th (and, so far, the 21st) century has dwarfed all previous progress in communication. What this means is that communication potential for science is now an order of magnitude greater than ever before, but the potential for miscommunication is equally great.

Miscommunication: A Definition

Merriam-Webster's online dictionary defines *communication* as "a process by which information is exchanged between individuals through a common system of symbols, signs, or behavior."[2] It follows that *miscommunication* is "a process by which information is *not* exchanged . . ." or, better yet, "a process by which information is exchanged in a faulty, incomplete, or incorrect way, resulting in a failure to understand on the part of the communication recipient." *Miscommunication* can also mean "a process by which incorrect information is communicated, perhaps a series of faulty research conclusions or findings that rest on a faulty research design, data collection process, or other research failure." If the recipient of the information misunderstands the truths purportedly being communicated, then the communication must be faulted.

Guidelines for communicating science have focused not only on communication practices themselves but also on strategies to avoid public misunderstanding of the supposed truths being communicated. The question that needs to be asked is not so much about the actual act of communicating the science, but rather, do the public audiences appropriately understand the scientific truths being communicated?

A number of good guidelines exist for best practices in communicating—that is, how to not miscommunicate. *Improving Public Understanding—Guidelines for Communicating Emerging Science on Nutrition, Food Safety, and Health*[3] from the International Food Information Council Foundation, for one, sets down some basic rules for ensuring that research results are understood, suggesting that scientists do a good deal of explaining when communicating their science: laying out, for example, all details of the study including the purpose, hypothesis, type and number of subjects, research design, methods of data collection and analysis, and the primary findings but also suggesting a kind of self-analysis somewhere in the written report analyzing the propriety of the methods of inquiry employed as well as any shortcomings or limitations of the research, including methods of data collection. We would like to focus on a key point in the guidelines not generally highlighted when science communication is discussed: *how consistent the study's findings are with the original purpose of the data collection.*

At a government-sponsored conference for science communicators several years ago, participants concluded that the simple skills of the past are no longer sufficient to communicate with contemporary audiences: "Today's science and technology communicators need a much broader array of skills. They need to understand both the technologies and the aesthetics of multimedia, interactivity, and the Web."[4] In this article, we would like to focus on 2 key points raised at the conference—points not normally highlighted in communication guidelines.

It is vital to tailor communications to a specific audience and remember the needs of the audience, not the needs of the researchers.

- There is no such thing as a "general audience" for science and technology communication; rather, there are many people with many different uses for science and technology information and many different levels of understanding. Communication programs should be designed to address and serve the needs of each group; there is no "one-size-fits-all" message or method of communication.
- Science and technology communication programs should be directed to addressing an audience's needs and interests, not by the research enterprise's ideas about what the public "should know."

A picture of how to best miscommunicate science is emerging: even if scientific protocol is followed, the study design is strong, the data collection is sound and sufficient, analysis is transparent, and so forth, it is still possible to transmit the findings in such a way that the public will fail to understand the truth.

Formula for Misunderstanding

- Operate from a preconceived idea of conclusions you want out of the research—forget about having a specific purpose for the formal data collection; you can see what pops up later in support of your preconception.
- Do not worry about targeting any specific audience for the research findings—the most famous scientific projects are the ones that seem earth shattering and universally applicable.
- Proceed with projects that have your desires and needs in mind (future research funding, book and television appearance potential, etc) rather than any public need—let Congress take care of public needs.
- In running the final analyses of your data, disregard any and all discrepancies that militate against your preconceived conclusions and cover yourself by including language disclaiming inaccuracies or apparent public policy implications of your work so that your work will appear above board.

You get the idea—this is just a short list of how miscommunication can erode good work or make less honest work seem credible.

It is possible to do unassailable research yet communicate it so inadequately that the public misses all the important points.

In fact, there is an inextricable association between how science is conducted and how it is communicated; is it possible to execute absolutely shoddy research yet communicate it perfectly so as to improve public understanding of the underlying truth? We think not. However, it is possible to do unassailable research yet communicate it so inadequately that the public misses all the important points. Most of us know of cases when the scientific community, in its zeal for creating correct protocol, may have forgotten to allow for communication to the public. Consider the following: there are formulas for submitting research papers; there is peer review to provide scientific feedback and appropriate editorial control; there are rules to safeguard ownership of intellectual discovery and rules to protect publishing rights. Yet, there is nothing in the protocols to guarantee public understanding in terms of the way we live, of emerging science.

Too often, the communication of science amounts to a battleground of would-be public policy advocacy, instead of public understanding. This, too, amounts to miscommunication, and what are the forces that promote miscommunication?

- sheer numbers
- sheer speed of transmission
- sheer velocity of calculation
- sheer greed (or, to put it less crudely, heightened competition for ownership)

Let us break these categories down.

Sheer numbers: sheer numbers of scientists competing for attention,[5] numbers of websites,[6] numbers of scientific journals,[7] number of scientific conferences[8]—the proliferation of all of these puts mounting pressure on good communication.

Sheer speed of transmission: sheer speed of transmission of scientific information, both at the university level and among professional scientists and science societies—what used to take weeks or months to get around is now transmitted electronically in minutes or seconds, offering markedly less time to catch errors or edit thoughtfully.

Sheer velocity of calculation: the speed at which scientists can run trials, calculate results, generate data, and reach mathematical conclusions—to offer just a crude example, early computers in 1942 were able to perform roughly 40 operations per second; the latest supercomputers work at a speed better than 6 trillion times faster.[9] This improvement in calculation speed came in just 65 years; before the invention of computers, human calculations were somewhat slower. The speed at which scientific conclusions can be reached adds to the pressure of communicating those results adequately.

Heightened opportunities for ownership: heightened opportunities and heightened demands for ownership of both information and the practical applications that derive from the information are enormous and increasing, placing ever greater challenges on the public communication of that science.

The Uncertain Road Ahead

Furthermore, in this Internet era, there is a widespread belief that information is or should be free and freely accessible; there is no hierarchy as to the accuracy of the thousands or millions of informational websites; news reports spread word of scientific discovery nearly instantaneously and often uncritically; communication often takes on the appearance of a battle for Internet eyeballs, nothing more. In other words, if you wish to miscommunicate your scientific research, it is now easier than it has ever been before.

In addition, that is not all—not just the communication of science but also the science itself is surely affected by the new speed, the new facility of research, calculation, and data analysis, as well communications. It is not necessary to dream up hypotheses to test when computer programs can be written to order up analysis of already available data and generate likely associations from which hypotheses can be inferred. The whole scientific process can now be stood on its ear, so to speak, and modern-day researchers can work backward, from computer-generated analyses to the hypotheses that used to be necessary before designing a study and collecting data (in effect, putting the scientific cart before the horse).

We would argue that publicizing such work amounts to miscommunication of science—miscommunication by computer—because the public is misled into thinking that the conclusions are the result of the normal scientific process.

The preceding comments are intended not to judge or cast aspersion on the current state of science communications but rather to bring attention to an issue that is growing more troubling by the day. If public understanding of science and, more importantly, emerging nutrition and health science is the objective, then the scientific community may be at a crucial crossroad—there needs to be a clear understanding not only of the best ways to communicate science but also of the increasing complexity of science miscommunication.

References

1. Brief History of the Society. The Royal Society website, http://royalsociety.org/page.asp?id=2176. Accessed February 10, 2008.
2. Merriam Webster.com. Definition of *communication.* www.merriam-webster.com/dictionary/communication. Accessed February 10, 2008.
3. International Food Information Council (IFIC) Foundation. www.ific.org/publications/brochures/guidelinesbroch.cfm. Accessed February 10, 2008.
4. Communicating the future: best practices for communication of science and technology to the public [proceedings summary]; National Institute of Standards and Technology (NIST): Gaithersburg, MD; March 6–8, 2002. www.nist.gov/public_affairs/bestpractices/conf_summary.htm. Accessed February 12, 2008.
5. Science Departments [Google search] (each listed agency presumably employing multiple scientists). Retrieved 13,000,000 listings. www.google.com/search?hl=en&rls=RNWE%2CRNWE%3A2006-40%2CRNWE%3Aen&q=science+departments&btnG=Search. Accessed February 13, 2008.
6. Science websites [Google search]. Retrieved 45,300,000 listings. www.google.com/search?hl=en&rls=RNWE%2CRNWE%3A2006-40%2CRNWE%3Aen&q=science+web+sites&btnG=Search. Accessed February 13, 2008.
7. Scientific journals [Google search]. Retrieved 4,420,000 listings. www.google.com/search?hl=en&rls=RNWE%2CRNWE%3A2006-40%2CRNWE%3Aen&q=2008+scientific+journals&btnG=Search. Accessed February 13, 2008.

8. 2008 Scientific conferences [Google search]. Retrieved 56,600 listings. www.google.com/search?sourceid=navelient& ie=UTF-8&rls=RNWE,RNWE:2006-40,RNWE:en&q= 2008+scientific+conferences. Accessed February 13, 2008.

9. Wikipedia. Definition of *supercomputer*. http://en.wikipedia .org/wiki/Supercomputer. Accessed February 13, 2008.

Critical Thinking

1. Who should scientists have in mind when writing manuscripts describing their research?

2. What are the driving factors that interfere with appropriate communication of science?

3. What is the purpose of the International Food Information Council?

SYLVIA ROWE, MA, is an adjunct professor at Tufts Friedman School of Nutrition Science and Policy and at the University of Massachusetts Amherst. She is also the president of SR Strategy, a health, nutrition, food safety, and risk communications and issue management consultancy located at Washington, DC. Previously, Ms Rowe served as president and chief executive officer of the IFIC and IFIC Foundation, nonprofit organizations that communicate science-based information of food safety and nutrition issues to health professionals, journalists, government officials, educators, and consumers. NICK ALEXANDER, BA, is former senior media counselor for the International Food Information Council Foundation, Washington, DC. He holds a Bachelor of Arts degree from Harvard University. A former network correspondent with ABC News, Mr Alexander has been, for the past 7½ years, tracking and writing about science communications issues and the evolving challenge to public acceptance of credible science.

UNIT 6

Food Safety and Technology

Unit Selections

Learning Outcomes

After reading this unit, you should be able to

- List the four most common biological contaminants (bacteria and viruses) found in our water supply.

- Describe how water from household faucets can be contaminated with bacteria by humans or pets.

- Explain how you can decrease the number of bacteria that you have on the surface of your faucets.

- List the detrimental effects of consuming lead, other than the well-known effects on the brain and nervous system.

- Identify four actions you should take to minimize your risk of exposure to environmental contaminants in your food.

- Describe how irradiation protects our food supply from international biological contamination.

- Discuss the pros and cons of irradiating fresh fruit and vegetables.

- Explain how antibiotic resistance develops in humans.

- List the steps you should take to prevent food-borne illness while processing meat and produce at home.

Student Website

www.mhhe.com/cls

Internet References

American Council on Science and Health (ACSH)
www.acsh.org
Centers for Disease Control and Prevention (CDC)
www.cdc.gov
FDA Center for Food Safety and Applied Nutrition
www.fda.gov/food/foodsafety/default.htm
Food Safety Project (FSP)
www.extension.iastate.edu/foodsafety
USDA Food Safety and Inspection Service (FSIS)
www.fsis.usda.gov

Food-borne disease constitutes an important public health problem in the United States. The U.S. Centers for Disease Control has reported 76 million cases of food-borne illness each year, out of which 5,000 end in death. The annual cost of losses in productivity ranges from $20 to 40 billion. Food-borne disease results primarily from microbial contamination (bacteria, viruses, and protozoa) and also from naturally occurring toxins, environmental contaminants, pesticide residues, and food additives.

The first Food and Drug Act was passed in 1906 and was followed by tighter control on the use of additives as possible carcinogens. In 1958, the Delaney Clause was passed and a list of additives that were considered as safe for human consumption (GRAS list) was developed. The Food and Drug Administration (FDA) controls and regulates procedures dealing with food safety, including food service and production. The FDA has established rules (Hazard Analysis and Critical Control Points) to improve the control of food safety practices and to monitor the production of seafood, meat, and poultry.

Agricultural trade between nations has led to a truly globalized food supply. This globalization meets the demand of wealthy nations for year-round access to foods grown in tropical environments and strengthens the economies of poorer, underdeveloped countries. One detriment of the global food supply is the translocation of biological contaminants via food. Less than 1 percent of foods imported into the United States are inspected each year. Although U.S. demand for a variety of foods has driven the worldwide food trade, our nation has not established an effective method to regulate the safety of foods shipped in from other countries. The current regulatory agency for U.S. food, the Food and Drug Administration, is faced with many challenges of trying to regulate the U.S. food and pharmaceutical industries, much less the newly introduced challenges of the safety of food imports.

Imported foods are not the only concern for biological contaminants. Changes in food production and farming in the United States have led to an increase in the spread of bacterial contamination of our foods. Many conventional poultry and livestock farms raise their animals in crowded, unsanitary conditions. The crowded conditions make the spread of bacteria very likely; therefore, conventional farmers must inoculate their animals with antibiotics to prevent bacteria from spreading throughout the entire stock. An example of the poor regulation of foods grown in the United States is the dramatic increase in *Salmonella* and *Campylobacter* bacteria in chickens over the past few years. Possible explanations for the increase in these two microorganisms could be due to the U.S. Department of Agriculture having no standards for *Campylobacter* and testing for *Salmonella* in a very small proportion of animals.

Surveys show that over 95 percent of the time people do not follow proper sanitation methods when working with food. Thus our best defense is to have safe food-handling practices at home. The U.S. government, therefore, launched the Food Safety Initiative program to minimize food-borne disease and to educate the public about safe-handling practices. An emphasis on improving food safety practices at home is also seen in the

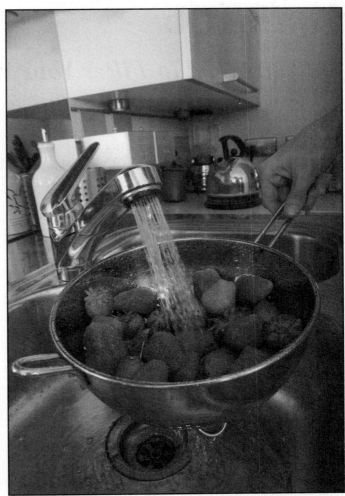

© Adam Gault/Getty Images

2010 Dietary Guidelines. In these latest guidelines the subcommittees of the USDA and HHS recommend creating and offering food safety education programs for children in schools and preschools, along with improving education efforts with adults.

Even though animal foods are more likely to be contaminated, there has been an increase in food-borne illness from fruit and vegetable consumption. Articles in this unit present and discuss why food-borne illnesses are on the rise, major outbreaks, and farming practices such as irrigation, animal husbandry, and feeding that may directly affect contamination. Food processors and growers are taking steps to eliminate new outbreaks. Meat products go through thermal treatment to kill bacteria and pathogens before consumption, but fresh fruits and vegetables are not treated and are often consumed raw. Irradiation could offer a solution to this problem, inactivating the pathogens on fresh produce. Different types of radiation and its positive and negative effects on different characteristics of produce are discussed.

H₂ Uh–Oh

Do You Need to Filter Your Water?

"For years, people said that America has the cleanest drinking water in the world," William K. Reilly, the Environmental Protection Agency's administrator under President George H. W. Bush, told *The New York Times* last year.

"That was true 20 years ago. But people don't realize how many new chemicals have emerged and how much more pollution has occurred. If they did, we would see very different attitudes."

Part of the problem: "The regulatory system is, frankly, slow to respond to emeriging threats to water safety," says Shane Snyder, a water-contaminant expert and professor of environmental engineering at the University of Arizona.

Here's some of what may be lurking in your tap water . . . and why you may not be able to rely on your local water utility to keep you safe.

Germs

"We estimate that 19.5 million illnesses occur each year in the United States that are caused by microorganisms in drinking water," says University of Arizona microbiologist Kelly Reynolds. Particularly vulnerable are older adults, young children, and people with weakened immune systems.

The culprits: viruses (primarily Norovirus), bacteria (like *Campylobacter, E. coli,* and *Shigella*), and cysts that are produced by protozoa like *Cryptosporidium* and *Giardia*. They can cause diarrhea, headaches, and, in rare cases, chronic conditions like reactive arthritis.

How do germs get into drinking water?

- **Contaminated surface water.** About two-thirds of Americans get their water from surface water sources like reservoirs, lakes, and rivers. "And all surface waters, no matter how pristine, contain water-borne pathogens from birds and animals, such as *Campylobacter* and *Salmonella*," notes Reynolds.

  Surface water can also harbor gastrointestinal germs that are flushed down the toilet by humans

when they're sick. How do they get into waterways? Blame it, at least in part, or the weather.

The water systems that serve some 40 million Americans—often older systems in the Northeast, the Great Lakes region, and the Pacific Northwest—carry sewage and storm water in the same pipes. When water from heavy or sustained rains overloads a system, the overflow—wastewater along with rainwater—is discharged into rivers and creeks to prevent it from backing up.

At least 40,000 sewage overflows occur each year in the United States. And that wastewater could become your drinking water after it's been treated by your local water utility. Since treatment plants can't eliminate 100 percent of the germs, some can get through to your tap.

Climate change will likely add to the stress on water utilities in the Northeast and Midwest if, as predicted, it results in more and heavier precipitation there. Researchers at Johns Hopkins University in Baltimore found that heavy downpours preceded half of the 548 reported water-borne disease outbreaks in the United States from 1948 to 1994.[1]

- **Contaminated groundwater.** "Historically, groundwater supplies were thought to be free of disease-causing microorganisms because the soil naturally filters them out," says Reynolds. But viruses and other microbes from contaminated septic tanks, landfill leaks, or inadequate disposal of animal waste or wastewater can end up in water beneath the surface.

  The Environmental Protection Agency now requires utilities to disinfect ground-water that has a history of contamination.

- **Leaks in the distribution pipes.** Disease-causing microorganisms can also get into drinking water after it leaves the treatment plant. About a quarter of the nation's water distribution pipes are in poor condition, with leaks, cracks, and corrosion. On average, a city loses 18 to 44 percent of its water from leaking pipes, notes Yale University microbiologist Stephen Edberg.

Those pipes are often buried in the same trenches as sewer pipes. Changes in water pressure can allow contaminants in the soil to be sucked into the water pipes, fouling the drinking water.

"The proportion of disease outbreaks linked to breaches in the water distribution has increased over the past decade," says Reynolds, "and it's going to be a continuing problem."

- **Plumbing.** In 2004, University of Arizona researchers measured bacteria in the tap water of seven Tucson homes. The EPA limits the amount of these bacteria—which in most cases are harmless—to no more than 500 per milliliter of drinking water. Tucson's public water averaged only about 50, so it was relatively clean.

Not so most of the homes. Water from kitchen and bathroom faucets in the seven houses averaged more than 3,000 bacteria per milliliter. Levels varied among homes (one had virtually none, while another had 13,000 bacteria), and from day to day within the same house. Bathroom tap water in two homes averaged 2,400 bacteria first thing in the morning, then dropped to 140 after running the water for 30 seconds.[2]

Where do the bacteria come from?

"If you have pets that lick the faucet, or children with dirty hands who play with the faucet, or if you handle raw meats arid then touch the faucet, bacteria can enter the pipes and grow," says Reynolds. "They get backwashed into the pipes, where they can form a layer, or biofilm."

Another potential source of bacteria is stagnant water sitting in pipes. "Maybe you're on vacation or maybe you have a second home," says Reynolds. "Bacteria can grow in pipes while you're gone, and then you can get a big dose when the water is turned back on again."

The antidote: "Flush out the system by letting the water run until it's as cold as it gets," suggests Reynolds. "That will certainly rinse out bacteria that haven't established a biofilm on the inside of the pipes."

If a bacteria biofilm has developed, it could loosen over time as the water faucet is used, says Reynolds, "and a chunk can break off and you can suddenly get exposed to a big dose of bacteria. It could be a significant health risk."

What to Do

Use a filter that has been certified for microbiological purification by the Water Quality Association (WQA), NSF International, or Underwriters Laboratories (UL).

Lead

It's clear that lead can damage the brains and nervous systems of children. But it may also cause high blood pressure, cataracts, decline in mental abilities, and kidney problems in adults. (See *Nutrition Action,* March 2005, cover story.)

"We're learning that older adults should also be concerned about lead poisoning," says researcher Marc Edwards, a professor of civil and environmental engineering at Virginia Tech University in Blacksburg.

"Recent studies have shown that low levels of lead in the blood that we once considered safe are causing health problems in adults. No one thinks to ever look for it in older people." (The most common symptoms are abdominal pain, headache, fatigue, muscular weakness, and pain, numbness, or tingling in the extremities.)

The evidence that lead affects the brain is troubling. In one study of nearly 600 women aged 47 to 74, those with higher levels of lead in their bones scored worse on memory and other cognitive tests than those with lower levels.[3] The women with higher lead had scores comparable to women who were three years older.

Where does lead in water come from?

"The lead or brass service lines that connect the community water supply from streets to homes in older cities can leach lead," says Edwards. So can the lead solder or brass and lead plumbing fixtures inside many buildings.

"Sometimes just one tap in a house might be providing water loaded with lead," notes Edwards. "It could be because some plumber had a bad day and did some sloppy soldering 40 years ago when your house was being built."

A case in point: The ex-mayor of a North Carolina town had suffered from chronic fatigue for years. "The kitchen tap in her apartment was perfectly clean," Edwards reports. "It was her bathroom faucet that had just outrageously high amounts of lead." All it took was an occasional drink of water from the bathroom tap.

Another potential source: hot tap water, which can contain high levels of dissolved lead.

"We're finding that there's quite a heavy use of hot tap water by the elderly to make tea, coffee, soup, and other foods," says Edwards. "And some devices that are used to heat water—like coffeemakers and those electric heating coils that are submerged directly into a cup of water—can dissolve high levels of lead into the water. It's safer to take cold water and heat it in a teapot on the stove."

What to Do

"People shouldn't panic, because the vast majority of taps in this country are safe," says Edwards. "Maybe only one out of 100 faucets is dispensing hazardous levels of lead into the water." That may not seem like many, says Edwards, "but if that's your family and that's your house, it's not good."

For about $20 per sample, you can have your water tested for lead. But testing isn't 100 percent reliable.

"We're discovering that little pieces of lead particles or solder, or lead rust that has corroded, can flake off the insides of pipes," says Edwards. "And that can deliver very, very high doses of lead" that a one-time test can miss.

The solution: a filter that removes lead at the faucet for all the water you use for cooking and drinking. "If there's a lead problem; it's probably coming from your plumbing, so you've got to treat it right at the end of the system," says Edwards.

Disinfection Byproducts

"Chlorine is an extremely good disinfectant for killing disease-causing bacteria and viruses in drinking water," says Paul Westerhoff director of Arizona State University's School of Sustainable Engineering and the Built Environment. "Plus, it's cheap."

That's why more than half the country's water treatment plants use chlorine. Another 30 percent use chloramine, a combination of chlorine and ammonia. Others use ozone. But there's a downside to those disinfectants.

"Chlorine combines with organic matter that is naturally found in water to form hundreds of compounds called disinfection byproducts, or DBPs," says Westerhoff. Chloramine and ozone produce smaller amounts of DBPs.

The EPA regulates the 11 most common and best-studied DBPs. Nine of the 11 cause cancer in laboratory animals.[4]

"This is an absolutely clear-cut case of humans' being exposed to chemicals that are known to be toxic in high doses," says David Savitz of the Mount Sinai School of Medicine in New York. "We all drink this water." (The EPA estimates that 94 percent of Americans consume foods and beverages that are made with chlorinated water.)

"The question is whether the DBPs are present at high enough levels to have measurable adverse effects on our health," Savitz explains. Researchers have focused on bladder cancer and pregnancy.

- **Bladder cancer.** "Using water with elevated levels of DBPs over years or decades does appear to be associated with a small increased risk of bladder cancer," says Savitz.

  A 2004 meta-analysis of studies pooled from the United States, Canada, France, Italy, and Finland found that men—but not women—whose tap water contained an average of more than 1 part per billion of DBPs (the legal limit is 80 ppb) had a 24 percent greater risk of being diagnosed with bladder cancer than men who had no more than 1 ppb in their water.[5]

  The EPA estimates that from 2 to 17 percent of the 56,000 new cases of bladder cancer each year in the United States may be caused by DBPs in

Is Bottled Water Better?

Is bottled water safer than tap water?

"There are not a lot of outbreaks associated with bottled water," notes the University of Arizona's Kelly Reynolds. But it's not clear whether that's because bottled water is less contaminated, or because it's harder to pin outbreaks on it.

"Bottled water gets distributed all over the country," says Reynolds. "If it caused an outbreak, that might be hard to identify."

In theory, *purified* bottled water should be safer. "Many bottled water companies start with tap water that has met all federal standards," notes Reynolds. "And the companies often add an additional treatment"—something like ultraviolet light or ozone to further disinfect the water or reverse osmosis to remove chemicals. "So you do sometimes get a higher standard of treatment."

The two big differences between tap and bottled water:

- The EPA, which regulates tap water, requires utilities to notify consumers when their water fails to meet legal standards. The FDA, which regulates bottled water, doesn't require bottlers to do the same. (The EPA's and FEA's standards are essentially the same.) So bottled-water drinkers are unlikely to know about any violations.
- Tap water doesn't come in plastic bottles that can end up in landfills.

BOTTLE BASICS

Purified Water: Most likely municipal tap water that has been distilled or treated with a process like deionization or reverse osmosis to remove impurities. The two major bottled drinking waters, Dasani and Aquafina, are purified water.

Spring Water: Comes from an underground formation from which water flows naturally to the surface of the earth. May be collected only at the spring or through a borehole tapping the underground formation that' feeds the spring.

Mineral Water: Contains not less than 250 parts per million total dissolved mineral solids when it emerges from its source. No minerals can be added.

Sparkling Bottled Water: Contains the same amount of carbon dioxide that it had as it emerged from its source. (Companies sometimes add CO_2 to replace what's lost during bottling.) Depending on the source, it may be labeled something like "sparkling drinking water," "sparkling mineral water," or "sparkling spring water."

Source: Adapted from the International Bottled Water Association (bottledwater.org/content/labeling-0).

drinking water. When the agency slightly lowered the maximum levels of some DBPs permitted in water in 2006, it estimated that the move would prevent about 275 cancer cases a year.

New research suggests that breathing in some DBPs and absorbing them through the skin could be more harmful than swallowing DBPs. Roughly half of our exposure to chlorinated water comes from washing with it and being near running water and flushing toilets, notes Savitz.

- **Pregnancy.** "Tap Water can Increase Risk of Miscarriages During First Trimester," warned the Associated Press headline in 1998. In a study of roughly 5,000 pregnant women in northern California, those who lived where the tap water contained more than 75 parts per billion of disinfection byproducts were nearly twice as likely to miscarry, but only if they drank at least five glasses of water a day.[6]

But a later study by Savitz found no link between DBPs and miscarriage in 2,400 pregnant women in Texas, Tennessee, and North Carolina.[7] "It was a pretty sophisticated study and it didn't corroborate the California research," says Savitz, then at the University of North Carolina in Chapel Hill.

Levels of the 11 regulated DBPs in drinking water have dropped by 60 to 90 percent since the early 1970s. "Their regulation has led to a huge improvement in drinking water quality," notes Westerhoff.

But there are more than 600 DBPs in water, and "new research over the last decade suggests that some of the unregulated ones that occur at very low concentrations are actually more genotoxic than the 11 regulated ones," he adds.

Genotoxic compounds damage DNA and can cause cancer. Among the metropolitan areas with the highest levels of the 11 regulated DBPs: Baltimore, Boston, Little Rock, Phoenix, and Washington, DC.

What to Do
Use a water filter that's certified to reduce volatile organic compounds (VOCs), which include DBPs.

Other Chemicals

"There's growing evidence that numerous chemicals in water are more dangerous than previously thought, but the EPA still gives them a clean bill of health," Linda Birnbaum, director of the government's National Institute of Environmental Health Sciences, told *The New York Times* in December 2009.

"These chemicals accumulate in body tissue. They affect developmental and hormonal systems in ways we don't understand." Some examples:

- **Atrazine.** It's the pesticide most often found in drinking water, especially in the Midwest, where it's applied to cornfields to kill weeds. It's also widely used on lawns, in parks, and on golf courses.

All of the watersheds monitored by the EPA, and some 40 percent of groundwater samples from agricultural areas, test positive for atrazine, according to the Natural Resources Defense Council.

In some studies, women living in areas with higher levels of atrazine in the drinking water were more likely to have lower-birth-weight babies. And in two studies, women in those areas were at higher risk of having babies with gastroschisis, a birth defect in which the intestines, stomach, or liver push through a hole in the abdominal wall.[8]

The EPA limits atrazine in drinking water to 3 parts per billion when averaged over an entire year. But people in agricultural areas may be exposed to much higher levels when use of the pesticide spikes during the growing season. The EPA says that it is reevaluating the safety of atrazirte, and will decide "whether new restrictions are necessary to better protect health and the environment."

- **Perchlorde.** It's an ingredient in solid fuels used for explosives, fireworks, road flares, and rocket motors. It also occurs naturally and is a byproduct that forms in bleach. And it can be detected in drinking water and groundwater in 35 states and in the urine of just about every American.[9]

In large amounts, perchlorate blocks iodine from reaching the thyroid gland, which can make it harder to produce thyroid hormone. Perchlorate may also block the transfer of iodine from mother to fetus, which can hinder normal growth.

California, Massachusetts, and New Jersey limit perchlorate levels in drinking water. In 2008, the EPA concluded that national perchlorate regulations wouldn't produce a great enough public health benefit. The agency now says that it's reevaluating its decision.

"It's extremely difficult for water utilities to remove perchlorate," says University of Arizona water expert Shane Snyder. "The only technologies available are ion exchange, which is extremely rare in water treatment systems, or a reverse osmosis system that's also rarely used because it is energy-intensive."

How to Choose a Water Filter

Point-of-use filters remove contaminants at the faucet, so they protect you from lead and other pollutants that may have gotten into your water after it left the treatment plant.

How do you go about choosing one for your home? "There's no one technology that takes everything out of water," says Joseph Harrison, former technical director at the Water Quality Association, a trade group of water filter manufacturers. Your choice generally narrows down to one or a combination of these basic types of filters:

Activated carbon: When water passes over the granular activated carbon or powdered carbon block, the negative ions of the contaminants are attracted to the slight positive charge of the carbon.

Reverse osmosis: A semipermeable membrane traps contaminants that activated carbon can't. Chlorine degrades the membranes, so most units contain activated carbon prefilters. Reverse osmosis is inefficient; it typically wastes three to five gallons of water for every gallon filtered. And it filters out good minerals like calcium and fluoride along with the contaminants.

Ion exchange: As water percolates through bead-like resins, ions in the water are swapped for ions on the beads. The system is used mostly to soften water.

Which filtration system is for you? That depends on what kind of protection you want and how much you're willing to spend:

1. **For basic protection.** Get an activated carbon filter that's certified to reduce lead, cysts, and volatile organic compounds (VOCs). Filtering VOCs should help protect you from disinfection byproducts (DBPs), atrazine and some other pesticides, and several dozen other contaminants. The filter should also be certified to eliminate the taste and smell of chlorine.

Check the filter's box or literature to make sure that the claims for lead, VOCs, and any other contaminants have been certified using NSF/ANSI Standard 53. Claims that the filter eliminates "aesthetic" contaminants (like taste, odor, or chlorine) should be certified using NSF/ANSI Standard 42.

The non-profit NSF International establishes standards for consumer goods and certifies products.

2. **To filter out bacteria and viruses.** Get a system that has been certified for micro-biological purification by the Water Quality Association (WQA), NSF International, or Underwriters Laboratories (UL). It could consist of an ultraviolet light to disinfect the water or a filter with pores so fine that microorganisms can't get through them.

3. **To target contaminants you know are in your water.** Have your tap water tested. Or get a copy of the Consumer Confidence Report that most water utilities are required to mail out by July 1 of every year. Many utilities also post the reports on their website. If your water has elevated levels of any contaminants, look for a filter that has been certified to reduce them.

4. **For the cleanest water on your block.** "Get a reverse osmosis system plus an activated carbon system," says Harrison. Then add a filter that has been certified for microbiological purification.

Before You Buy Any Filter

Check the website of the California Department of Public Health (cdph.ca.gov/certlic/device/Pages/WTD2009Directory.aspx). If the filter you're looking at is sold in California, the website will tell you whether its claims have been verified by independent, state-approved laboratories.

The website lists all approved models and what they are certified to remove, and has separate lists of filters that have been certified to remove arsenic, *Cryptosporidium* and *Giardia* cysts, fluoride, chromium, lead, bacteria and viruses, MTBE (a gasoline additive), nitrates, perchlorate, radium, and volatile organic compounds (VOCs) like disinfection byproducts (DBPs) and atrazine.

For basic information on the water supply and the effectiveness of different kinds of filters, see the EPA's booklet "Water on Tap" (www.epa.gov/safewater/wot/pdfs/book_waterontap_full.pdf). For questions about your drinking water, you can call the EPA's Safe Drinking Water Hotline (800-426-4791).

- **Drugs.** When you take an aspirin, or birth control pills, or Lipitor, or another drug, tiny amounts end up in the toilet bowl, where they're flushed into the sewage system and, eventually, into a wastewater treatment plant.

"Conventional wastewater plants typically remove more than 90 percent of these compounds," explains Snyder. "But even if you have 99.99 percent removal, that still leaves parts per trillion in the water which is subsequently discharged into rivers and streams." And that water, with its drug residues, can eventually end up coming out of your tap.

While the traces of drugs in drinking water are one-ten-thousandth to one-hundred-thousandth the amount in any therapeutic dose, "I don't know that we can completely dismiss the impact on human health," says Snyder, "because we don't know much about the toxicity of mixtures of drugs. But based on the concentrations of the individual compounds, harm to humans doesn't appear to be likely."

What to Do

- **Atrazine.** Use a filter that's certified to reduce levels of volatile organic compounds (VOCs), which include atrazine.

- **Perchlorate.** Only reverse osmosis and ion exchange filters reduce perchlorate.
- **Drugs.** Claims that filters reduce drug residues are based on the manufacturers' own tests. Official standards to verify the tests are in the works, though.

Notes

1. *Am. J. Public Health 91:* 1194, 2001
2. *Int. J. Food Microbiol. 92:* 289, 2004.
3. *Environ. Health Perspect. 117:* 574, 2009.
4. *Mutation Research 636:* 178, 2007.
5. *Epidemiology 15:* 357, 2004.
6. *Epidemiology 9:* 134, 1998.
7. *Epidemiology 19:* 729 and 738, 2008.
8. *Am. J. Obstet. Gynecol. 202:* 241, 2010.
9. *J. Expo. Sci. Environ. Epidemiol. 17:* 400, 2007.

Critical Thinking

1. What are the four most common biological contaminants (bacteria and viruses) found in our water supply?

2. How can water from household faucets be contaminated with bacteria by humans or pets?

3. What are the detrimental effects of consuming lead, other than the well-known effects on the brain and nervous system?

Produce Safety: Back to Basics for Producers and Consumers

Feeling a little uneasy these days about the health-promoting properties of those fresh fruits and vegetables? Have we learned to love the invisible army of phytonutrients, vitamins, and minerals fighting the good fight for our long-term health, only to be reminded of the insidious presence of an equally invisible army of foodborne bacteria with the potential to make us sick?

According to the Centers for Disease Control and Prevention, there are approximately 76 million cases of foodborne illness reported in the United States each year. To reduce the incidence of foodborne illness, the actions taken to prevent produce contamination must be diligent and consistent, beginning on the farm and continuing through the entire food-handling process to consumer preparation.

Although proper cooking will kill most pathogens that may be present in or on a food, recent outbreaks in the United States have involved fresh produce that was not cooked before being consumed. Nevertheless, the consumption of raw fresh fruits and vegetables provides numerous valuable dietary nutrients. Therefore, it is important to consider ways to enhance the safety of these foods so that consumers can continue to enjoy fresh produce, whether it is cooked or uncooked.

Consumers want to reduce the risk in food; therefore, food producers and government regulators work tirelessly to do this as much as possible. There are also steps that consumers can take to reduce that risk. Still, an absolute absence of risk, even for food, simply is not possible.

Many factors can contribute to the risk of foodborne illness. Pathogens (any disease-producing agent) may be introduced by the exposure of foods to improperly processed manure used as fertilizer or to manure from animals on the farm. Exposure to foodborne pathogens may also occur because of the use of bad-quality water in irrigation or as a result of poor worker hygiene. Inferior storage and preparation practices, such as the storage of food at improper temperatures and cross-contamination among foods, can also further the growth of pathogens that are already present.

Food producers and suppliers, including farmers, processors, distributors, grocery stores, and restaurants that prepare and sell food to consumers, all play a significant role in reducing foodborne illness risk. Foods must be grown, harvested, packed, processed, and distributed in a manner that minimizes microbial contamination.

Produce growers and processors have recognized the importance of preventing contamination at each step from farm to fork, as the pathogens present on these foods are difficult to remove. For example, the natural curve and curling characteristics of lettuce and leafy greens provide a safe haven for microbial stowaways.

What Are Food Producers and Regulators Doing to Protect Consumers?

The actions that industry and government regulators have taken to protect consumers from foodborne illness can be broken down into four categories: (1) preventing contamination; (2) minimizing actual harm to the public if contamination has occurred; (3) improving communications among food producers, regulators, and the public; and (4) research into how and where foodborne illnesses arise in produce, and identify actions that can be taken to reduce these risks.

Numerous local actions have been ramped up as the result of the recent outbreaks. In January 2007, the produce industry—supported by industry representatives in the processing, distribution, and retail industries—called for the application of mandatory, strong, consistent, science-based, safety standards to both domestic and imported produce.

What Can Consumers Do to Protect Themselves?

It is important to remember that we do not live in a world free from risk. Thus, although consumers must understand that foodborne illness is a real risk, health care professionals can convey that prevention is possible and provide them with specific steps to prevent the consumption of foodborne pathogens. The Fight-BAC! campaign, managed by the Partnership for Food Safety Education is an excellent resource for consumer guidance for safe food handling procedures (www.fightbac.org). The four steps are simple and memorable:

- Clean: Wash hands and surfaces often
- Separate: Don't cross-contaminate
- Cook: Cook to proper temperature
- Chill: Refrigerate promptly

The FightBAC! website, as well as the International Food Information Council Foundation's brochure *A Consumer's Guide to Food Safety Risks* (http://ific.org/publications/other/consumersguideom.cfm), provide specific guidance for each step.

Fresh fruits and vegetables should be rinsed under running tap water. Fruits and vegetables with firm skins should be rubbed under running tap water or scrubbed with a clean cloth or paper towel. The use of detergent or bleach to wash produce is unnecessary and potentially hazardous, but even foods that will be peeled should be washed first. If pathogens are camped out on the rind of a cantaloupe, a perfectly clean knife could transfer the pathogen from the rind to the edible flesh with one slice.

Tips to Keep Your Kitchen Clean

Always wash all surfaces and utensils that come into contact with food with soap and hot water after each use. To kill bacteria, sanitize surfaces and utensil that come into contact with food with a solution of one to three tablespoons of household chlorine bleach per gallon of water, let stand two minutes; rinse, and allow the surface to air dry.

Creating and Sustaining Change

The incidence of foodborne illness can be reduced significantly, and consumers can play a leading role in making that happen. Together, the integrated actions of consumers, food suppliers, and regulators not only will reduce the incidence of foodborne illness, but also will sustain the wholesomeness of the food that we eat.

Critical Thinking

1. How many cases of food-borne illness are reported in the United States each year?

2. How are bacteria, viruses, and protozoa introduced into foods?

3. What are the four steps of the FightBAC! Campaign?

Reprinted from *Food Insight,* March/April 2007, published by the International Food Information Council Foundation. www.ific.org

Irradiation of Fresh Fruits and Vegetables

Irradiation could provide a kill step to enhance safety of fresh and fresh-cut produce, but challenges remain for full commercial application.

Xuetong Fan, Brendan A. Niemira, and Anuradha Prakash

Consumption of fresh and fresh-cut fruits and vegetables in the United States has increased every year in the past decade, because of their convenience and nutritional benefits. Unfortunately, the increasing consumption of fresh produce has been accompanied with an increase in the number of outbreaks and recalls due to contamination with human pathogens.

Fresh fruits and vegetables carry the potential risk of contamination because they are generally grown in open fields with potential exposure to enteric pathogens from soil, irrigation water, manure, wildlife, or other sources. Unlike meat and meat products to which a kill step (thermal treatment) is applied before being consumed, fresh produce is often consumed without cooking or other treatments that could eliminate pathogens that may be present.

The recent *Escherichia coli* O157:H7 illness outbreaks and product recalls of spinach, lettuce, and other leafy greens, most notably in 2006 and 2007, have gained much media attention and raised public concerns over produce safety. The fresh produce industry is in need of a kill step to ensure the safety of produce. Ionizing radiation is known to effectively eliminate human pathogens such as *E. coli* O157:H7 on fresh produce.

This article reviews the latest knowledge about irradiation inactivation of human pathogens on and in fresh-cut produce and its impact on the quality of produce. It also highlights current developments in irradiation regulation and labeling, the challenge and opportunity for commercial application, and research needs.

Types of Ionizing Radiation

Radiation is in every part of our lives, and we encounter it every day in the natural environment. Common types of radiation include radio frequency, visible light, infrared light, microwave, and ultraviolet light. More energetic forms of radiation, such as gamma-ray, X-ray, and electron beams are called ionizing radiations because they are capable of producing ions, electronically charged atoms or molecules. All three types of ionizing radiation have the same mechanisms in terms of their effects on foods and microorganisms.

Water is the principal target of ionizing radiation. The radiolysis of water generates free radicals, and these radicals, in turn, attack other components such as DNA in microorganisms.

Water is the principal target of ionizing radiation. The radiolysis of water generates free radicals, and these radicals, in turn, attack other components such as DNA in microorganisms. Each type of ionizing radiation has its own advantages and disadvantages. For example, gamma rays and X-rays have higher penetration ability than electron beams. However, gamma rays are emitted by radioactive materials, such as cobalt-60 and cesium-137, while generation of X-rays is a relatively inefficient and energy-intensive process. Most energy (about 90%) is lost to heat during the conversion of electron beams into X-rays. Electron beams have a low penetration ability, even though the electron beam generators can be switched on and off and do not involve radioactive materials.

Effectiveness in Inactivating Pathogens

Historically, the high radiation doses used in attempts to produce a sterile or shelf-stable fruit or vegetable commodity have resulted in unpalatable products. Of specific interest within the context of modern produce processing is the potential for incorporating lower irradiation doses, lower than 3 kGy, as one of several "hurdles" in an otherwise conventional produce processing system. Recent research has consistently shown that irradiation effectively kills bacterial pathogens on fresh and fresh-cut produce (Smith and Pillai, 2004; Niemira and Fan, 2005). This efficacy holds for human bacterial pathogens such as *E. coli* O157:H7, *Salmonella,* and *Listeria monocytogenes,* as well as for bacterial phytopathogens and spoilage organisms.

Irradiation doses that will result in a 1-log reduction in bacterial pathogens are typically in the range of 0.2–0.8 kGy. In contrast, pathogenic viruses and fungi are generally more resistant to irradiation, often requiring 1–3 kGy to achieve 1-log reduction (Niemira and Fan, 2005). To achieve meaningful reductions of viruses and fungi, the doses required are typically above what most produce will tolerate.

In terms of food safety, it should be noted that on an annual basis, the majority of minor foodborne illnesses are caused by viruses (67%), while the majority of serious foodborne illnesses resulting in hospitalizations and deaths (60% and 72%, respectively) stem from bacterial pathogens (Mead et al., 1999). As an intervention, irradiation is thus most suited for elimination of the most serious safety threats for consumers of fruits and vegetables.

The antimicrobial efficacy of irradiation is influenced by a number of factors, including the pathogen being targeted as the primary safety concern, the type of produce being treated, the condition of the fruit or vegetable (whole vs cored, peeled, cut, chopped, etc.), the atmosphere in which it is packaged, and other commodity-specific factors (Niemira and Fan, 2005). Like any other industrial food processing technology, the methodological details of time, temperature, handling, and irradiation protocols must undergo process validation for the product being treated. For example, irradiation protocols developed for elimination of *E. coli* O157:H7 from leafy greens may not achieve the required food safety and quality benchmarks if applied for the elimination of *Salmonella* from tomatoes.

One area of recent research focuses on determining the ability of irradiation to kill internalized, biofilm-associated, or otherwise protected pathogens. These protective environments dramatically reduce the efficacy of chemicals and other conventional treatment options, often by orders of magnitude (Niemira and Fan, 2005). Initial data in this emerging field of research suggest that *Salmonella* and *E. coli* O157:H7 in biofilms are effectively eliminated by irradiation, although the specific response depends on the pathogen type and maturity (Niemira, 2007).

Cells of *E. coli* O157:H7 that are internalized appear to be more resistant to irradiation than surface-associated cells (Table 1). At 1 kGy, pathogens such as *E. coli* O157:H7 on the surface of fresh-cut produce can be reduced by 3–8 logs, while internalized pathogens are only reduced by 2–3 logs. Additional research is needed to more fully understand the influence of internalization on pathogens, and on the efficacy of irradiation and other treatments.

Table 1 Dose Required to Achieve a 1 Log Reduction for *E. coli* O157:H7 Inoculated on or in Fresh-Cut Produce, Then Irradiated with Gamma Rays

| Product | D_{10} Value (kGy) | |
	On Surface	Inside
Iceberg lettuce	0.14	0.30
Boston lettuce	0.14	0.45
Red leaf lettuce	0.12	0.35
Green leaf lettuce	0.12	0.37
Romaine lettuce	0.21	0.39
Baby spinach	0.24	0.45
Green onion, long cut	0.26	0.42
Green onion, short cut	0.28	0.42

From Niemira and Fan (2007).

Quality of Irradiated Fresh Produce

At low dose levels (1 kGy or less), most fresh-cut vegetables show little change in appearance, flavor, color, and texture, although some products can lose firmness. As an example, the appearance of irradiated spinach was similar to that of the non-irradiated samples after 14 days storage at 4°C. Some vegetables such as fresh-cut cilantro can tolerate 3.85 kGy of radiation (Foley et al., 2004). In fact, the destruction of spoilage organisms increases the shelf life of most fresh and fresh-cut vegetables (Prakash and Foley, 2004; Niemira and Fan, 2005). The response to irradiation is specific to product, and even similar varieties, as shown in studies on various lettuce types (Niemira et al., 2002), exhibit differences in texture and respiration rates.

Irradiation's effect on permeability and functionality of cell membranes can result in electrolyte leakage and loss of tissue integrity.

Appearance and leakage. Irradiation's effect on permeability and functionality of cell membranes can result in electrolyte leakage and loss of tissue integrity. These effects are limited at dose levels below 1 kGy, but at higher dose levels, electrolyte leakage may cause a soggy and wilted appearance. The increase in electrolyte leakage varies among vegetables (Table 2). In a study of 13 vegetables, Fan and Sokorai (2005) observed that red cabbage, broccoli, and endive had the lowest increases in electrolyte leakage, while celery, carrot, and green onion had the most increases in leakage.

Texture. Irradiation may induce the loss of firmness (softening) in some fruits (Gunes et al., 2000; Palekar et al., 2004).

Table 2 Electrolyte Leakage of Fresh-Cut Vegetables as a Function of Radiation Dose[a]

Vegetable	Leakage (%)							
	0 kGy	0.5	1	1.5	2.0	2.5	3.0	LSD$_{0.05}$[b]
Broccoli	0.6	0.7	0.7	0.8	0.7	1.2	1.1	0.4
Endive	1.5	1.7	1.8	2.3	2.2	3.2	3.1	0.6
Red cabbage	1.3	1.4	1.4	1.9	1.8	2.0	2.5	0.5
Green leaf lettuce	2.5	3.1	3.9	3.4	3.2	4.4	4.8	0.8
Parsley	2.1	2.1	2.6	3.0	3.7	3.7	4.7	1.1
Romaine lettuce	1.4	2.8	3.3	4.1	3.8	5.7	5.1	1.5
Iceberg lettuce	1.4	1.9	2.4	2.6	3.2	3.8	4.3	1.1
Spinach	2.8	3.4	3.3	3.8	4.1	5.4	6.2	1.2
Red leaf lettuce	3.5	3.7	4.6	5.0	5.0	6.8	8.5	1.3
Celery	2.1	3.4	3.3	4.9	6.9	8.4	9.8	1.3
Cilantro	1.4	1.8	2.1	2.4	3.1	4.3	4.1	0.9
Green onion	3.8	5.2	7.1	7.0	9.5	12.5	12.4	1.6
Carrots	2.8	3.1	3.8	4.4	5.7	6.1	8.6	1.0

[a]Vegetables were irradiated with 0, 0.5, 1.0, 1.5, 2.0, 2.5, and 3.0 kGy of gamma radiation at 5°C in air, then electrolyte leakage was measured.
[b]Least significant difference at $P<0.05$.
Modified from Fan and Sokorai (2005).

Irradiation-induced loss of firmness is related to partial depolymerization of cell-wall polysaccharides, cellulose, and pectin and to changes in activity of the cell-wall enzymes pectinmethylesterase and polygalacturonase that act on pectic substrates. However, the loss of firmness can be mitigated by dipping diced tomatoes and fresh-cut apples in a calcium solution prior to irradiation (Gunes et al., 2000; Prakash et al., 2007) and by storing the products in modified-atmosphere packaging (Boynton et al., 2006).

Irradiated (1 kGy) cilantro (Fan et al., 2003a) and lettuce (Fan et al., 2003b) showed some softening, but after a few days of storage, there was no significant difference between irradiated and non-irradiated samples. Other products, such as celery (Prakash et al., 2000), mushroom slices (Koorapati et al., 2004), and shredded carrots (Hagenmaier and Baker, 1998), also showed no change in firmness.

Flavor and aroma. At low dose levels (≤1 kGy), few if any effects on flavor and aroma are observed in fresh and fresh-cut vegetables. A decrease in characteristic aroma of cilantro (Fan et al., 2003a) and off-flavor of Bell peppers (Masson, 2002) has been observed at doses of ≥3 kGy. Changes in flavor and aroma of fresh vegetables are highly correlated with microbial spoilage. Thus, irradiation generally inhibits or delays development of off-flavors related to growth of spoilage organisms.

At low dose levels (≤1 kGy), few if any effects on flavor and aroma are observed in fresh and fresh-cut vegetables.

Nutritional quality. At low dose levels (≤1 kGy), the effects on nutritional quality are minimal. Irradiation can reduce ascorbic acid (vitamin C) in some vegetables, but the decrease is generally insignificant, given the natural variation observed in fresh produce, and does not exceed the decrease seen during storage (Fan and Sokorai, 2002). Irradiation converts ascorbic acid to dehydroascorbic acid, both of which exhibit biological activity and are readily interconvertible. Irradiation can also increase phenolic content of certain vegetables, thus increasing their antioxidant capacity (Fan, 2005). However, since phenolic compounds are also responsible for the browning reactions in vegetables, their increase is not a desired outcome.

In general, the effect of irradiation on quality of fresh and fresh-cut vegetables is minimal. In those cases where significant changes are seen at effective dose levels, effects on texture, color, or browning can be minimized by combining irradiation with other technologies such as calcium dips, modified-atmosphere packaging, or antibrowning agents.

Regulatory Approval, Labeling, and Safety

Currently in the U.S., irradiation of whole fruits and vegetables is approved only for insect control and shelf-life extension, with a maximum allowable dose of 1 kGy (Table 3). The use of irradiation for the purpose of enhancing microbial food safety has not been approved by the Food and Drug Administration. However, FDA is evaluating a petition, filed by the Food Irradiation Coalition, asking for the use of irradiation to enhance safety of fresh-cut produce at doses up to 4.5 kGy.

Table 3 Foods Permitted to Be Irradiated

Type of Food	Purpose	Maximum Dose (kGy)
Fresh, non-heated processed pork	Control of *Trichinella spiralis*	1
Fresh produce	Growth and maturation inhibition	1
Fresh produce	Arthropod disinfection	1
Dry or dehydrated enzyme preparations	Microbial disinfection	10
Dry or dehydrated spices/seasonings	Microbial disinfection	30
Fresh or frozen, uncooked poultry products	Pathogen control	3
Frozen packaged meats (solely NASA)	Sterilization	44
Refrigerated, uncooked meat products	Pathogen control	4.5
Frozen uncooked meat products	Pathogen control	7
Fresh shell eggs	Control of *Salmonella*	3.0
Seeds for sprouting	Control of microbial pathogens	8.0
Fresh or frozen molluscan shellfish	Control of *Vibrio* species and other foodborne pathogens	5.5

From FDA (2007c).

Under current FDA rules, foods that have been irradiated must bear both a "Radura" logo and a statement that the food has been "treated with radiation" or "treated by irradiation." Earlier last year, FDA proposed a change in the labeling of irradiated foods (FDA, 2007b). Under the proposed rule, only irradiated foods in which irradiation causes a material change in the food would need to be labeled with the Radura logo and either of those statements. The term "material change" refers to a change in the organoleptic, nutritional, or functional properties of a food. In addition, FDA would allow petitions for the use of alternative labeling, such as "pasteurized" or "pasteurization," for a food that has been treated by irradiation, where the irradiation results in the same level of pathogen reduction as thermal pasteurization. These changes are still under consideration by FDA, and a final ruling has not yet been made.

In multi-generational studies, animals fed irradiation-sterilized foods throughout their life were healthy and nutritionally satisfied, with no evidence of any negative nutritional or developmental effects. More recently, FDA has investigated the possibility that furan, a possible carcinogen present in canned meats, soups, and many other conventional thermally processed foods, might also be produced during irradiation. Studies demonstrated that irradiation at 5 kGy did not induce detectable levels of furan in most fresh-cut fruits and vegetables. In those few fruits where furan was detectable after irradiation, the levels were much lower than those in many thermally processed foods (Fan and Sokorai, 2007).

Consumer Acceptance

Adoption of irradiation for food applications has been a slow process. The limited number of foods approved by regulatory agencies, cost, consumer reluctance to accept irradiated foods, and the public's uncertainty of this technology may contribute to its minimal commercialization.

Studies on marketing of irradiated foods have demonstrated that consumers are more willing to buy irradiated foods after they are provided information about the process (Bhumiratana et al., 2007). Typically, fewer than half will buy the irradiated food if given a choice between an irradiated product and the non-irradiated product. If consumers are first educated about food irradiation and food safety, most of them will buy the product in these marketing tests.

In a survey conducted by *The Packer* (Anonymous, 2007), 63% of growers/shippers believe that the produce industry should push for irradiation or similar treatments if produce is not damaged in the process; 40% of packers think the industry should push for irradiation or similar treatments, with the same percentage undecided; more than 30% of growers/shippers think consumers are ready to buy irradiated produce, particularly leafy greens; but only 25% of retailers think consumers are ready to buy irradiated produce, leafy greens in particular—about 7% of retailers stock irradiated produce.

It seems that enthusiasm about the commercial application of irradiation on fresh produce decreases from growers/shippers, to packers, to retailers, and to consumers. Therefore, educating retailers and consumers about irradiation processing may be needed to advance the commercial applications of this technology.

Packaging

Packaging is another important aspect of food irradiation. FDA has approved about 10 polymeric packaging materials for use during irradiation of prepackaged foods. Package materials currently used by the produce industry are diversified. Most polymeric packaging materials that are used by the produce industry have been approved by FDA. The agency allows industry to submit requests for exemption from regulation if the use of the substance in the food-contact article results in a dietary concentration at or below 0.5 ppb. As a result, Proveit, on behalf of Sadex Inc., has successfully petitioned FDA to expand the packaging materials for irradiated foods (FDA, 2007a).

Specifically, FDA allows the use of all approved packaging materials to package food being irradiated, provided that the packaged food is already permitted by FDA, the packaging materials are subjected to radiation doses not exceeding 3 kGy, and the packaged food is irradiated in an oxygen-free environment or while the food is frozen and contained under vacuum.

Unfortunately, the exemptions cannot be applied for fresh-cut produce because fresh-cut produce cannot be frozen or processed in an oxygen-free environment (even though nitrogen is used for flushing some packages of leafy vegetables). Fresh-cut produce is usually packaged with oxygen levels of 1–20% and therefore does not qualify under the exemption.

The majority of fresh-cut produce is packaged in polyolefin film bags, which themselves are mostly approved under 21 CFR 179.45 without any limitation on oxygen environment. However, these polyolefins may contain additives that have not been approved for use during irradiation. Therefore, packaging materials intended for irradiation of prepackaged fresh-cut produce in the presence of oxygen may still need premarket approval.

In addition, packaging materials are very complex, and emerging new packaging materials present a challenge to FDA. For example, polyethylene terephthalate (PET) films are approved by FDA under 21 CFR 179.45, but rigid and semi-rigid PET polymers are not (Komolprasert, 2007). New materials such as degradable and antimicrobial packages, adjuvants (antioxidants, stabilizers, etc.), plasticizers, colorants, and adsorbent pads may need more research before being evaluated and approved by FDA (Komolprasert, 2007).

Additional Research Needed

More studies on sensory analysis of irradiated fresh produce are needed. In addition, similar to studies on consumer acceptance of ground beef and chicken, consumer acceptance of irradiated produce needs to be evaluated, especially within the context of recent outbreaks related to produce.

Fresh produce is unique because fresh-cut fruits and vegetables are promoted as fresh and nutritious. However, it is unknown whether the word "irradiation" will affect the consumer perception of "freshness" of irradiated produce. In its recent proposal of labeling changes, FDA (2007b) expressed interest in receiving information on whether the control of foodborne pathogens changes the characteristics of food in a way outside of normal variation, which would therefore require additional labeling to inform the consumer of such changes. Thus, studies are needed to determine irradiation conditions that would minimize changes in organoleptic, nutritional, or functional properties, if any, that would constitute a material change to the consumer.

Because the response of each type (cultivar, species, whole vs fresh-cut, etc.) of fruits and vegetables to irradiation varies, process validation is required for each. While much work has been done already, it is important to prioritize future studies and products that need to be evaluated by their implication in outbreaks and/or volume of consumption.

As mentioned above, radiation resistance of pathogens is influenced by their environment. More research is needed to determine radiation resistance of internalized and biofilm-associated pathogens. In addition, radiation resistance of pathogens is mostly determined by artificially inoculating fresh-cut produce to high populations before irradiation. Ideally, radiation resistance of pathogens should be determined using naturally contaminated produce and levels of pathogens similar to those found in naturally contaminated produce.

Furthermore, the effect of modified-atmosphere packaging on radiation resistance of pathogens requires more investigation. In most studies on determining radiation resistance of pathogens, the inoculated samples were irradiated in air, whereas many fresh-cut produce are packaged in modified atmosphere. The modified atmosphere (low O_2 and high CO_2 levels) may alter the radiation resistance of pathogens. Other areas, such as packaging materials, may need approval and research before irradiation is fully applied by the produce industry.

Thus, low-dose irradiation is a reliable technology capable of killing human pathogens such as *E. coli* O157:H7 and *Salmonella* by 2–8 logs without causing significant deterioration in product quality. There are many challenges ahead for commercial application of irradiation for fresh and fresh-cut produce, including regulatory approval, packaging materials, consumer acceptance, and lack of premarket studies.

References

Anonymous. 2007. Produce pulse. *The Packer* 114(6): A1, A4.

Bhumiratana, N., Belden, L.K., and Bruhn, C.M. 2007. Effect of an educational program on attitudes of California consumers toward food irradiation. *Food Protection Trends* 27: 744–748.

Boynton, B.B., Welt, B.A., Sims, C.A., Balaban, M.O., Brecht, J.K., and Marshall, M.R. 2006. Effects of low-dose electron beam irradiation on respiration, microbiology, texture, color, and sensory characteristics of fresh-cut cantaloupe stored in modified-atmosphere packages. *J. Food Sci.* 71: S149–S155.

Fan, X. 2005. Antioxidant capacity of fresh-cut vegetables exposed to ionizing radiation. *J. Sci. Food Agric.* 85: 995–1000.

Fan, X. and Sokorai, K.J.B. 2002. Sensorial and chemical quality of gamma irradiated fresh-cut iceberg lettuce in modified atmosphere packages. *J. Food Protect.* 65: 1760–1765.

Fan, X. and Sokorai, K.J.B. 2005. Assessment of radiation sensitivity of fresh-cut vegetables using electrolyte leakage measurement. *Postharvest Biol. Technol.* 36: 191–197.

Fan, X. and Sokorai, K.J.B. 2007. Formation of furan from fresh fruits and vegetables due to ionizing radiation. *J. Food Sci.* (in press).

Fan, X., Niemira, B.A., and Sokorai, K.J.B. 2003a. Sensorial, nutritional and microbiological quality of fresh cilantro leaves as influenced by ionizing irradiation and storage. *Food Res. Intl.* 36: 713–719.

Fan, X., Toivonen, P.M.A., Rajkowski, K.T., and Sokorai, K.J.B. 2003b. Warm water treatment in combination with modified atmosphere packaging reduced undesirable effects or irradiation on the quality of fresh-cut iceberg lettuce. *J. Agric. Food Chem.* 50: 1231–1236.

FDA. 2007a. Threshold of regulation exemptions. Food and Drug Admin. www.cfsan.fda.gov/~dms/opa-torx.html, accessed Oct. 25.

FDA. 2007b. Irradiation in the production, processing and handling of food. Proposed rules. Fed. Reg. 72: 16291–16306. www.cfsan.fda.gov/~lrd/ fr070404.html, accessed Oct. 25.

FDA. 2007c. Foods permitted to be irradiated under FDA's regulations (21 CFR 179.26). www.cfsan.fda.gov/~dms/irrafood.html, accessed Oct. 25.

FDA. 2007d. Packaging materials listed in 21 CFR 179.45 for use during irradiation of prepackaged foods. www.cfsan.fda.gov/~dms/irrapack.html, accessed Oct. 25.

Foley, D., Euper, M., Caporaso, F., and Prakash, A. 2004. Irradiation and chlorination effectively reduces *Escherichia coli* O157:H7 inoculated on cilantro (*Coriandrum sativum*) without negatively affecting quality. *J. Food Protect.* 67: 2092–2098.

Gunes, G., Watkins, C.B., and Hotchkiss, J.H. 2000. Effects of irradiation on respiration and ethylene production of apple slices. *J. Sci. Food Agric.* 80: 1169–1175.

Hagenmaier, R.D., and Baker, R.A. 1998. Microbial population of shredded carrot in modified atmosphere packaging as related to irradiation treatment. *J. Food Sci.* 63: 162–164.

Komolprasert, V. 2007. Packaging for foods treated with ionizing radiation. In "Packaging for Non-Thermal Processing of Food," ed. J.H. Han, pp. 87–116. Blackwell Publishing, Ames, Iowa.

Koorapati, A., Foley, D., Pilling, R., and Prakash, A. 2004. Electron-beam irradiation preserves the quality of white button mushroom (*Agaricus bisporus*) slices. *J. Food Sci.* 69: S25–S29.

Masson, S. 2002. Effects of gamma irradiation on the shelf-life and quality characteristics of diced bell peppers. M.S. thesis. Chapman Univ., Orange, Calif.

Mead, P.S., Slutsker, L., Dietz, V., McCaig, L.F., Bresee, J.S., Shapiro, C., Griffin, P.M., and Tauxe, R.V. 1999. Food-related illness and death in the United States. *Emerg. Infect. Dis.* 5: 607–625.

Niemira, B.A. 2007. Irradiation sensitivity of planktonic and biofilm-associated *Escherichia coli* O157:H7 isolates is influenced by culture conditions. *Appl. Environ. Microbiol.* 73: 3239–3244.

Niemira, B.A., and Fan, X. 2005. Low-dose irradiation of fresh and fresh-cut produce: Safety, sensory and shelf life. In "Food Irradiation Research and Technology," ed. C. Sommers and X. Fan, pp. 169–181. Blackwell Publishing and the Institute of Food Technologists, Ames, Iowa.

Niemira, B.A., and Fan, X. 2007. Ionizing radiation enhances microbial safety of fresh and fresh-cut fruits and vegetables while maintaining product quality. Abstract# 042-03 Institute of Food Technologists Ann. Mtg., Chicago, IL.

Niemira, B.A., Sommers, C.H., and Fan, X. 2002. Suspending lettuce type influences recoverability and radiation sensitivity of *Escherichia coli* O157:H7. *J. Food Protect.* 65: 1388–1393.

Palekar, M.P., Cabrera-Diaz, E., KalbasiAshtari, A., Maxim, J.E., Miller, R.K., Cisneros-Zevallos, L., and Castillo, A. 2004. Effect of electron beam irradiation on the bacterial load and sensorial quality of sliced cantaloupe. *J. Food Sci.* 69: M267–M273.

Prakash, A., and Foley, D. 2004. Improving safety and extending shelf-life of fresh-cut fruits and vegetables using irradiation. In "Irradiation of Food and Packaging: Recent Developments," ed. V. Komolprasert and K.M. Morehouse, pp. 90–106. American Chemical Soc., Washington, D.C.

Prakash, A., Chen, P.C., Pilling, R., Johnson, N., and Foley, D. 2007. 1% Calcium chloride treatment in combination with gamma irradiation improves microbial and physicochemical properties of diced tomatoes. *Foodborne Pathogens Dis.* 4(1): 89–97.

Smith, J.S., and Pillai, S. 2004. Irradiation and food safety. An IFT Scientific Status Summary. *Food Technol.* 58(11): 48–55.

Critical Thinking

1. Why do fresh fruits and vegetables have a strong potential to carry microorganisms and cause food-borne illness?
2. What role does water play in the destruction of microorganisms by ionizing radiation?
3. Why is radiation more effective at destroying bacteria as opposed to viruses or fungi?

Xuetong Fan (xuetong.fan@ars.usda.gov) and **Brendan A. Niemira** (brendan.niemira@ars.usda.gov) are, respectively, Research Food Technologist and Microbiologist, U.S. Dept. of Agriculture, Agricultural Research Service, Eastern Regional Research Center, 600 E. Mermaid Ln., Wyndmoor, PA 19038. **Anuradha Prakash** (prakash@chapman.edu) is Professor, Chapman University, One University Dr., Orange, CA 92866. The authors are Professional Members of IFT. Send reprint requests to Xuetong Fan.

Is Your Food Contaminated?

New approaches are needed to protect the food supply.

MARK FISCHETTI

Given the billions of food items that are packaged, purchased and consumed every day in the U.S., let alone the world, it is remarkable how few of them are contaminated. Yet since the terrorist attacks of September 11, 2001, "food defense" experts have grown increasingly worried that extremists might try to poison the food supply, either to kill people or to cripple the economy by undermining public confidence. At the same time, production of edible products is becoming ever more centralized, speeding the spread of natural contaminants, or those introduced purposely, from farms or processing plants to dinner tables everywhere. Mounting imports pose yet another rising risk, as recent restrictions on Chinese seafood containing drugs and pesticides attest.

Can the tainting of what we eat be prevented? And if toxins or pathogens do slip into the supply chain, can they be quickly detected to limit their harm to consumers? Tighter production procedures can go a long way toward protecting the public, and if they fail, smarter monitoring technologies can at least limit injury.

Tighten Security

Preventing a terrorist or a disgruntled employee from contaminating milk, juice, produce, meat or any type of comestible is a daunting problem. The food supply chain comprises a maze of steps, and virtually every one of them presents an opportunity for tampering. Blanket solutions are unlikely because "the chain differs from commodity to commodity," says David Hennessy, an economics professor at Iowa State University's Center for Agricultural and Rural Development. "Protecting dairy products is different from protecting apple juice, which is different from protecting beef."

Even within a given supply chain there are few technology-based quick fixes. Preventing contamination largely comes down to tightening physical plant security and processing procedures at every turn. Each farmer, rancher, processor, packager, shipper, wholesaler and retailer "has to identify every possible vulnerability in the facility and in their procedures and close up every hole," says Frank Busta, director of the National Center for Food Protection and Defense at the University of Minnesota. The effort begins with standard facility access controls, which Busta often refers to as "gates, guns and guards," but extends to thoroughly screening employees and carefully sampling products at all junctures across the facility at all times.

That advice seems sound, of course, but the challenge for operators is how best to button down procedures. Several systems for safeguarding food production have been rolled out in recent years. Though these are not required by any regulatory agency, Busta strongly recommends that producers implement them. In the U.S., that impetus has been made stronger by legislation such as the 2002 Bioterrorism Act and a 2004 presidential directive, both of which require closer scrutiny of ingredient suppliers and tighter control of manufacturing procedures.

The primary safeguard systems Busta recommends borrow from military practices. The newest tool, which the FDA and the U.S. Department of Agriculture are now promoting, carries the awkward name of CARVER + Shock. It is being adapted from Defense Department procedures for identifying a military service's greatest vulnerabilities. "CARVER + Shock is essentially a complete security audit," says Keith Schneider, associate professor at the University of Florida's department of food science and human nutrition. The approach analyzes every node in the system for factors that range from the likely success of different kinds of attacks to the magnitude of public health, economic and psychological effects (together, the "shock" value) that a given type of infiltration could cause.

Track Contaminants

No matter how tightly procedures are controlled, determined perpetrators could still find ways to introduce pathogens or poisons. And natural pathogens such as salmonella are always a

Detect, Track and Trace

If a natural pathogen, or a perpetrator, contaminates food, lives will be saved if the tainted product can be quickly detected, then traced back to its point of origin so the rest of the batch can be tracked down or recalled. The following technologies, in development, could help:

- **Microfluidic Detectors**—Botulinum bacteria produce the most poisonous toxin known. They and similar agents, such as tetanus, could be detected during food processing by microfluidic chips—self-contained diagnostic labs the size of a finger. The University of Wisconsin–Madison is crafting such a chip, lined with antibodies held in place by magnetic beads, that could detect botulism during milk production. The chip could sample milk before or after it was piped into tanker trucks that leave the dairy and before or after it was pasteurized at a production plant. Other chips could detect other toxins at various fluid-processing plants, such as those that produce apple juice, soup or baby formula.

- **Active Packaging**—*E. coli,* salmonella and other pathogens could be detected by small windows in packaging, such as the cellophane around meat or the plastic jar around peanut butter. The "intelligent" window would contain antibodies that bind to enzymes or metabolites produced by the microorganism, and if that occurred the patch would turn color. The challenge is to craft the windows from materials and reactants that can safely contact food. Similar biosensors could react if the contents reached a certain pH level or were exposed to high temperature, indicating spoilage. And they could sense if packaging was

tampered with, for example, by reacting to the pressure imposed by a syringe or to oxygen seeping in through a puncture hole.

- **RFID Tags**—Pallets or cases of a few select foods now sport radio-frequency identification (RFID) tags that, when read by a scanner, indicate which farm or processing plant the batch came from. Future tokens that are smaller, smarter and cheaper could adorn individual packages and log every facility they had passed through and when. The University of Florida is devising tags that could be read through fluid (traditional designs cannot) and thus could be embedded inside the wall of sour cream or yogurt containers. The university is also developing active tags that could record the temperatures a package had been exposed to.

- **Edible Tags**—Manufacturers often combine crops from many growers, such as spinach leaves, into a retail package, so tags affixed to bags might not help investigators track contamination back to a specific source. ARmark Authentication Technologies can print microscopic markers that indicate site of origin directly onto a spinach leaf, apple or pellet of dog food using a spray made from edible materials such as cellulose, vegetable oil or proteins. Also, the tiny size would be hard for terrorists to fake, making it harder for them to sneak toxin-laced counterfeit foods past inspectors and into the supply. As an alternative, DataLase can spray citrus fruits or meats with an edible film in a half-inch-diameter patch that is then exposed to a laser beam that writes identification codes within the film.

concern. Detecting these agents, tracing them back to the spot of introduction, and tracking which grocery stores and restaurants ended up with tainted products are therefore paramount. Putting such systems in place "is just as important as prevention," Schneider says.

Here new technology does play a major role, with various sensors applied at different points along the chain. "You can't expect one technology to counter all the possible taintings for a given food," notes Ken Lee, chairman of Ohio State University's department of food science and technology.

A variety of hardware is being developed [see box on top of this page], although little has been deployed commercially thus far. Radio-frequency identification (RFID) tags are furthest along, in part because the Defense Department and Wal-Mart have required their main suppliers to attach the tokens to pallets or cases of foodstuffs. The Metro AG supermarket chain in Germany has done the same. The ultimate intent is for automated readers to scan the tags at each step along the supply chain—from farm, orchard, ranch or processor, through

packaging, shipping and wholesale—and to report each item's location to a central registry. That way if a problem surfaces, investigators can quickly determine where the batch originated and which stores or facilities might have received goods from that batch and when. Retailers can also read the tags on their items to see if they have received a product later identified as suspicious.

As RFID tags get smaller and cheaper, they will be placed directly on individual items—on every bag of spinach, jar of peanut butter, container of shrimp and sack of dog food. "That way if a recall is issued, the items can be found as they run past a scanner at the checkout counter," says Jean-Pierre Émond, professor of agricultural and biological engineering at the University of Florida.

Universities and companies are developing all kinds of other tags, some that are very inexpensive and others that cost more but supply extensive information. Some tokens, for example, can sense if food has been exposed to warm temperatures and thus might be more likely to harbor *Escherichia coli* or

Intentional Poisonings

U.S., 1984,
salmonella in salad bars, by Rajneeshees cult,
751 sickened

China, 2002,
rat poison in breakfast foods, by competitor to the vendor,
400 sickened, over 40 killed

U.S., 2002,
nicotine sulfate in ground beef, by disgruntled worker,
111 sickened

salmonella. Other tags could track how long items spent in transit from node to node in the supply chain, which could indicate unusually long delays that might raise suspicion about tampering. So-called active packaging could detect contamination directly and warn consumers not to eat the product they are holding.

The big impediment for any marker, of course, is the price. "Right now it costs 25 cents to put an RFID tag on a case of lettuce," Émond notes. "But for some growers, that equals the profit they're going to make on that case."

To be embraced widely, therefore, he says tags will have to provide additional value to suppliers or buyers. His university has been conducting an ongoing project with Publix Super Markets and produce suppliers in Florida and California to assess the possibilities. In initial trials, tags tracked crates and pallets that were shipped from the growers to several of Publix's distribution centers. Information gleaned from scanning tags at various points was available to all the companies via a secure Internet site hosted by VeriSign, the data security firm. The compilation allowed the participants to more quickly resolve order discrepancies, to log how long food sat idle, and to reveal ways to raise shipping efficiency. The group plans to extend the test to retail stores.

The U.S. imports 50 percent more food than it did just five years ago.

Control Suppliers

Costs will not drop until new technologies are widely deployed, but food defense analysts say adoption is unlikely to occur until clear, streamlined regulations are enacted. That prospect, in turn, will remain remote until the highest levels of government are reformed. "There are more than a dozen different federal agencies that oversee some aspect of food safety," Lee points out, noting that simple coordination among

Making Imports Safer

Alarming warnings about Chinese products in recent months have shown how dangerous imported edibles can be. In March some 100 brands of pet food were recalled after they were found to contain melamine, a toxic chemical used as a cheap replacement for wheat gluten. Then in June the U.S. Food and Drug Administration issued alerts about five types of seafood that contained antibiotic residues, pesticides and salmonella.

After the seafood scare, Senator Charles Schumer of New York declared that the federal government should establish an import czar. He blamed poor control of imports on a lack of inspection and poor regulation, telling the *Washington Post* that "neither the Chinese or American government is doing their job."

Regardless of how safe domestic production is, "imports are our Achilles' heel," says Ken Lee, chairman of Ohio State University's department of food science and technology. "There is no global food regulator. If the Chinese want to put an adulterant into food, they can do it until they get caught. I'll wager it will happen again, because it's driven by the profit motive."

Realistically, no technology can ensure that imports are safe. The food in every shipping container entering a U.S. port or border crossing could be pulled and irradiated, and some comestibles such as spices are already processed this way. But industry says the step would add significant cost for producers and shipping delays for middlemen. And the public continues to be wary of the technology. Furthermore, although irradiation would kill pathogens, it would have no effect on poisons or adulterants.

Inspecting all incoming food would also require vast increases in FDA and U.S. Department of Agriculture budgets; the agencies currently inspect a meager 1 percent of imports. As a partial alternative, in June the FDA said it intended to conduct more inspections of products from countries it deems to have poorer food-safety controls, such as China, offset by fewer inspections of products from countries with stronger standards, such as Britain and Canada. The agency also said it might require importers and U.S. manufacturers that use imported ingredients to provide more detailed information about production processes at foreign suppliers.

The best recourse, Lee says, is for companies to insist that suppliers impose strict standards and that the companies send inspectors overseas to verify compliance. Other experts agree, adding that government edicts are not as effective. "Too often import requirements are used as trade barriers, and they just escalate," says David Hennessy, an economics professor at Iowa State University. "The food companies themselves have a lot to lose, however. When they source a product in a country, they ought to impose tough procedures there."

—M.F.

The Vigilant Kitchen

If contaminated food does make it into your grocery bag, smart appliances could still prevent it from reaching your mouth. Innovations that could reach commercial introduction are described here by Ken Lee of Ohio State University. "None of this technology would be visually obtrusive," he says, "and all of it would be easy to clean."

Pulsed Light

When homeowners are asleep, fixtures underneath cabinets emit pulses of ultraviolet light that kill germs on counter-tops and other surfaces.

Microwave

An infrared sensor gauges internal food temperature and compares it with safety guidelines, indicating when the proper value has been reached. Instead of entering a cooking time, a user enters the food type or target temperature.

Refrigerator

A built-in reader scans RFID tags on food and checks for recalls over a wireless Internet connection. (A homeowner could hold nonrefrigerator items under it, too.) The reader also notes expiration dates written into the tags and tracks when containers such as milk cartons are removed and put back, to see if they have been out for too long and therefore might be spoiled. A red light warns of trouble.

and plant pathology at Oklahoma State University. "The requirements for organic farmers are different from those for nonorganic farmers."

Spurred by recent recalls, members of Congress have called for streamlining the regulation system. Illinois Senator Richard Durbin and Connecticut Representative Rosa DeLauro are advocating a single food-safety agency, but turf wars have hampered any progress toward that goal.

Concerned that more effective government is a long shot, experts say the responsibility for improved vigilance falls largely on food suppliers. "The strongest tool for stopping intentional contamination is supply-chain verification," says Shaun Kennedy, deputy director of the National Center for Food Protection and Defense. That means a brand-name provider such as Dole or a grocery store conglomerate such as Safeway must insist that every company involved in its supply chain implement the latest security procedures and detection, track and trace technologies or be dropped if it does not. The brand company should also validate compliance through inspections and other measures. The impetus falls on the brand-name provider because it has the most to lose. If a natural or man-made toxin is found in, say, a bag of Dole spinach or a container of Safeway milk, consumers will shun that particular label. "If a brand-name company wants to protect its products," Kennedy says, "it should validate every participant in the chain, all the way back to the farm."

Critical Thinking

1. What is the purpose of CARVER + Stock audit technique? Which government agencies/departments are supporting the use of this technique in the U.S. food supply chain?

2. What is RFID? How could the use of this technology be beneficial to the food supply?

3. Why is food safety more of a concern now than 50 years ago?

them is difficult enough, and efficient approval of sensible requirements is even harder to come by. The FDA regulates pizza with cheese on it, but the USDA regulates pizza if it has meat on it, quips Jacqueline Fletcher, professor of entomology

UNIT 7

Hunger, Nutrition, and Sustainability

Unit Selections

Learning Outcomes

After reading this unit, you should be able to

- Explain why creating ammonia from nitrogen gas is considered the most significant inventions to public health in human history.

- List the detrimental effects of synthetic fertilizers on the atmosphere, rivers, and oceans.

- Explain why a plant-based diet will lead to less destruction of the atmosphere and pollutants of our water supplies.

- Define perennial grain crops and explain how perennial grain crops differ from annual grain crops.

- Assess the pros and cons of creating perennial grain crops.

- Evaluate the pros and cons of continuing to produce annual grain crops.

- Identify the three grain crops that provide 70 percent of the calories for human consumption worldwide.

- List five steps you can take to conserve water.

- Describe where tap water comes from.

- Explain why there is a risk for a shortage of drinkable water.

Student Website

www.mhhe.com/cls

Internet References

Food and Agriculture Organization of the United Nations (FAO)
www.fao.org/economic/ess/food-security-statistics/en

Population Reference Bureau
www.prb.org

US Sustainable Agriculture Research and Education Program, University of California-Davis
www.sarep.ucdavis.edu/concept.htm

World Health Organization (WHO)
www.who.int/en

Malnutrition is the main culprit for lowered resistance to disease, infection, and death, especially in children. The malnutrition–infection combination results in stunted growth, lowered mental development in children, lowered productivity, and higher incidence of degenerative disease in adulthood. This directly affects the economies of developing countries. Over 1 billion people globally suffer from micronutrient malnutrition frequently called "hidden hunger." In addition, partnerships between the public and private sectors may prove valuable in combating malnutrition. Solutions to these problems such as building sustainability through indigenous knowledge and practices that are community based and environmentally friendly with emphasis on biofortification and dietary diversification may combat hunger and nutrient deficiencies in the future.

Nutrient deficiencies magnify the effect of disease, resulting in more severe symptoms and greater complications in countries with developing economies. For example, vitamin A deficiency leads to blindness in about 250,000–300,000 children annually and exacerbates the symptoms of measles. Iron deficiency, which is widespread among pregnant women and those in the child-bearing years in developing countries, increases the risk of death from hemorrhage in their offspring and reduces physical productivity and learning capacity. Finally, iodine deficiency causes brain damage and mental retardation. It is estimated that 1.5 billion people are at risk for iodine deficiency disorders.

Malnutrition not only affects children and adults in developing countries, but it is also prevalent in the United States. Thirty million Americans (including 11 million children), experience food insecurity and hunger. In a country where one-fifth of the food is wasted and 130 pounds of food per person is disposed of, it is unacceptable that Americans go hungry. Gleaning is an initiative that is growing in popularity to make use of excess crops that lay unpicked in the fields. Gleaning programs locate excess produce from farms, harvest the produce, and distribute it to food-insecure communities primarily with volunteer labor.

The primary nutrient deficiencies in this country, as in developing countries, are iron deficiency anemia, common in infants, young children, and teens, and lead toxicity. Undernourished pregnant women give birth to low-weight babies who suffer developmental delays and increases in mortality rate. Another group in the United States that experiences health problems due to hunger is the elderly.

Food security is now critical to consumers worldwide. The movement for purchasing local and seasonal foods with regard for the environment attempts to reconnect the consumer to the farmer, producer, or purveyor. In response to consumer demands, food companies are finding ways to improve the sustainability of their processing and packaging operations and be more environmentally conscious. From energy efficient processing plants to reducing or modifying packaging material,

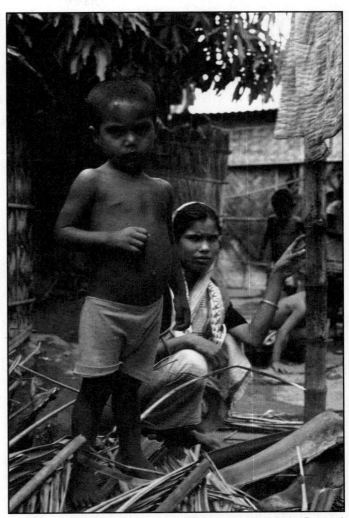

"In Search of Sustainability" by Karen Nachay informs you on how these companies are trying to deal with the problems faced by our environment.

Another alarming issue is that the earth's supply of fresh water is declining. Water tables all over the world are being depleted at a very fast rate. What many people don't realize is that with a shortage of water also comes a shortage of food; water is necessary to raise livestock and grow crops. "Draining Our Future: The Growing Shortage of Freshwater" reveals just how serious the world's water crisis is and makes suggestions on how we can resolve the problem.

Fixing the Global Nitrogen Problem

Humanity depends on nitrogen to fertilize croplands, but growing global use is damaging the environment and threatening human health. How can we chart a more sustainable path?

ALAN R. TOWNSEND AND ROBERT W. HOWARTH

Billions of people today owe their lives to a single discovery now a century old. In 1909 German chemist Fritz Haber of the University of Karlsruhe figured out a way to transform nitrogen gas—which is abundant in the atmosphere but nonreactive and thus unavailable to most living organisms—into ammonia, the active ingredient in synthetic fertilizer. The world's ability to grow food exploded 20 years later, when fellow German scientist Carl Bosch developed a scheme for implementing Haber's idea on an industrial scale.

Over the ensuing decades new factories transformed ton after ton of industrial ammonia into fertilizer, and today the Haber-Bosch invention commands wide respect as one of the most significant boons to public health in human history. As a pillar of the green revolution, synthetic fertilizer enabled farmers to transform infertile lands into fertile fields and to grow crop after crop in the same soil without waiting for nutrients to regenerate naturally. As a result, global population skyrocketed from 1.6 billion to six billion in the 20th century.

But this good news for humanity has come at a high price. Most of the reactive nitrogen we make—on purpose for fertilizer and, to a lesser extent, as a by-product of the fossil-fuel combustion that powers our cars and industries—does not end up in the food we eat. Rather it migrates into the atmosphere, rivers and oceans, where it makes a Jekyll and Hyde style transformation from do-gooder to rampant polluter. Scientists have long cited reactive nitrogen for creating harmful algal blooms, coastal dead zones and ozone pollution. But recent research adds biodiversity loss and global warming to nitrogen's rap sheet, as well as indications that it may elevate the incidence of several nasty human diseases.

Today humans are generating reactive nitrogen and injecting it into the environment at an accelerating pace, in part because more nations are vigorously pursuing such fertilizer-intensive endeavors as biofuel synthesis and meat production (meat-intensive diets depend on massive growth of grain for animal feed). Heavy fertilizer use for food crops and unregulated burning of fossil fuels are also becoming more prevalent in regions such as South America and Asia. Not surprisingly then, dead zones and other nitrogen-related problems that were once confined to North America and Europe are now popping up elsewhere.

At the same time, fertilizer is, and should be, a leading tool for developing a reliable food supply in sub-Saharan Africa and other malnourished regions. But the international community must come together to find ways to better manage its use and mitigate its consequences worldwide. The solutions are not always simple, but nor are they beyond our reach.

The world is capable of growing MORE FOOD with LESS FERTILIZER.

Too Much of a Good Thing

Resolving the nitrogen problem requires an understanding of the chemistry involved and a sense of exactly how nitrogen fosters environmental trouble. The element's ills—and benefits—arise when molecules

Nitrogen's Dark Side

Doubled up as N_2 gas, the most abundant component of the earth's atmosphere, nitrogen is harmless. But in its reactive forms, which emanate from farms and fossil-fuel-burning factories and vehicles, nitrogen can have a hand in a wide range of problems for the environment and human health.

1. The nitrogen produced during fossil-fuel combustion can cause severe air pollution . . .
2. Before it then combines with water to create nitric acid in rain . . .
3. And joins with nitrogen leaking from fertilized fields, farm animal excrement, human sewage and leguminous crops.
4. When too much nitrogen enters terrestrial ecosystems, it can contribute to biodiversity decline and perhaps to increased risk for several human illnesses.
5. A single nitrogen atom from a factory, vehicle or farm can acidify soil and contaminate drinking water before entering rivers . . .
6. Where it can travel to the oceans and help fuel toxic algal blooms and coastal dead zones.
7. At any point along this chain, bacteria may transform the rogue atom into nitrous oxide, a potent greenhouse gas that also speeds the loss of protective stratospheric ozone. Only bacteria that convert the atom back to innocuous N_2 gas can halt its ill effects.

of N_2 gas break apart. All life needs nitrogen, but for the vast majority of organisms, the biggest reservoir—the atmosphere—is out of reach. Although 78 percent of the atmosphere consists of N_2, that gas is inert. Nature's way of making nitrogen available for life relies on the action of a small group of bacteria that can break the triple bond between those two nitrogen atoms, a process known as nitrogen fixation. These specialized bacteria exist in free-living states on land and in both freshwater and saltwater and in symbiotic relationships with the roots of legumes, which constitute some the world's most important crops. Another small amount of nitrogen gas is fixed when lightning strikes and volcanic eruptions toast it.

Before humanity began exploiting Haber-Bosch and other nitrogen-fixation techniques, the amount of reactive nitrogen produced in the world was balanced by the activity of another small bacterial group that converts reactive nitrogen back to N_2 gas in a process called denitrification. In only one human generation, though, that delicate balance has been transformed completely. By 2005 humans were creating more than 400 billion pounds of reactive nitrogen each year, an amount at least double that of all natural processes on land combined.

At times labeled nature's most promiscuous element, nitrogen that is liberated from its nonreactive state can cause an array of environmental problems because it can combine with a multitude of chemicals and can spread far and wide. Whether a new atom of reactive nitrogen enters the atmosphere or a river, it may be deposited tens to hundreds of miles from its source, and even some of the most remote corners of our planet now experience elevated nitrogen levels because of human activity. Perhaps most insidious of all: a single new atom of reactive nitrogen can bounce its way around these widespread environments, like a felon on a crime spree.

Reaping the Consequences

When nitrogen is added to a cornfield or to a lawn, the response is simple and predictable: plants grow more. In natural ecosystems, however, the responses are far more intricate and frequently worrisome. As fertilizer-laden river waters enter the ocean, for example, they trigger blooms of microscopic plants that consume oxygen as they decompose, leading later to so-called dead zones. Even on land, not all plants in a complex ecosystem respond equally to nitrogen subsidies, and many are not equipped for a sudden embarrassment of riches. Thus, they lose out to new species that are more competitive in a nutrient-rich world. Often the net effect is a loss of biodiversity. For example, grasslands across much of Europe have lost a quarter or more of their plant species after decades of human-created nitrogen deposition from the atmosphere. This problem is so widespread that a recent scientific assessment ranked nitrogen pollution as one of the top three threats to biodiversity around the globe, and the United Nations Environment Program's Convention on Biological Diversity considers reductions of nitrogen deposition to be a key indicator of conservation success.

The loss of a rare plant typically excites little concern in the general public or among those who forge policy. But excess nitrogen does not just harm other species—it can threaten our own. A National Institutes of Health review suggests that elevated nitrate concentrations in drinking water—often a product of water pollution from the high nitrate levels in common fertilizers—may contribute to multiple health problems, including several cancers. Nitrogen-related air pollution, both particulates and ground-level ozone, affects hundreds of millions of people, elevating the incidence of cardiopulmonary ailments and driving up overall mortality rates.

Ecological feedbacks stemming from excess nitrogen (and another ubiquitous fertilizer chemical, phosphorus) may be poised to hit us with a slew of other health threats as well. How big or varied such

responses will become remains to be seen, but scientists do know that enriching ecosystems with nitrogen changes their ecology in myriad ways. Recent evidence suggests that excess nitrogen may increase risk for Alzheimer's disease and diabetes if ingested in drinking water. It may also elevate the release of airborne allergens and promote the spread of certain infectious diseases. Fertilization of ragweed elevates pollen production from that notorious source, for instance. Malaria, cholera, schistosomiasis and West Nile virus show the potential to infect more people when nitrogen is abundant.

These and many other illnesses are controlled by the actions of other species in the environment, particularly those that carry the infective agent—for example, mosquitoes spread the malaria parasite, and snails release schistosomes into water. Snails offer an example of how nitrogen can unleash a chain reaction: more nitrogen or phosphorus run-off fuels greater plant growth in water bodies, in turn creating more food for the snails and a larger, faster-growing population of these disease-bearing agents. The extra nutrients also fuel an exponentially increasing effect of having each snail produce more parasites. It is too soon to tell if, in general, nutrient pollution will up the risk of disease—in some cases, the resulting ecological changes might lower our health risks. But the potential for change, and thus the need to understand how it will play out, is rising rapidly as greater use of fertilizers spreads to disease-rich tropical latitudes in the coming decades.

Mounting evidence also blames reactive nitrogen for an increasingly important role in climate change. In the atmosphere, reactive nitrogen leads to one of its major unwanted by-products—ground-level ozone—when it occurs as nitric oxide (NO) or as nitrogen dioxide (NO_2), collectively known as NO_x. Such ozone formation is troubling not only because of its threat to human health but also because at ground level, ozone is a significant greenhouse gas. Moreover, it damages plant tissues, resulting in billions of dollars in lost crop production every year. And by inhibiting growth, ozone curtails plants' ability to absorb carbon dioxide (CO_2) and offset global warming.

Reactive nitrogen is an especially worrisome threat to climate change when it occurs as nitrous oxide (N_2O)—among the most powerful of greenhouse gases. One molecule of N_2O has approximately 300 times the greenhouse warming potential of one molecule of CO_2. Although N_2O is far less abundant in the atmosphere than CO_2 is, its current atmospheric concentration is responsible for warming equivalent to 10 percent of CO_2's contribution. It is worth noting that excess nitrogen can at times counteract warming—by combining with other airborne compounds to form aerosols that reflect incoming radiation, for example, and by stimulating plants in nitrogen-limited forests to grow faster and thus scrub more CO_2 out of the atmosphere. But despite uncertainties regarding the balance between nitrogen's heating and cooling effects, most signs indicate that continued human creation of excess nitrogen will speed climate warming.

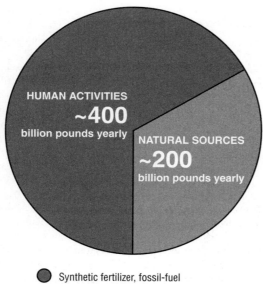

HUMAN ACTIVITIES
~400
billion pounds yearly

NATURAL SOURCES
~200
billion pounds yearly

● Synthetic fertilizer, fossil-fuel combustion, industrial uses of ammonia (plastics, explosives, etc.), cultivation of soybeans and other leguminous crops

● Nitrogen-fixing bacteria on land, lightning, volcanoes

HUMAN ACTIVITIES have tripled the amount of reactive nitrogen released into terrestrial environments and coastal oceans every year.

Global Perspectives
Shifting Hotspots

Regions of greatest nitrogen use were once limited mainly to Europe and North America. But as new economies develop and agricultural trends shift, patterns in the distribution of nitrogen are changing rapidly. Recent growth rates in nitrogen use are now much higher in Asia and in Latin America, whereas other regions—including much of Africa—suffer from fertilizer shortages.

- **Southern Brazil:** Rapid population growth and industrialization around Sao Paulo, poor civic sewage treatment and vibrant sugar cane production all contribute to this new South American nitrogen hotspot.
- **North China Plain:** More vigorous application of fertilizer has produced stunning increases in maize and wheat production, but China now has the highest fertilizer inputs in the world.

What to Do

Although fertilizer production accounts for much of the nitrogen now harming the planet—roughly two thirds of that fixed by humans—abandoning it certainly is not an option. Fertilizer is too important for feeding the world. But an emphasis on efficient use has to be a part of the solution, in both the wealthy and the developing nations.

It's up to You

Making certain personal choices will reduce your carbon and nitrogen footprints simultaneously:

- Support wind power, hybrid cars and other policies designed to reduce fossil-fuel consumption.
- Choose grass-fed beef and eat less meat overall.
- Buy locally grown produce.

Wealthy countries have blazed a path to an agricultural system that is often exceptionally nitrogen-intensive and inefficient in the use of this key resource. Too often their use of nitrogen has resembled a spending spree with poor returns on the investment and little regard for its true costs. Elsewhere, a billion or more people stand trapped in cycles of malnutrition and poverty. Perhaps best exemplified by sub-Saharan Africa, these are regions where agricultural production often fails to meet even basic caloric needs, let alone to provide a source of income. Here an infusion of nitrogen fertilizers would clearly improve the human condition. Recent adoption of policies to supply affordable fertilizer and better seed varieties to poor farmers in Malawi, for example, led to substantial increases in yield and reductions in famine.

But this fertilizer does not need to be slathered on injudiciously. The proof is out there: studies from the corn belt of the U. S. Midwest to the wheat fields of Mexico show that overfertilization has been common practice in the breadbaskets of the world—and that less fertilizer often does not mean fewer crops. The simple fact is that as a whole, the world is capable of growing more food with less fertilizer by changing the farming practices that have become common in an era of cheap, abundant fertilizer and little regard for the long-term consequences of its use. Simply reducing total application to many crops is an excellent starting point; in many cases, fertilizer doses are well above the level needed to ensure maximum yield in most years, resulting in disproportionately large losses to the environment. In the U.S., people consume only a little more than 10 percent of what farmers apply to their fields every year. Sooner or later, the rest ends up in the environment. Estimates vary, but for many of our most common crops, a quarter to half immediately runs off the field with rainwater or works its way into the atmosphere.

Precision farming techniques can also help. Applying fertilizer near plant roots only at times of maximum demand is one example of methods that are already in play in some of the wealthier agricultural regions of the planet. By taking advantage of Global Positioning System technology to map their fields, coupled with remotely sensed estimates of plant nutrient levels, farmers can refine calculations of how much fertilizer a crop needs and when. But the high-tech equipment is costly, prohibitively so for many independent farmers, and so such precision farming is not a panacea.

The solutions are not all high tech. Cheaper but still effective strategies can include planting winter cover crops that retain nitrogen in a field instead of allowing a field to lie bare for months, as well as maintaining some form of plant cover in between the rows of high-value crops such as corn. Simply applying fertilizer just before spring planting, rather than in the fall, can also make a big difference.

The world can also take advantages of changes in meat production. Of the nitrogen that ends up in crop plants, most goes into the mouths of pigs, cows and chickens—and much of that is then expelled as belches, urine and feces. Although a reduction in global meat consumption would be a valuable step, meat protein will remain an important part of most human diets, so efficiencies in its production must also improve. Changing animal diets—say, feeding cows more grass and less corn—can help on a small scale, as can better treatment of animal waste, which, like sewage treatment facilities for human waste, converts more of the reactive nitrogen back into inert gas before releasing it into the environment [see "The Greenhouse Hamburgerr" by Nathan Fiala; *Scientific American*, February 2009].

On the energy side, which represents about 20 percent of the world's excess nitrogen, much reactive nitrogen could be removed from current fossil-fuel emissions by better deployment of NO_X-scrubbing technologies in smokestacks and other sources of industrial pollution. Beyond that, a sustained global effort to improve energy efficiency and move toward cleaner, renewable sources will drop nitrogen emissions right alongside those for carbon. Removing the oldest and least-efficient power plants from production, increasing vehicle emission standards and, where possible, switching power generation from traditional combustion to fuel cells would all make a meaningful difference.

Of course, one source of renewable energy—biofuel made from corn—is generating a new demand for fertilizer. The incredible increase in the production of ethanol from corn in the U.S.—a nearly fourfold rise since 2000—has already had a demonstrable effect on increased nitrogen flows down the Mississippi River, which carries excess fertilizer to the Gulf of Mexico, where it fuels algal blooms and creates dead zones. According to a report last April by the Scientific Committee on Problems of the Environment (then part of the International Council for Science), a business-as-usual approach to biofuel production could exacerbate global warming, food security threats and human respiratory ailments in addition to these familiar ecological problems.

How to Get It Done

Society already has a variety of technical tools to manage nitrogen far more effectively, retaining many of its benefits while greatly reducing the risk. As for our energy challenges, a switch to more sustainable nitrogen use will not come easily, nor is there a silver bullet. Furthermore, technological know-how is not enough: without economic incentives and other policy shifts, none of these solutions will likely solve the problem.

The speed at which nitrogen pollution is rising throughout the world suggests the need for some regulatory control. Implementing or strengthening environmental standards, such as setting total maximum daily loads that can enter surface waters and determining the reactive nitrogen concentrations allowable in fossil-fuel emissions, is probably

essential. In the U.S. and other nations, regulatory policies are being pursued at both national and regional scales, with some success [see "Reviving Dead Zones," by Laurence Mee; *Scientific American*, November 2006]. And as much needed policy changes bring fertilizer to those parts of the world largely bypassed by the green revolution, those areas should employ sustainable solutions from the outset—to avoid repeating mistakes made in the U.S. and elsewhere.

Promising improvements could occur even without the regulatory threat of monetary fines for exceeding emissions standards. Market-based instruments, such as tradable permits, may also be useful. This approach proved remarkably successful for factory emissions of sulfur dioxide. Adoption of similar approaches to NO_X pollution are already under way, including the U.S. Environmental Protection Agency's NO_X Budget Trading Program, which began in 2003. Such policies could be extended to fertilizer runoff and livestock emissions as well—although the latter are more difficult to monitor than the smokestacks of a coal-burning power plant.

Other approaches to the problem are also beginning to take hold, including better use of landscape design in agricultural areas, especially ensuring that crop fields near bodies of water are fringed by intervening wetlands that can markedly reduce nitrogen inputs to surface waters and the coastal ocean. Protected riparian areas, such those promoted by the U.S. Conservation Reserve Program, can do double duty: not only will they reduce nitrogen pollution, but they also provide critical habitat for migratory birds and a host of other species.

Substantial progress may also require a rethinking of agricultural subsidies. In particular, subsidies that reward environmental stewardship can bring about rapid changes in standard practice. A recent not-for-profit experiment run by the American Farmland Trust shows promise. Farmers agreed to reduce their fertilizer use and directed a portion of their cost savings from lowered fertilizer purchases to a common fund. They then fertilized the bulk of the crop at reduced rates, while heavily fertilizing small test plots. If such plots exceeded the average yield of the entire field, the fund paid out the difference.

As one of us (Howarth) reported in a Millennium Ecosystem Assessment in 2005, such pay-outs would rarely be required, given the current tendency to overfertilize many crops. The average farmer in the breadbasket of the upper U.S. Midwest (the source of the great majority of nitrogen pollution fueling the Gulf of Mexico dead zones) typically uses 20 to 30 percent more nitrogen fertilizer than agricultural extension agents recommend. As predicted, farmers who participated in this and similar experiments have applied less fertilizer with virtually no decrease in crop yield and have saved money as a result, because what they paid into the fund is less than the amount they saved by buying less fertilizer. As a result, such funds grow with no taxpayer subsidy.

Finally, better public education and personal choice can play critical roles. In much the way that many individuals have begun reducing their own energy consumption, so, too, can people from all walks of life learn how to select a less nitrogen-intensive lifestyle.

One big improvement would be for Americans to eat less meat. If Americans were to switch to a typical Mediterranean diet, in which average meat consumption is one sixth of today's U.S. rates, not only would Americans' health improve, the country's fertilizer use would be cut in half. Such shifts in dietary and agricultural practices could simultaneously lower environmental nitrogen pollution and improve public health: nitrogen-intensive agricultural practices in wealthier nations contribute to overly protein-rich, often unbalanced diets that link to health concerns from heart disease and diabetes to childhood obesity.

Making personal choices designed to reduce an individual's carbon footprint can help—not just on the industrial side, as in supporting wind power and hybrid cars, but on the agricultural side as well. Eating less meat, eating locally grown food and eating grass-fed rather

---

Solutions Are within Reach

- Industry can install more NO_X-scrubbing technologies in smokestacks and other sources of pollution.
- Farmers can use less fertilizer. For many crops, applying less fertilizer would not sacrifice yield.
- Community officials can ensure that crop fields are fringed by wetlands that can absorb nitrogen-laden runoff before it enters streams or lakes.
- Nations can institute farm subsidies that reward environmental stewardship.

Where Fertilizer *Shortage* Is the Problem

Synthetic fertilizer has been, and will continue to be, critical to meeting world food demands, particularly in malnourished regions, such as sub-Saharan Africa, where increased fertilizer use is one of the leading strategies for developing a reliable food supply.

Humans already produce more than enough fertilizer to feed the world, but inequitable and inefficient distribution means that excessive use is causing problems in some places while poverty-stricken regions are mired in a cycle of malnutrition. Making synthetic fertilizer available to those who typically cannot afford it has clearly played a role in bettering food security and the human condition in parts of rural sub-Saharan Africa, where wide-spread malnutrition stems directly from nutrient depletion and soil erosion.

Fertilizer subsidies are one pillar of the African Millennium Villages Project, an ambitious proof-of-concept project in which coordinated efforts to improve health, education and agricultural productivity are now under way in a series of rural villages across Africa. Launched in 2004, the project was implemented on a national scale in Malawi. After a decade of repeated food shortages and famine, Malawi created subsidies that provided poor farmers with synthetic fertilizer and improved seed varieties. Although better climate conditions played a role, the approach clearly worked: Malawi went from a 43 percent food deficit in 2005 to a 53 percent surplus in 2007.

—*A.R.T. and R.W.H.*

More to Explore

Nutrient Management. R. W. Howarth et al. in *Ecosystems and Human Well-Being: Policy Responses.* Millennium Ecosystem Assessment. Island Press, 2005.
Transformation of the Nitrogen Cycle: Recent Trends, Questions, and Potential Solutions. James N. Galloway et al. in *Science,* Vol. 320, pages 889–892; May 16, 2008.
Biofuels: Environmental Consequences and Interactions with Changing Land Use. Edited by R. W. Howarth and S. Bringezu. *Proceedings of the SCOPE International Biofuels Project Rapid Assessment,* Cornell University, April 2009. http://cip.cornell.edu/biofuels
Nutrient Imbalances in Agricultural Development. P. M. Vitousek et al. in *Science,* Vol. 324, pages 1519–1520; June 19, 2009.

nitrogen production continuing to rise, we will face a future in which the enormous benefits of Fritz Haber's discovery become ever more shrouded by its drawbacks.

Still, as we have argued here, nitrogen cycle problems could be significantly reduced with current technology at relatively affordable costs. We can and must do better. It will take immediate and ongoing effort, but a sustainable nitrogen future is entirely achievable.

Critical Thinking

1. How did the creation of nitrogen-based synthetic fertilizers change agricultural production?

2. How do synthetic fertilizers affect the atmosphere, rivers, and oceans?

3. Why does raising animals for consumption require more fertilizer than raising vegetable, fruit, legumes, and grain crops for consumption?

ALAN R. TOWNSEND is incoming director of the Environmental Studies Program at the University of Colorado at Boulder and is a professor in the university's Institute of Arctic and Alpine Research and department of ecology and evolutionary biology. He studies how changes in climate, land use and global nutrient cycles affect the basic functioning of terrestrial ecosystems. **ROBERT W. HOWARTH**, who is David R. Atkinson Professor of Ecology and Environmental Biology at Cornell University, studies how human activities alter ecosystems, with an emphasis on fresh water and marine locales.

than corn-fed beef all tackle the carbon and nitrogen problems simultaneously. Individual choices alone are unlikely to solve the problems, but history shows they can spur societies to move down new paths. The well-known trade-offs between climate and energy production that were long ignored as hypothetical now appear everywhere from presidential speeches to roadside billboards to budding regulatory schemes.

Unfortunately, the nitrogen problem is in one critical way tougher than the carbon problem. In solving the latter, it is reasonable to work toward a future of one day producing energy without CO_2-emitting fossil fuels. But it is not possible to envision a world free of the need to produce substantial amounts of reactive nitrogen. Synthetic fertilizer has been, and will continue to be, critical to meeting world food demands. Yet if we stay on a business-as-usual trajectory, with

Perennial Grains
Food Security for the Future

Developing perennial versions of our major grain crops would address many of the environmental limitations annuals while helping to feed an increasingly hungry planet.

JERRY D. GLOVER AND JOHN P. REGANOLD

Colorful fruits and vegetables piled to overflowing at a farmer's market or in the produce aisle readily come to mind when we think about farming and food production. Such images run counter to those of environmental destruction and chronic hunger and seem disconnected from the challenges of climate change, energy use, and bio-diversity loss. Agriculture, though, has been identified as the greatest threat to biodiversity and ecosystem function of any human activity. And because of factors including climate change, rising energy costs, and land degradation, the number of "urgently hungry" people, now estimated at roughly 1 billion, is at its highest level ever. More troubling, agriculture-related problems will probably worsen as the human population expands—that is, unless we reshape agriculture.

The disconnect between popular images of farming and its less rosy reality stems from the fact that fruits and vegetables represent only a sliver of farm production. Cereal, oilseed, and legume crops dominate farming, occupying 75% of U.S. and 69% of global croplands. These grains include crops such as wheat, rice, and maize and together provide more than 70% of human food calories. Currently, all are annuals, which means they must be replanted each year from seed, require large amounts of expensive fertilizers and pesticides, poorly protect soil and water, and provide little habitat for wildlife. Their production emits significant greenhouse gases, contributing to climate change that can in turn have adverse effects on agricultural productivity.

These are not the inevitable consequences of farming. Plant breeders can now, for perhaps the first time in history, develop perennial versions of major grain crops. Perennial crops have substantial ecological and economic benefits. Their longer growing seasons and more extensive root systems make them more competitive against weeds and more effective at capturing nutrients and water. Farmers don't have to replant the crop each year, don't have to add as much fertilizer and pesticide, and don't burn as much diesel in their tractors. In addition,

soils are built and conserved, water is filtered, and more area is available for wildlife. Although perennial crops such as alfalfa exist, there are no commercial perennial versions of the grains on which humans rely. An expanding group of plant breeders around the world is working to change that.

Although annual grain crops have been with us for thousands of years and have benefited from many generations of breeding, modern plant breeding techniques provide unprecedented opportunities to develop new crops much more quickly. During the past decade, plant breeders in the United States have been working to develop perennial versions of wheat, sorghum, sunflowers, and legumes. Preliminary work has also been done to develop a perennial maize, and Swedish researchers see potential in domesticating a wild mustard species as a perennial oilseed crop. Relatively new breeding programs in China and Australia include work to develop perennial rice and wheat. These programs could make it possible to develop radically new and sustainable farming systems within the next 10 to 20 years.

Currently, these efforts receive little public funding in marked contrast to the extensive public support for cellulosic ethanol technologies capable of converting perennial biomass crops into liquid fuels. Yet perennial grain crops promise much larger payoffs for the environment and food security and have similar timelines for widespread application. Public research funds distributed through the U.S. Department of Agriculture (USDA) and the National Science Foundation (NSF) could greatly expand and accelerate perennial grain breeding programs. Additionally, the farm bill could include support for the development of perennial breeding programs.

The Rise of Annuals

Since the initial domestication of crops more than 10,000 years ago, annual grains have dominated food production. The agricultural revolution was launched when our Neolithic ancestors began harvesting and sowing wild seed-bearing plants. The earliest cultivators had long collected seed from both annual and perennial plants; however, they found the annuals to be better adapted to the soil disturbance and annual sowing they had adopted in order to maintain a convenient and steady supply of grains harvested from the annual plants.

Although some of the wild annuals first to be domesticated, such as wheat and barley, were favored because they had large seeds, others had seeds comparable in size to those of their wild perennial counterparts. With each year's sowing of the annuals, desirable traits were selected for and carried on to the next generation. Thus, selection pressure was applied, albeit unintentionally, to annual plants but not to perennials. Evidence indicates that selection pressures on wild annuals quickly resulted in domesticated plants with more desirable traits than their wild relatives. The unchanged wild perennials probably would have been ignored in favor of the increasingly large, easily harvested seeds of the modified annual plants.

The conversion of native perennial landscapes to the monocultures of annual crops characteristic of today's agriculture has allowed us to meet our increasing food needs. But it has also resulted in dramatic changes. Fields of maize and wheat require frequent, expensive care to remain productive. Compared to perennials, annuals typically grow for shorter lengths of time each year and have shallower rooting depths and lower root densities, with most of their roots restricted to the surface foot of soil or less. Even with crop management advances such as no-tillage practices, these traits limit their access to nutrients and water, increase their need for nutrients, leave croplands more vulnerable to degradation, and reduce soil carbon inputs and provisions for wildlife. These traits also make annual plants less resilient to the increased environmental stress expected from climate change.

Even in regions best suited for annual crops, such as the Corn Belt, soil carbon and nitrogen levels decreased by 40 to 50% or more after conversion from native plants to annuals. Global data for maize, rice, and wheat indicate that they take up only 20 to 50% of the nitrogen applied in fertilizer; the rest is lost to surrounding environments. Runoff of nitrogen and other chemicals from farm fields into rivers and then coastal waters has triggered the development of more than 400 "dead zones" that are depleted of fish and other sea dwellers.

Annual crops do, however, have some advantages over perennial crops in terms of management flexibility. Because they are short-lived, they offer farmers opportunities to quickly change crops in response to changing market demands as well as environmental factors such as disease outbreaks. Thus, annual grain production will undoubtedly be important far into the future. Still, the expanded use of perennial grain crops on farms would provide greater biological and economic diversity and yield additional environmental benefits.

Perennial Advantages

Developing new crop species capable of significantly replacing annuals will require a major effort. During the past four decades, breeders have had tremendous success in doubling,

tripling, and even quadrupling the yields of important annual grains, success that would seem to challenge the notion that a fundamental change in agriculture is needed. Today, however these high yields are being weighed against the negative environmental effects of agriculture that are increasingly seen around the world. And with global grain demand expected to double by 2050, these effects will increase.

The development of perennial crops through breeding would help deal with the multiple issues involving environmental conservation and food security in a world of shrinking resources. We know that perennials such as alfalfa and switchgrass are much more effective than annuals in maintaining topsoil. Soil carbon may also increase 50 to 100% when annual fields are converted to perennials. With their longer growing seasons and deeper roots, perennials can dramatically reduce water and nitrate losses. They require less field attention by the farmer and less pesticide and fertilizer inputs, resulting in lower costs. Wildlife benefit from reduced chemical inputs and from the greater shelter provided by perennial cover.

There are other benefits as well. Greater soil carbon storage and reduced input requirements mean that perennials have the potential to mitigate global warming, whereas annual crops tend to exacerbate the problem. With more of their reserves protected belowground and their greater access to more soil moisture, perennials are also more resilient to temperature increases of the magnitude Predicted by some climate change models. Although perennials may not offer farmers the flexibility of changing crops each year, they can be planted on more-marginal lands and can be used to increase the economic and biological diversity of a farm, thereby increasing the flexibility of the farming system. Perhaps most important in a crowded world with limited resources, perennials are more resilient to social, political, health, and environmental disruptions because they don t rely on annual seedbed preparation and planting. A farmer suffering from illness might be unable to harvest her crop one season, but a new crop would be ready the next season when she recovers. Meanwhile, the soil is protected and water has been captured.

The increased use of perennials could also slow, reverse, or prevent the increased planting of annuals on marginal lands, which now support more than half the world's population. Because marginal lands are by their nature fragile and subject to rapid degradation, large areas of these lands now being planted with annuals are already experiencing declining productivity. This will mean that additional marginal lands will be cultivated. This troubling reality makes the development of crops that can be more sustainably produced a matter of necessity. Developing perennial versions of our major grain crops would address many of the environmental limitations of annuals while helping to feed an increasingly hungry planet.

Perennial Possibilities

Recent advances in plant breeding, such as the use of marker-assisted selection, genomic in situ hybridization, transgenic technologies, and embryo rescue, coupled with traditional breeding techniques, make the development of perennial grain crops possible in the next 10 to 20 years. Two traditional approaches to developing these crops are direct domestication and wide hybridization, which have led to the wide variety of crops on which humans now rely. To directly domesticate a wild perennial, breeders select desirable plants from large populations of wild plants with a range of characteristics. Seeds are collected for replanting in order to increase the frequency of genes for desirable traits, such as large seed size, palatability, strong stems, and high seed yield. In wide hybridization, breeders cross an annual grain such as wheat with one of its wild perennial relatives, such as intermediate wheatgrass. They manage gene flow by making a large number of crosses between the annual and perennial plants, selecting offspring with desirable traits and repeating this cycle of crossing and selection multiple times. Ten of the 13 most widely grown grain and oilseed crops are capable of hybridization with perennial relatives.

The idea that plants can build and maintain perennial root systems and produce sufficient yields of edible grains seems counterintuitive. After all, plant resources, such as carbon captured through photosynthesis, must be allocated to different plant parts, and more resource allocation to roots would seem to mean that less can be allocated to seeds. Fortunately for the breeder, plants are relatively flexible organisms that are responsive to selection pressures, able to change the size of their resource "pies" depending on environmental conditions, and able to change the size of the slices of the resource pie. For example, when plant breeders take the wild plant out of its resource-strapped natural environment and place it into a managed environment with greater resources, the plant's resource pie can suddenly grow bigger, typically resulting in a larger plant.

Many perennial plants, with their larger overall size, offer greater potential for breeders to reallocate vegetative growth to seed production. Additionally, for a perennial grain crop to be successful in meeting our needs, it may need to live for only 5 to 10 years, far less than the lifespan of many wild perennials. In other words, the wild perennial is unnecessarily overbuilt for a managed agricultural setting. Some of the resources allocated to the plant's survival mechanisms, such as those allowing it to survive infrequent droughts or pest attacks, could be reallocated to seed production, and the crop would still persist in normal years.

Breeders see several other opportunities for perennials to achieve high seed yield. Perennials have greater access to resources over a longer growing season. They also have greater ability to maintain, over longer periods of time, the health and fertility of the soils in which they grow. Finally, the unprecedented success of plant breeders in recent decades in selecting for the simultaneous improvement of two or more characteristics that are typically negatively correlated with one another (meaning that as one characteristic increases, the other decreases, as is typical of seed yield and protein content) can be applied to perennial crop development.

Although current breeding efforts focused on developing perennial grain crops have been under way for less than a decade, the idea isn't new. Soviet researchers abandoned their attempts to develop perennial wheat through wide hybridization in the 1960s, in part because of the inherent difficulties of developing new crops at the time. California plant scientists in the 1960s also developed perennial wheat lines with yields similar to the then-lower-yielding annual wheat cultivars. At the time, large yield increases achieved in annuals overshadowed the modest success of these perennial programs, and the widespread environmental problems of annual crop production were not generally acknowledged.

In the late 1970s, Wes Jackson at the Land Institute revisited the possibility of developing perennial grain crops in his book *New Roots for Agriculture*. In the 1990s, plant breeders at the Land Institute initiated breeding programs for perennial wheat, sunflowers, sorghum, and some legumes. Some preliminary genetics work and hybridization research have also focused on perennial maize. Washington State University scientists have initiated a perennial wheat breeding program to address the high rates of erosion resulting from annual wheat production in eastern Washington. In 2001, some of those perennial wheat lines yielded 64% of the of the yield produced by the annual wheat cultivars grown in the region. Scientists at Kansas State University, the Kellogg Biological Station at Michigan State, the University of Manitoba, Texas A&M, and the University of Minnesota are carrying out additional plant breeding, genetics, or agronomic research on perennial grain crops.

The potential for perennial crops to tolerate or prevent adverse environmental conditions such as drought or soil salinity has attracted interest in other parts of the world. The conversion of native forests for annual wheat production in southwest Australia resulted in the rise of subsurface salts to the surface. This salinization threatens large areas of this non-irrigated, semi-arid agricultural region, and scientists there believe perennial crops would use more subsurface water, which would keep salts from rising to the surface and produce high-value crops. During the past decade, Australian scientists have been working to develop perennial wheat through wide hybridization and to domesticate a wild perennial grass for the region. More recently, plant breeders at the Food Crops Research Institute in Kunming, China, initiated programs to develop perennial rice to address the erosion problems associated with upland rice production. It is believed that perennial rice would also be more tolerant of the frequent drought conditions of some lowland areas. Scientists at the institute have also been evaluating perennial sorghum, sunflower, and intermediate wheatgrass for their potential as perennial grain crops.

Vision of a New Agriculture

The successful development of perennial grain crops would have different effects on the environment, on life at the dinner table, and on the farm. Producing grains from perennials rather than from annuals will have large environmental implications, but the consumer will see little if any difference at the dinner table. On the farm, whether mechanically harvested from large fields or hand-harvested in the parts of the world where equipment is prohibitively expensive, perennial grains 20 to 50 years from now will also look much the same to the farmer. The addition, however, of new high-value perennial crops to the farm would increase farmers' flexibility.

Farmers could use currently available management practices, such as no-till or organic approaches, but with a new array of high-value perennial grain crops. These would give farmers more options to have long rotations of perennial crops or rotations in which annuals are grown for several years followed by several years of perennials. Crop rotation aids in managing pests, diseases, and weeds but is often limited by the number of profitable crops from which farmers can choose. There are also opportunities to simultaneously grow annual and perennial grain crops or to grow multiple species of perennials together because of differences in rooting characteristics and growth habits. And because perennial grains regrow after seed harvest, livestock can be integrated into the system, allowing for greater use of the crops and therefore greater profit.

Although the environmental and food-security benefits of growing perennial grain crops are attractive, much work remains to be completed. For the great potential of perennial grain crops to be realized, more resources are needed to accelerate plant breeding programs with more personnel, land, and technological capacity; expand ecological and agronomic research on improved perennial germplasm; coordinate global activities through germplasm and scientist exchanges and conferences; identify global priority crop-lands; and develop training programs for young scientists in ecology, perennial plant breeding, and crop management.

Where, then, should the resources come from to support these objectives? The timeline for widespread production of perennials, given the need for extensive plant breeding work first, discourages private-sector investment at this point. As has occurred with biofuel production R&D, large-scale funding by governments or philanthropic foundations could greatly accelerate perennial grain crop development. As timelines for the release and production of perennial grain crops shorten, public and philanthropic support could increasingly be supplanted by support from companies providing agricultural goods and services. Although perennial grain crops might not initially interest large agribusinesses focused on annual grain crop production, the prospect of developing a suite of new goods and services, including equipment management consulting, and seeds, would be attractive to many entrepreneurial enterprises.

Although public support for additional federal programs is problematic given the current economic conditions, global conditions are changing rapidly. Much of the success of modern intensive agricultural production relies on cheap energy, a relatively stable climate, and the public's willingness to overlook widespread environmental problems. As energy prices increase and the costs of environmental degradation are increasingly appreciated, budgeting public money for long-term projects that will reduce resource consumption and depletion will probably become more politically popular. Rising food and fuel prices, climatic instability that threatens food production, and increased concern about the degradation of global ecological systems should place agriculture at the center of attention for multiple federal agencies and programs.

The USDA has the greatest capability to accelerate perennial grain crop development. Most important would be the use of research funds for the rapid expansion of plant breeding programs. Funds for breeding could be directed through the Agricultural Research Service and the competitive grant programs. Such investments directly support the objectives of the National Institute of Food and Agriculture (NIFA), created by the Food, Conservation and Energy Act of 2008, which will be responsible for awarding peer-reviewed grants for agricultural research. Modeled on the National Institutes of Health, NIFA objectives include enhancing agricultural and environmental sustainability and strengthening national security by improving food security in developing countries.

As varieties of perennial grain crops become available for more extensive testing, additional funds will be needed for agronomic and ecological research at multiple sites in the United States and elsewhere. This would include support for the training of students and scientists in managing perennial farming systems. Currently, less than $1.5 million directly supports perennial grain R&D projects around the world. USDA funds will provide less than $300,000 annually over the next few years through competitive grant awards, primarily for the study and development of perennial wheat and wheatgrass. Much of the rest is provided by the Land Institute.

Once the suitability of a perennial grain crop is well established, support from federal programs for farmers might be needed to encourage the initial adoption of new crops and practices. Farm subsidies, distributed through the USDA and which now primarily support annual cropping systems, could be used to encourage fundamental changes in farming practices, such as those offered by perennial grain crop development. Public funds supporting the Conservation Reserve Program (CRP) could be redirected toward transitioning CRP lands, once the federal contracts have expired, to perennial grain production. The CRR initially established in the 1985 farm bill, pays farmers to remove highly erodible croplands from production and to plant them for 10 years with grasses, trees, and other long-term cover to stabilize the soil. Some 36 million acres are enrolled in the program, and most are unsuitable or marginal for annual grain crop production but would be suitable for the production of perennials.

One obstacle to supporting programs necessary to achieve such long-term goals is the short timeframes of current policy agencies. The farm bill is revisited every five years and focuses primarily on farm exports, commodities, subsidies, food programs, and some soil conservation measures. Thus, it is poorly suited to deal with long-term agendas and larger objectives. The short-term objectives can change with changes in the political fortunes of those in charge of approving the bill. The Land Institute's Jackson has proposed a 50-year farm bill to serve as compass for the five-year bills. This longer-term agenda would focus on the larger environmental issues and on rebuilding and preserving farm communities. In the near term, Jackson proposes that, during an initial buildup phase, the federal government should fund 80 plant breeders and geneticists who would develop perennial grain, legume, and oilseed crops, and 30 agricultural and ecological scientists to develop the necessary agronomic systems. They would work on six to eight major crop species at diverse locations. Budgeting $400,000 per scientist-year for salaries and research costs would add less than $50 million annually to the farm bill, a blip in a bill that will cost taxpayers $288 billion between 2008 and 2012.

Some limited federal money has already been awarded for research related to perennial grain through the USDAs, competitive grants programs. Most recently, researchers at Michigan State University received funding to study the ecosystem services and performance of perennial wheat lines obtained from Washington State University and the Land Institute. The Green Lands Blue Waters Initiative, a multistate network of universities, individual scientists, and nonprofit research organizations, is also advocating the development of perennial grain crops, along with other perennial forage, biofuel, and tree crops.

Although agriculture has traditionally been primarily the concern of the USDA, it now plays an increasingly important role in how we meet challenges—international food security, environmental protection, climate change, energy supply, economic sustainability, and human health—beyond the primary concerns of that agency. Public programs intended to address these challenges should consider the development of perennial grain crops a priority. For example, programs at the NSF, Department of Energy (DOE), Environmental Protection Agency, and the National Oceanic and Atmospheric Administration and U.S. international assistance and development programs could provide additional incentives through research programs or subsidies.

Currently, no government funding agencies, including the USDA, specifically target the development of perennial crops as they do for biofuels. In the 2009 federal economic stimulus package alone, the DOE was appropriated $786.5 million in funds to accelerate biofuels research and commercialization. The displacement of food crops by biofuel crops recently played a significant role in the rise of global food prices and resulted in increased hunger and social unrest in many parts of the world. Although some argue that biofuel crops should be grown only on marginal lands unsuited for annual food crops, perennial crops have the potential to be grown on those same lands and be used for food, feed, and fuel.

Substantial public funding of perennial grain crops need not be permanent. As economically viable crops become widely produced, farmers and businesses will have opportunities to market their own seeds and management inputs just as they do with currently available crops. Although private-sector companies may not profit as much from selling fertilizers and pesticides to farmers producing perennial grains, they will probably adapt to these new crops with new products and services. The ability of farmers to spread the initial planting costs over several seasons rather that meet these costs each year opens up opportunities for more expensive seed with improved characteristics.

Although the timelines for development and widespread production of perennial grain crops may seem long, the potential payoffs stretch far into the future, and the financial costs are low relative to other publicly funded agricultural expenditures. Adding perennial grains to our agricultural arsenal will give farmers more choices in what they can grow and where, while sustainably producing food for the growing population.

Adding perennial grains to our agricultural arsenal will give farmers more choices in what they can grow and where, while sustainably producing food for the growing population.

Recommended Reading

T. S. Cox, J. D. Glover, D. L. Van Tassel, C. M. Cox, and L. R. DeHaan, "Prospects for Developing Perennial Grain Crops," *BioScience* 56 (2006): 649–659.

J. D. Glover, C. M. Cox, and J. P. Reganold, "Future Farming: A Return to Roots?" *Scientfic American* 297 (2007): 66–73.

Green Lands, Blue Waters, *A Vision and Roadmap for the Next Generation of Agricultural Systems* (www.greenlandsbluewaters.org).

W. Jackson, *New Roots for Agriculture* (Lincoln, NE: University of Nebraska, 1980).

W. Jackson, *A 50-year Farm Bill* (www.landinstitute.org/pages/50yrfb-booklet_7-29-09.pdf).

N. Jordan, G. Boody, W. Broussard, J. D. Glover, D. Keeney, B. H. McCown, G. McIsaac, M. Muller, H. Murray, J. Neal, C. Pansing, R. E. Turner, K. Warner, and D. Wyse, "Sustainable Development of the Agricultural Bio-Economy," *Science* 316 (2007): 1570–1571.

Critical Thinking

1. Are the current grains that feed the world annual crops or perennial crops?

2. How do perennial grain crops differ from annual grain crops?

3. What are the advantages and disadvantages of creating perennial grain crops?

4. Identify the three grain crops that provide 70 percent of calories for human consumption worldwide.

JERRY D. GLOVER is an agroecologist with the Land Institute in Salina, Kansas. **JOHN P. REGANOLD** (reganold@wsu.edu) is a Regents professor in the Department of Crop and Soil Sciences at Washington State University in Pullman, Washington.

Draining Our Future

The Growing Shortage of Freshwater

Global demand for freshwater has tripled in the last half century and will continue to grow along with population increases and economic development. Shrinking water supplies endanger not only the natural environment, but also food and energy supplies and even statehood and international stability.

Lester R. Brown

The world is incurring a vast water deficit—one that is largely invisible, historically recent, and growing fast. Globally, demand for water has tripled over the last half century, and millions of irrigation wells have been drilled, pushing water withdrawals beyond recharge rates. In other words, we're now mining groundwater.

Governments have failed to limit pumping to the sustainable yield of aquifers. The result: Water tables are now falling in countries that contain more than half the world's people, including the big three grain producers—China, India, and the United States.

The link between water and food is strong: We each drink on average nearly four liters of water per day in one form or another, while 500 times as much water is required to produce our daily food totals. Seventy percent of all water use is for irrigation, compared with 20% used by industry and 10% used for residential purposes. With the demand for water growing in all three categories, competition among sectors is intensifying—and agriculture almost always loses. While most people recognize that the world is facing a future of water shortages, not everyone has connected the dots to see that this also means a future of food shortages.

World's Water Tables Are Dropping

Scores of countries are overpumping aquifers as they struggle to satisfy their growing water needs. Most aquifers are replenishable, but when they are depleted—as may happen in India, for instance—the maximum rate of pumping will be automatically reduced to the rate of recharge.

Fossil aquifers, however, are not replenishable. If the vast U.S. Ogallala aquifer or the Saudi aquifer, for example, become depleted, pumping comes to an end. Farmers who lose their irrigation water have the option of returning to lower-yield dryland farming if rainfall permits. But in more arid regions, such as in the southwestern United States or the Middle East, the loss of irrigation water means the end of agriculture.

Falling water tables are already adversely affecting harvests in some countries, including China, which rivals the United States as the world's largest grain producer. A 2001 groundwater survey revealed that the water table is falling fast under the North China Plain—an area that produces more than half of the country's wheat and a third of its corn. Overpumping has largely depleted the shallow aquifer, forcing well drillers to turn to the region's deep aquifer, which is not replenishable.

The World Bank warns, "Anecdotal evidence suggests that deep wells [drilled] around Beijing now have to reach 1,000 meters [more than half a mile] to tap fresh water, adding dramatically to the cost of supply." In unusually strong language for a Bank report, it foresees "catastrophic consequences for future generations" unless water use and supply can quickly be brought back into balance.

Falling water tables, the conversion of cropland to nonfarm uses, and the loss of farm labor in provinces that are rapidly industrializing are combining to shrink China's grain harvest. The wheat crop, grown mostly in semiarid northern China, is particularly vulnerable to water shortages. After peaking at 123 million tons in 1997, the harvest has fallen, coming in at 105 million tons in 2007, a drop of 15%.

According to the World Bank, China is mining underground water in three adjacent river basins in the north—those of the Hai, the Yellow, and the Huai. Since it takes 1,000 tons of water to produce one ton of grain, the Hai basin's shortfall of nearly 40 billion tons of water per year means that, when the aquifer is depleted, the grain harvest will drop by 40 million tons—enough to have fed 120 million Chinese.

As serious as water shortages are in China, they are even more serious in India, where the margin between food consumption and survival is so precarious. India's grain harvest, squeezed both by water scarcity and the loss of cropland to nonfarm uses, has plateaued since 2000. This helps explain why India reemerged as a leading wheat importer in 2006. Some 15% of India's food supply is produced by mining groundwater, the World Bank reports. In other words, 175 million Indians are fed with grain produced with water from irrigation wells that will soon go dry.

As water tables fall, the energy required for pumping rises. In both India and China, the rising electricity demand from irrigation is satisfied largely by building coal-fired power plants.

In the United States, according to the Department of Agriculture, the underground water table has dropped by more than 30 meters (100 feet) in parts of Texas, Oklahoma, and Kansas—three leading grain-producing states. As a result, wells have gone dry on thousands of farms in the southern Great Plains, forcing farmers to return to lower-yielding dryland farming. Although this mining of underground water is taking a toll on U.S. grain production, irrigated land accounts for only one-fifth of the U.S. grain harvest, compared with close to three-fifths of the harvest in India and four-fifths in China.

Other countries affected by falling water tables include:

- **Pakistan,** where future irrigation water cutbacks as a result of aquifer depletion will undoubtedly reduce grain harvest.
- **Iran,** which is overpumping its aquifers by an average of 5 billion tons of water per year, the water equivalent of one-third of its annual grain harvest. Villages in eastern Iran are being abandoned as wells go dry, generating a flow of "water refugees."
- **Saudi Arabia,** which is as water-poor as it is oil-rich. With plunging fossil water reservoirs, irrigated agriculture in Saudi Arabia could last for another decade or so and then will largely vanish.
- **Yemen,** with a water table falling by roughly 2 meters a year as water use outstrips the sustainable yield of aquifers. With its population growing at 3% a year and water tables falling everywhere, Yemen is fast becoming a hydrological basket case. Its grain production has fallen by two-thirds over the last 20 years, and it now imports four-fifths of its grain supply.
- **Israel,** which is depleting both of its principal aquifers, despite being a pioneer in raising irrigation water productivity. Because of severe water shortages, Israel has banned the irrigation of wheat. Conflicts between Israelis and Palestinians over the allocation of water are ongoing.
- **Mexico,** where population is projected to reach 132 million by 2050 and where demand for water is outstripping supply. More than half of all the water extracted from underground is from aquifers that are being overpumped.

Since the overpumping of aquifers is occurring in many countries more or less simultaneously, the depletion of aquifers and the resulting harvest cutbacks could come at roughly the same time. And the accelerating depletion of aquifers means this day may come soon, creating potentially unmanageable food scarcity.

Rivers Running Dry and Lakes Shrinking

Falling water tables are largely hidden, but we can see rivers that are drained dry or reduced to a trickle before they reach the sea. The Colorado—the major river in the southwestern United States—and the Yellow—the largest river in northern China—are two rivers where this phenomenon can be seen. Others include the Nile, the lifeline of Egypt; the Indus, which supplies most of Pakistan's irrigation water; and the Ganges in India's densely populated Gangetic basin. Many smaller rivers have disappeared entirely.

Compounding the growing demand for water is the demand for hydroelectric power, which has grown even faster. Dams and diversions of river water have drained many rivers dry. As water tables have fallen, the springs that feed rivers have gone dry, reducing river flows.

Since 1950, the number of large dams (more than 15 meters high) has increased from 5,000 to 45,000. Each dam deprives a river of some of its flow. Engineers like to say that dams built to generate electricity take only a river's energy, not its water, but this is not entirely true. Reservoirs increase evaporation. The annual loss of water from a reservoir in arid or semiarid regions, where evaporation rates are high, is typically equal to 10% of its storage capacity.

The Colorado River now rarely makes it to the sea. With the states of Colorado, Utah, Arizona, Nevada, and California depending heavily on the Colorado's water, there is little, if any, water left when it reaches the Gulf of California. This excessive demand for water is destroying the river's ecosystem, including its fisheries.

Pakistan, like Egypt, is essentially a river-based civilization, heavily dependent on the Indus. This river, originating in the Himalayas and flowing southwestward to the Indian Ocean, not only provides surface water, but it also recharges aquifers that supply the irrigation wells dotting the Pakistani countryside. In the face of Pakistan's growing population and water demand, the Indus, too, is starting to run dry in its lower reaches.

The same problem exists with the overused Tigris and Euphrates rivers, which originate in Turkey and flow through Syria and Iraq en route to the Persian Gulf. Large dams erected in Turkey and Iraq have reduced water flow to the once "fertile crescent," helping to destroy 80% of the vast wetlands that formerly enriched the delta region.

In river systems such as the Colorado, the Yellow, the Nile, and many others around the world, virtually all the water in the basin is being used. Inevitably, if people upstream get more water, those downstream will get less. Allocating water among competing interests, within and among societies, is part of an emerging politics of resource scarcity.

Lakes, too, are shrinking or even disappearing, including some of the world's best known: Lake Chad in Central Africa, the Aral Sea in Central Asia, and the Sea of Galilee (also known as Lake Tiberias).

With the Jordan's flow further diminished as it passes through Israel, the Dead Sea is shrinking even faster than the Sea of Galilee. Over the past 40 years, its water level has dropped by some 25 meters (nearly 80 feet). It could disappear entirely by 2050.

Of all the shrinking lakes and inland seas, none has gotten as much attention as the Aral Sea. Its ports, once centers of commerce, are now abandoned, looking like the ghost mining towns of the American West. Once one of the world's largest freshwater bodies, the Aral has lost four-fifths of its volume since 1960, as Soviet planners diverted water from its feeding rivers to an expanding cotton and textile industry. By 1990, an aerial view of the dry, salt-covered seabed resembled the surface of the Moon.

As the sea shrank, the salt concentrations climbed until the fish died. The thriving fishery that once yielded 50,000 tons of seafood per year disappeared, as did the jobs on the fishing boats and in the fish processing factories.

Lakes are disappearing on every continent and for the same reasons: excessive diversion of water from rivers and over-pumping of aquifers. No one knows exactly how many lakes have disappeared over the last half century, but we do know that thousands of them now exist only on old maps.

Farmers Losing to Cities

Water tensions among countries are more likely to make the headlines, but it is the jousting for water between cities and farms within countries that preoccupies local political leaders. The economics of water use do not favor farmers in this competition, simply because it takes so much water to produce food. For example, while it takes only 14 tons of water to make a ton of steel worth $560, it takes 1,000 tons of water to grow a ton of wheat worth $200. In countries preoccupied with expanding the economy and creating jobs, agriculture becomes the residual claimant.

Many of the world's largest cities are located in water-sheds where all available water is being used. Cities in such watersheds—Mexico City, Cairo, and Beijing, for example—can increase their water consumption only by importing water from other basins or taking it from agriculture. Increasingly, the world's cities are meeting their growing needs by taking irrigation water from farmers. Among the U.S. cities doing so are San Diego, Los Angeles, Las Vegas, Denver, and El Paso.

The competition between farmers and cities for underground water resources is intensifying throughout India. Nowhere is this more evident than in Chennai (formerly Madras), a city of 7 million on the east coast of south India. The government has failed to supply water for some of the city's residents, so a thriving tank-truck industry has emerged to bring in water that it buys from farmers.

For farmers surrounding the city, the price of water far exceeds the value of the crops they can produce with it. Unfortunately, the 13,000 tankers hauling the water to Chennai are mining the underground water resources. Water tables are falling and shallow wells have gone dry. Eventually even the deeper wells will go dry, depriving these communities of both their food supply and their livelihood.

Chinese farmers along the Juma River downstream from Beijing discovered in 2004 that the river had suddenly stopped flowing. A diversion dam had been built near the capital to take river water for Yanshan Petrochemical, a state-owned industry. The farmers protested bitterly, but it was a losing battle. For the 120,000 villagers downstream from the diversion dam, the loss of water could cripple their ability to make a living from farming.

Literally hundreds of cities in other countries are meeting their growing water needs by taking the water that farmers count on. In western Turkey, for example, the historic city of Izmir now relies heavily on well fields (a network of wells connected by pipe) from the neighboring agricultural district of Manisa.

In the U.S. southern Great Plains and Southwest, where virtually all water is now spoken for, the growing water needs of cities and thousands of small towns can be satisfied only by taking water from agriculture.

Colorado has one of the world's most active water markets. Fast-growing cities and towns in a state with high immigration are buying irrigation water rights from farmers and ranchers. And in 2003, San Diego made a 75-year deal to buy annual rights to 247 million tons of water from farmers in the nearby Imperial Valley—the largest farm-to-city water transfer in U.S. history. Without irrigation water, the highly productive land owned by these farmers is wasteland. The farmers who are selling their water rights would like to continue farming, but city officials are offering far more for the water than the farmers could possibly earn by irrigating crops.

Whether it is outright government expropriation, farmers being outbid by cities, or cities simply drilling deeper wells than farmers can afford, the world's farmers are losing the water war. They are faced with not only a shrinking water supply in many situations, but also a shrinking share of that shrinking supply. Slowly but surely, fast-growing cities are siphoning water from the world's farmers even as they try to feed some 70 million more people each year.

Scarcity Crosses National Borders

Water scarcity has historically been a local issue. It was up to national governments to balance water supply and demand. Now, scarcity crosses national boundaries via the international grain trade. It takes a thousand tons of water to produce one ton of grain, so importing grain is the most efficient way to import water. In effect, countries are using grain to balance their water books. Similarly, trading in grain futures is in a sense trading in water futures.

After China and India, there is a second tier of smaller countries with large water deficits. Algeria, Egypt, and Mexico already import much of their grain. Pakistan, too, may soon turn to world markets for grain, with a population outgrowing its water supply.

From Morocco to Iran, the Middle East and North Africa region has become the world's fastest-growing grain import market. The demand for grain is driven both by rapid population growth and by rising affluence, thanks largely to oil exports. Virtually every country in the region is pressing against its water limits, so the growing urban demand for water can be satisfied only by taking irrigation water from agriculture.

Egypt has become a major importer of wheat in recent years, vying with Japan for the top spot as the world's leading wheat importer. Egypt now imports close to 40% of its total grain supply, a dependence that reflects a population that is outgrowing the grain harvest produced with the Nile's water. And Algeria imports well over half of its grain.

The water now required to produce a year's worth of grain and other farm products imported into the Middle East and North Africa nearly equals the annual flow of the Nile River at Aswan. In effect, the region's water deficit can be thought of as another Nile flowing into the region in the form of imported food.

It is often said that future wars in the Middle East will more likely be fought over water than oil, but in reality the competition for water is taking place in world grain markets. The countries that are financially the strongest, not necessarily those that are militarily the strongest, will fare best in this competition.

Knowing where grain deficits will be concentrated tomorrow requires looking at where water deficits are developing today. Thus far, the countries importing much of their grain have been smaller ones. Now we are looking at fast-growing water deficits in both China and India, each with more than a billion people.

As noted earlier, overpumping is a way of satisfying growing food demand that virtually guarantees a future drop in food production when aquifers are depleted. Many countries are essentially creating a "food bubble economy"—one in which food production is artificially inflated by the unsustainable mining of groundwater. At what point does water scarcity translate into food scarcity?

David Seckler and his colleagues at the International Water Management Institute, the world's premier water research group, summarized this issue well: "Many of the most populous countries of the world—China, India, Pakistan, Mexico, and nearly all the countries of the Middle East and North Africa—have literally been having a free ride over the past two or three decades by depleting their groundwater resources. The penalty for mismanagement of this valuable resource is now coming due and it is no exaggeration to say that the results could be catastrophic for these countries and, given their importance, for the world as a whole."

Water Scarcity Yields Political Stresses

We typically measure well-being in economic terms—in income per person—but water well-being is measured in cubic meters or tons of water per person. A country with an annual supply of 1,700 cubic meters of water per person is well supplied with water, able to comfortably meet agricultural, industrial, and residential needs. Below this level, stresses begin to appear. When water supply drops below 1,000 cubic meters per person, people face scarcity. Below 500 cubic meters, acute scarcity, they suffer from hydrological poverty—living without enough water to produce food or, in some cases, even for basic hygiene.

The world's most severe water stresses are found in North Africa and the Middle East. While Morocco and Egypt have fewer than 1,000 cubic meters per person per year, Algeria, Tunisia, and Libya have fewer than 500. Some countries, including Saudi Arabia, Yemen, Kuwait, and Israel, have less than 300 cubic meters per person per year. A number of sub-Saharan countries are also facing water stress, including Kenya and Rwanda.

While national averages indicate an adequate water supply in each of the world's three most populous countries—China, India, and the United States—regions within these countries also suffer from acute water shortages. Water is scarce throughout the northern half of China. In India, the northwestern region suffers extreme water scarcity. For the United States, the southwestern states from Texas to California are experiencing acute water shortages.

Although the risk of international conflict over water is real, so far there have been remarkably few water wars. Water tensions tend to build more within societies, particularly where water is already scarce and population growth is rapid. Recent years have witnessed conflicts over water in scores of countries, such as the competition between cities and farmers in countries like China, India, and Yemen. In other countries, the conflicts are between tribes, as in Kenya, or between villages, as in India and China, or between upstream and downstream water users, as in Pakistan or China. In some countries, local water conflicts have led to violence and death, as in Kenya, Pakistan, and China.

In Pakistan's arid southwest province of Balochistan, water tables are falling everywhere as a fast-growing local population swelled by Afghan refugees is pumping water far faster than aquifers can recharge. The provincial capital of Quetta is facing a particularly dire situation. And Iraq is concerned that dam building on the Euphrates River in Turkey and Syria will leave it without enough water to meet its basic needs. The flow into Iraq of the Euphrates River has shrunk by half over the last few decades.

Many of the countries high on the list of failing states are those where populations are outrunning their water supplies.

At the global level, most of the projected population growth of nearly 3 billion by 2050 will come in countries where water tables are already falling. The states most stressed by the scarcity of water tend to be those in arid and semiarid regions, with fast-growing populations and a resistance to family planning. Many of the countries high on the list of failing states are those where populations are outrunning their water supplies: Sudan, Iraq, Somalia, Chad, Afghanistan, Pakistan, and Yemen, for instance. Unless population can be stabilized in these countries, the continually shrinking supply of water per person will put still more stress on already overstressed governments.

Although spreading water shortages is a daunting problem, we have the technologies needed to raise water use efficiency, thus buying time to stabilize population size. Prominent among these technologies are those for more water-efficient irrigation, industrial water recycling, and urban water recycling.

Raising Water Productivity

Raising irrigation efficiency is central to raising water productivity overall. Using more water-efficient irrigation technologies and shifting to crops that use less water permit the expansion of irrigated area even with a fixed water supply. Eliminating water and energy subsidies that encourage wasteful water use allows water prices to rise to market levels. Higher water prices encourage all water users to use water more efficiently. In many countries, local rural water users associations that directly involve users in water management have raised water productivity.

Evaporation, percolation, and runoff also reduce irrigation's efficiency. In surface water projects—that is, dams that deliver water to farmers through a network of canals—crop usage of irrigation water never reaches 100%. Water policy analysts Sandra Postel and Amy Vickers found that "surface water irrigation efficiency ranges between 25% and 40% in India, Mexico, Pakistan, the Philippines, and Thailand; between 40% and 45% in Malaysia and Morocco; and between 50% and 60% in Israel, Japan, and Taiwan." In hot arid regions, the evaporation of irrigation water is far higher than in cooler humid regions.

In 2004, China's Minister of Water Resources Wang Shucheng shared details of China's plans to raise irrigation efficiency from 43% in 2000 to 55% in 2030. The steps included raising the price of water, providing incentives for adopting more irrigation-efficient technologies, and developing the local institutions to manage this process. Reaching these goals, he felt, would assure China's future food security.

Raising irrigation water efficiency typically means shifting from the less-efficient flood or furrow system to overhead sprinklers or drip irrigation, the gold standard of irrigation efficiency. Switching from flood or furrow to low-pressure sprinkler systems reduces water use by an estimated 30%, while switching to drip irrigation typically cuts water use in half.

A few small countries—Cyprus, Israel, and Jordan—rely heavily on drip irrigation. Among the big three agricultural producers, this more efficient technology is used on 1%–3% of irrigated land in India and China and on roughly 4% in the United States.

In recent years, small-scale drip-irrigation systems—virtually a bucket with flexible plastic tubing to distribute the water—have been developed to irrigate small vegetable gardens with roughly 100 plants (covering 25 square meters). Somewhat larger drum systems irrigate 125 square meters. In both cases, the containers are elevated slightly, so that gravity distributes the water. Large-scale drip systems using plastic lines that can be moved easily are also becoming popular. These simple systems can pay for themselves in one year. By simultaneously reducing water costs and raising yields, they can dramatically raise incomes of smallholders.

In the Punjab, with its extensive double cropping of wheat and rice, fast-falling water tables led the state farmers' commission in 2007 to recommend a delay in transplanting rice from May to late June or early July. This would reduce irrigation water use by roughly one-third, since transplanting would coincide with the arrival of the monsoon. This reduction in groundwater use would help stabilize the water table, which has fallen from 5 meters below the surface to 30 meters in parts of the state.

Institutional shifts—specifically, moving the responsibility for managing irrigation systems from government agencies to local water users associations—can facilitate the more efficient use of water. In many countries, farmers are organizing locally so they can assume this responsibility. Since they have an economic stake in good water management, they tend to do a better job than a distant government agency.

Mexico is a leader in developing water users associations. As of 2002, farmers associations managed more than 80% of Mexico's publicly irrigated land. One advantage of this shift for the government is that the cost of maintaining the irrigation system is assumed locally, reducing the drain on the treasury. This means that associations often need to charge more for irrigation water, but for farmers the production gains from managing their water supply themselves more than outweigh this additional outlay.

Low water productivity is often the result of low water prices. In many countries, subsidies lead to irrationally low water prices, creating the impression that water is abundant when in fact it is scarce. As water becomes scarce, it needs to be priced accordingly.

What is needed now is a new mind-set, a new way of thinking about water use. For example, shifting to more water-efficient crops wherever possible boosts water productivity. Rice production is being phased out around Beijing because rice is such a thirsty crop. Similarly, Egypt restricts rice production in favor of wheat.

Any measures that raise crop yields on irrigated land also raise the productivity of irrigation water. Similarly, any measures that convert grain into animal protein more efficiently in effect increase water productivity.

For people consuming unhealthy amounts of livestock products, moving down the food chain reduces water use. In the United States, where annual consumption of grain as food and feed averages some 800 kilograms (four-fifths of a ton) per person, a modest reduction in the consumption of meat, milk, and eggs could easily cut grain use per person by 100 kilograms. For 300 million Americans, such a reduction would cut grain use by 30 million tons and irrigation water use by 30 billion tons.

Reducing water use to the sustainable yield of aquifers and rivers worldwide involves a wide range of measures not only in agriculture but throughout the economy. The more obvious steps, in addition to more water-efficient irrigation practices and more water-efficient crops, include adopting more water-efficient industrial processes and using more water-efficient household appliances. Recycling urban water supplies is another obvious step to consider in countries facing acute water shortages.

Unless we commit to a plan for restoring water security, our water planet's future will be thirstier, hungrier, and more precarious. The good news is that momentum is building to reverse the damaging environmental and resource trends that we ourselves have set in motion.

Critical Thinking

1. Identify the nations that are at greatest risk of depleting their water supply. Within the United States, which states are at greatest risk of depleting their water supply?

2. What is causing underground water tables to decline, rivers to shrink or dry up, and lakes levels to decline?

3. What type of arrangements are being made between governments and farmers to ensure water is available for cities?

LESTER R. BROWN is president of the Earth Policy Institute, 1350 Connecticut Avenue, N.W., Suite 403, Washington, D.C. 20036. Website www.earthpolicy.org.

In Search of Sustainability

Seeking to reduce energy costs and to protect the environment, companies are exploring 'green' manufacturing practices and sustainable/renewable packaging applications.

KAREN NACHAY

Skyrocketing energy costs are hitting our pocketbooks, and a growing awareness of environmental issues is affecting our lifestyles. As a result, members of both the public and business communities are examining ways to reduce costs and promote their environmental consciousness by using renewable or sustainable sources of energy rather than nonrenewable sources like fossil fuels. As people reduce the number of miles they drive and switch from plastic to paper, or better yet, reusable cloth bags, they are also looking toward business to make sound changes. And many businesses are responding by installing technologies to help reduce energy usage and costs, redesigning packaging to use less material, or engineering innovative processing methods.

"It is no longer enough to create a quality product," said John Z. Blazevich, CEO of Contessa Premium Foods, Los Angeles, Calif., which opened the doors to a fully energy-efficient, eco-friendly frozen food plant earlier this year. "How you produce it is now the most important thing. Consumers are concerned about global warming and many blame big business for its role in it."

Companies are learning that this not only makes good sense for the environment, it makes good business sense, too. Information Resources Inc. recently conducted a survey that asked 22,000 U.S. consumers about their purchasing habits of products marketed as sustainable or green in four categories: eco-friendly products, eco-friendly packaging, organic, and fair treatment of employees and suppliers. The results revealed that about 30% of consumers look for eco-friendly products and packaging when choosing between brands. Consumers age 55 and older were much more likely to take these four categories into consideration when making a purchase. (See sidebar, "Green Products Gain Market Share," on page 166 for more information about the purchasing habits of consumers.)

"It's a new reality that manufacturers and retailers will need to address with new products and unique assortments to tap into emerging growth potential," said Andrew Salzman, Chief Marketing Officer, IRI. "Safeguarding the environment in whatever small way is becoming a consumer priority. And all successful consumer packaged goods industry mainstays live by one basic fact of life: The consumer's priorities are the industry's priorities."

Developing and implementing environmentally friendly initiatives and sourcing sustainable ingredients and raw materials are not always easy, as the process often requires a large investment, both financially and in the commitment from the company, its employees, and, quite often, the community. This article will provide information about what some food companies—both large and small—have done to improve the sustainable and eco-friendly nature of their processing and packaging operations.

Green Plants Save Energy

The food industry requires energy and water for processing, storage, and transport of food and beverage products, and the cost can be quite burdensome. Food processors, realizing the need to reduce their energy costs, as well as to lower greenhouse gas emissions, are harnessing the power of the wind and sun—sources of renewable energy—as well as recycling and reusing water from processing streams, installing energy-efficient equipment, and designing buildings with improved ventilation systems and more natural light. And even food by-products and organic food waste become sources of energy as part of companies' solid waste management and recycling efforts. For example, H.J. Heinz Co., Pittsburgh, Pa., in May announced plans to reduce greenhouse gas emissions through a series of initiatives, among them converting potato peels from its Ontario, Ore., facility into biofuel that will be sold to a local natural gas pipeline grid. And Miller Brewing Co., Milwaukee, Wis., operates a brewery in Irwindale, Calif., where brewery wastewater is recycled to generate bio-gas used to power electrical generators (Miller, 2008).

Frito-Lay, Plano, Texas, a division of PepsiCo, let the sun shine in earlier this year when it flipped the switch on a field of solar concentrators at its Modesto, Calif., *SunChips* manufacturing facility. Here, 54,000 sq ft of concave mirrors absorb sunlight while 192 solar collectors generate steam used to heat the cooking oil for the chips, thereby helping the company reduce its use of natural gas and the cost associated with it. The California Energy Commission provided a grant and the National Renewable Energy Laboratory, part of the U.S. Dept. of Energy, reviewed the design. Last year, the company installed a photovoltaic solar electric power system on

Fair Trade Helps More than the Environment

Check the packages of many different food products and you will see phrases such as "sustainably produced" and "fair trade" listed. These apply to a variety of products, including coffee, chocolate, tea, certain fruits, seafood, and wine. Both terms fall under the umbrella of sustainable agriculture, which refers to farming that does not irreversibly damage the land while at the same time improves or enhances the lives of farmers and members of their communities. Generally speaking, the farming methods employed minimize soil erosion and balance the amount of water used in irrigation with the amount that would be replenished naturally, all while reducing the amount of nonrenewable sources used to accomplish this. The 1990 Farm Bill describes sustainable agriculture as "an integrated system of plant and animal production practices having a site-specific application that will, over the long term, satisfy human food and fiber needs; enhance environmental quality and the natural resource base upon which the agricultural economy depends; make the most-efficient use of nonrenewable resources and on-farm resources and integrate, where appropriate, natural biological cycles and controls; sustain the economic viability of farm operations; and enhance the quality of life for farmers and society as a whole" (FACTA, 1990).

The goal of fair trade is to address global poverty by paying a fair price to farmers in Central and South America, Africa, and Asia for growing and harvesting such crops as coffee and cocoa. Food companies often work directly with farmers, suppliers, and exporters. According to the International Fair Trade Association (IFTA), a network of fair trade organizations from around the world, a fair price "covers not only the costs of production but enables production which is socially just and environmentally sound."

Paying farmers/producers a fair price is one of 10 standards that IFTA says fair trade organizations must follow. The others cited by the organization include creating economic opportunities for producers; improving transparency and accountability; helping producers to build their independence; promoting fair trade; promoting gender equity; ensuring safe and healthy working conditions; following child labor laws and regulations; respecting and protecting the environment; and maintaining trade relations. IFTA issues a certification mark to registered organizations that follow these fair trade standards.

A second organization, Fairtrade Labelling Organizations International (FLO), issues a certification mark for products that meet fair trade standards, as well as sets standards for 20 labeling initiatives such as Max Havelaar and TransFair USA used in 21 countries to label fair trade products.

Companies such as Starbucks, Cargill, Sara Lee, Hain Celestial Group, and many more that buy and sell coffee, cocoa, and other commodities participate in sustainable agriculture programs. Ingredients like vanilla can be certified as fair trade, and within the past several years, flavor manufacturers Virginia Dare and David Michael & Co. began offering it. At this year's IFT Annual Meeting and Food Expo in New Orleans, La., David Michael showcased its fair trade vanilla, which is certified by TransFair USA, in a *Double Bourbon and Cola* beverage made with vanilla ice cream.

Datamonitor predicts growth of 15.7% in the global sales of fair trade products for 2007–12. FLO reported that in the largest markets—the UK and the United States—sales of fair trade products grew by 72% and 46%, respectively, in 2007. The fastest-growing markets—Sweden and Norway—had sales increases of 166% and 110%, respectively.

the roof of its Arizona Service Center in Phoenix. The system produces no emissions and generates about 350,000 kWh of electricity to meet the daytime energy requirements for the facility, which is Frito-Lay's largest U.S. distribution center.

Other companies such as Decas Cranberry Products Inc., Carver, Mass., are investigating the use of wind as a way to generate energy. First used to grind grain and pump water, today's modern windmills—called wind turbines—are viewed as sustainable instruments in energy production. Decas in May began operating a wind turbine that should produce 3,279,000 kWh—or about half of the energy that the company uses per year. Ice cream manufacturer Mackie's, Aberdeenshire, Scotland, uses three wind turbines at its facility to meet about half of its total energy use of 3,000,000 kWh/year. A wind turbine icon and the phrase "made with 100% renewable energy" appear on the cartons of ice cream as a way, according to the company, to show its commitment to functioning as a carbon-neutral facility.

Certifying Green Buildings

Utilizing sustainable ways to generate energy recently earned Kettle Foods, Salem, Ore., a gold level certification for Leadership in Energy and Environmental Design (LEED) from the U.S.

Green Building Council (USGBC) for its new potato chip factory in Beloit, Wis. USGBC is a nonprofit organization with more than 15,000 members from across the building industry dedicated to sustainable construction. According to Jim Green, Kettle Foods spokesman, the company's goal was to be the first U.S. food manufacturing facility to earn the LEED gold certification, and it worked with engineers and architects who had experience with green building practices.

The company's 73,000-sq-ft building, which USGBC called "the greenest food manufacturing plant in the United States," contains energy-efficient equipment to reduce the use of natural gas and electricity and has the capacity to filter and reuse 1.65 million gallons of water used in the potato washers. The 18 wind turbines generate enough energy to produce 56,000 bags of potato chips per year and offset 100% of the building's electricity use. The company sourced more than 35% of building materials from within 500 miles of the facility's site. Even improving and protecting the indoor air quality was addressed by using zero-volatile organic compounds paints and increasing the ventilation for fresh air.

"The plant is green from the carpet, counters, and paint to the rooftop wind turbines and sophisticated water reclamation system that recycles potato wash water into gray water used to flush toilets," Green said.

Green Products Gain Market Share

Both manufacturers and consumers are embracing the green movement, according to data from market research company Mintel.

The percentage of consumers who purchased products made with recycled packaging and/or manufactured in an energy-efficient, environmentally friendly way jumped from 12% in August 2006 to 36% in December 2007 (Mintel, 2008b).

"We're seeing the green movement rapidly transition from niche to mainstream," said Colleen Ryan, Senior Analyst, Mintel, in a statement. "Major companies have jumped on board, promotional messages have changed, and the American public is increasingly looking at green products as a normal part of everyday life."

Mintel also reported that 328 products boasting an eco-friendly claim were launched in 2007. Compare that to only five of these product introductions in 2002 (Mintel, 2008a).

Mintel noted that while some of the food products labeled as eco-friendly were organic and natural, others focused on different environmental issues such as Green Energy Credits logos on packaging or support for health associations.

European consumers, too, are purchasing more products positioned as eco-friendly, including those that feature reduced packaging, are made with biodegradable packaging, and are labeled certified organic and/or fair trade. About 27% of European consumers bought these products in 2006, and in Europe, more than 60% of new product launches in 2007 were of these environmentally friendly products (Dodds, 2007).

USGBC also awarded LEED certification to Contessa for its "Green Cuisine Plant," the first LEED-certified frozen food facility in the world. The plant features a solar power system to generate electricity and a loading dock that prevents the loss of refrigerated air. But the biggest challenge the company faced was in trying to design an energy-efficient 4,000,000-cu-ft frozen food plant (almost entirely temperature-controlled). At that size, it is similar to running 200,000 refrigerators at the same time in the same place, said Blazevich, so it took plenty of creative thinking to design a plant that uses the least amount of energy possible. To accomplish this, the company installed a heat-redirection system that captures waste heat in the form of gas from refrigeration compressors and redirects the gas to a heat exchanger where it is condensed to a liquid that then heats water in a circulation system.

Plans are underway to maintain and improve the energy-efficient features of the plant. "We have an ongoing mission to fine tune the systems and features of our new Green Cuisine plant so that we can reduce water and energy consumption and even further reduce our greenhouse gas emissions," said Blazevich.

Although it cost the company an extra $6 million to improve the energy efficiency of the building, Blazevich said that it was the right thing to do for the sustainability of the planet.

"Two years ago, I converted my home to use geothermal energy, so I thought to myself, why not transfer this into the plant? I saw this as a great opportunity to address my business's output of greenhouse gases. If we don't do something about them, in 30 years we won't be living in the same place we have been."

Blazevich's efforts have not gone unrecognized. In addition to receiving the LEED certification, the company has fielded questions from and provided advice to companies seeking more information about energy-efficient building design. "From university engineers and major food manufacturers to major retailers, we have been approached to share our innovative patented technologies and processes," said Blazevich. "Food manufactures of all sizes will soon be expected to show that their back-end operations are as clean and responsible as the face they show the public."

Packing an Environmental Punch

Individuals trying to live a green lifestyle often urge companies to review the types of materials used to package products, develop ways to reduce packaging material, or adopt new material altogether. For example, after working closely with the Environmental Defense Fund (EDF) to address solid waste issues and develop ways to reduce and recycle, McDonald's discontinued the use of polystyrene foam "clamshell" boxes and switched to paper-based packaging for its sandwiches. EDF and McDonald's formed a task force in 1989, and EDF reported that in 1999, McDonald's eliminated 150,000 tons of packaging by redesigning or reducing the amount of material used to make a variety of items, including sandwich packaging, cups, napkins, and straws.

For the most part, processed food products need to be packaged in some type of package, be it paper, paperboard, plastic, or a combination of these. Even fresh produce, which is displayed unpackaged at the retail level, is transported from the point of origin to stores in crates, bags, and other containers. Packaging helps to keep food fresh, protect it from adulteration, and minimize damage and breakage due to shipping and handling. It also communicates important information about the product, how to prepare it, and what the nutrient content is.

Even though food manufacturers cannot eliminate packaging, they can redesign packages to reduce the amount of material used or to incorporate newly developed materials such as biodegradable plastic in their products' packaging. This is particularly important in the European Union where many countries are considering tougher legislation to encourage the use of less packaging material (Dodds, 2007). Reducing the weight of the package can also have a positive affect by reducing the amount of energy required to transport the products.

Other companies such as Nestlé and Tetra Pak support and encourage recycling efforts or use recyclable materials to produce their packages and products. In a number of countries around the world, Tetra Pak, Lausanne, Switzerland, has established plants to recycle its aseptic carton packages and campaigns to encourage recycling. Additionally, some packaging manufacturers are becoming more aware of depleting natural resources and opting to use materials from renewable sources.

According to Tetra Pak, about 75% of its raw material use in 2006 was for paperboard, which is used in the company's aseptic carton packaging material. To help ensure that the raw materials are sustainably sourced, the company collaborates with environmental organizations and nonprofit groups such as World Wildlife Fund, Forest Stewardship Council, ProForest, Global Forest and Trade Network, and High Conservation Value Resource Network. Forest Stewardship Council (FSC) certifies forests and forest management around the world according to 10 principles and 57 criteria that address such issues as indigenous rights, labor rights, and environmental impact (FSC, 1996). The importance of the latter is to help maintain the integrity of the entire forest ecosystem: trees and other plant life, water, and soil.

"We have a corporate policy that more trees are planted than harvested in the process of making our packaging, and we conduct independent audits of our paper manufacturers to ensure this," said Laurens Van de Vijver, Vice President, Marketing and Product Placement, Tetra Pak U.S. & Canada.

These efforts, along with an initiative that encourages recycling, have allowed the company to position its packages as tools that, as Van de Vijver explained, help food and beverage companies meet their own sustainability goals and meet their own energy- and cost-savings goals. Also, since the packaging is lighter than plastic, glass, or steel, is non-breakable, and can be stacked closely during transport and storage, less fuel is required to transport the packages. All of this is increasingly important because rising costs of energy are quickly cutting into companies' bottom line.

"Industries across sectors are feeling the economic strain of rising fossil fuel and gas prices," said Van de Vijver. "This means that the availability of plastic packaging—made from petroleum—is less stable than the availability of feedstocks such as paper, which can be renewed through responsible harvesting and reforestation programs. Given this, it is important to look at beverage packaging options that minimize fossil fuel inputs by using fewer materials made from nonrenewable resources."

Bigger May Not Be Better

Choosing raw materials that are sourced or produced in ways that minimally affect the environment is a step that companies can take to become green. Designing packages to use more environmentally friendly material or use less material overall is another step. Unilever has made changes to product packaging, including *Knorr* vegetable mix and *Knorr Recipe Secrets* soup pouch (eliminated outer carton), *Lipton* soup (reduced the width of the outer box), and *Bertolli* frozen meal pouches (reduced the height of the package). According to the company, the changes have helped Unilever reduce the amount of corrugated material and other packaging matter as well as the number of pallets and trucks used to transport the products.

Two of the world's beverage industry giants recently announced environmental initiatives that include design changes to bottles.

PepsiCo Inc., Purchase, N.Y., reduced the plastic content of its new 500-mL bottles for noncarbonated beverages by 20%. Introduced in May, the bottle is used for *Lipton Iced Tea, Tropicana* juice drinks, *Aquafina FlavorSplash,* and *Aquafina Alive* products. Additionally, the company reduced by 10% the label size and by 5% the shrink wrap film used to wrap multipacks.

It's Not Easy Being Green

Today's consumers are confronted with a barrage of advertising from companies touting their green products, celebrities exclaiming how they are reducing their carbon footprint, or officials telling us how we can reduce global warming by switching to compact fluorescent light bulbs. As more manufacturers promote their environmentally friendly products and sustainable business initiatives, some consumers are becoming confused and downright skeptical of what these companies are doing.

The Federal Trade Commission this year has held three public hearings and workshops in a series that will review its environmental marketing guidelines called the Green Guides. The guides, last updated in 1998, address eco-friendly marketing claims such as biodegradability, recyclability, and others and "help marketers avoid making environmental claims that are unfair or deceptive under Section 5 of the FTC Act, 15 U.S.C. 45" (CFR, 2007). The guides do not address new claims such as renewable energy certificates, carbon offsets, green packaging, green building claims, and sustainability. Since companies are using more and more ecofriendly marketing claims, especially these newer ones, on their products, FTC decided to move up the review process from 2009 to the beginning of this year.

"Consumers today have the option to purchase products and use them in ways that were unforeseen 15 years ago, when we first developed our guides, and consumer perceptions of old green claims may have evolved significantly over time," said Deborah Platt Majoras, FTC Chairman, at the hearing in January 2008. "Our robust review of these guides will allow us to explore emerging consumer protection issues and provide better direction to green marketers."

FTC will use the information gathered from these meetings to decide what modifications to the Green Guides are needed, particularly those that will benefit consumers and businesses, as well as deciding what steps should be taken to define the new green marketing claims.

"When such claims are used to sell products, consumer perception and substantiation issues may arise," reported FTC. "Also, in recent years, there has been an increase in the use of environmental seals and third-party certification programs purporting to verify the positive environmental impact of product packaging. Consumers may have varying interpretation of such seals and programs."

Taking on an effort like this is not as simple as one might think. According to Robert Lewis, Vice President of Worldwide Beverage Packaging and Equipment Development, PepsiCo, a team of employees from across the company took one year to complete the project, which included developing a bottle that was lighter and able to provide the same shelf life while withstanding the manufacturing and distribution process as well as the heavier bottle. The team submitted more than 30 bottle designs for consumer testing to determine the most aesthetically pleasing ones.

Coca-Cola Co., Atlanta, Ga., too, has redesigned some of its bottles for its carbonated and noncarbonated beverages. It introduced in 2007 a newly designed 20-oz polyethylene terephthalate (PET) contour bottle for its *Coca-Cola* brands. The bottle has 5% less PET than the previous bottle. The company also reduced the plastic used in its *Dasani* bottles by 30%.

Earlier this year, the company announced a long-term plan to recycle or reuse 100% of the aluminum beverage cans it sells in the U.S. This followed an announcement last year that the company plans to invest more than $60 million to build the world's largest plastic bottle-to-bottle recycling plant to help meet its goal of recycling or reusing 100% of the company's PET plastic bottles in the U.S. The plant will be located in Spartanburg, S.C. When it is fully operational in 2009, it is expected that the plant will produce about 100 million lb of food-grade recycled PET plastic for reuse each year. Coca-Cola has invested in other recycling facilities in Austria, Switzerland, Mexico, and the Philippines.

One Word: Bioplastics

Environmentalists heavily criticize the use of plastic grocery bags and, more recently, plastic water bottles, so much so that natural and organic foods retailer Whole Foods Market—in conjunction with this year's Earth Day celebration on April 22—eliminated the use of plastic grocery bags in its 270 stores in the U.S., Canada, and the UK. Over the years, environmentalists and scientists studying environmental issues have said that plastic bags and bottles, particularly those that are petroleum-based, take up space in landfills and pollute the landscape. But developments in biodegradable ingredients now make it possible for more manufacturers to produce plastic bags, bottles, and packages made from bioplastics.

NatureWorks LLC, Minnetonka, Minn., a joint venture between Cargill Inc., and Teijin Ltd., produces the *NatureWorks* PLA (polyactide) line of polymers that are derived from the starch of standard field corn. The polymers are said to biodegrade when packages that are made from them are composted. Moisture and heat in the compost pile break the PLA polymer chains to smaller chains, and then ultimately to lactic acid. Microorganisms in the compost consume the lactic acid for nourishment.

Other biodegradable corn starch-based ingredients, these from Plantic Technologies Ltd., Melbourne, Australia, are used in plastic trays for some Marks & Spencer and Cadbury confectionery products. Last year, the company and DuPont Packaging and Industrial Polymers, Wilmington, Del., announced that they will collaborate to develop and sell renewably sourced polymers based on Plantic's technology.

While some bioplastics are made from crops like corn, wheat, and sugar cane, there are others that are made from petrochemical sources.

Bioplastics are both blessed and cursed, though. While producing the polymers uses less fuel and generates fewer greenhouse gases than petroleum-based polymers, they are still farmed industrially, which means that fuel is needed to operate the farming equipment and chemicals are used to fertilize the crops. Most bioplastics will degrade under the right conditions in composts to produce benign lactic acid, but will degrade very little, if at all, in tightly packed landfills in the absence of oxygen. If they do break down slightly in the landfill, they produce methane, a greenhouse gas. One additional drawback is the fact that bioplastics cannot be recycled with traditional plastics because of contamination issues.

Sustaining the Green Movement

So what does the future hold for eco-friendly practices, sustainably produced products, and the like? If companies continue to see value in these, i.e., consumers continue to purchase products that are promoted as eco-friendly or sustainable, they will produce more of these products as well as invest in corporate sustainable/environmental practices. Americans and Europeans lead the world as purchasers of eco-friendly products. Entering new markets may extend the reach of these products as well as educate consumers and those who work for government agencies and food companies on developing government policies and company initiatives that address environmental issues. Or will consumers who are dealing with the high costs for fuel, food, and other products decide that paying a premium for eco-friendly products is not worth it and retreat from purchasing these products?

Any single solution offered by the companies mentioned in this article will not immediately solve the problems faced by our environment; try as they might, the companies can only do so much, and there are still challenges that they must overcome. Remember, it's not easy being green. But perhaps these are the changes that need to take place to compel more people and companies to save precious resources and protect our environment.

References

CFR. 2007. Guides for the use of environmental marketing claims. Code of Federal Regulations 16CFRPart260. Nov. 27. 72: 66091-66093.

Dodds, A. 2007. The Future of Ethical Food and Drinks: Growth Opportunities in Organic and Sustainable Products and Packaging. Business Insights Ltd., London, UK.

FACTA. 1990. Food, Agriculture, Conservation, and Trade Act of 1990. Public Law 101-624, Title XVI, Subtitle A, Section 1603. NAL Call #KF1692.A31 1990.

FSC. 1996. FSC International Standard FSC Principles and Criteria for Forest Stewardship. FSC-STD-01-001 (version 4-0) EN. Forest Stewardship Council, Bonn, Germany.

Miller. 2008. Live Sustainably: The 2008 Sustainable Development Report. Miller Brewing Co., Milwaukee, Wis.

Mintel. 2008a. Mintel finds more new products boasting environmentally friendly claims. Press Release, Mintel, London, UK, April 9.

Mintel. 2008b. Americans go three shades greener in 16 months. Press Release, Mintel, London, UK, March.

Critical Thinking

1. According to the 1990 Farm Bill, what is the definition of sustainable agriculture?

2. What is the goal of fair trade? What types of food are commonly offered as fair trade products?

3. Give examples of how companies such as Heinz, Miller Brewing, PepsiCo, and Decas Cranberry Products are using green technology to produce their products.

KAREN NACHAY, a Member of IFT, is Assistant Editor of *Food Technology* magazine (knachay@ift.org).

Test-Your-Knowledge Form

We encourage you to photocopy and use this page as a tool to assess how the articles in *Annual Editions* expand on the information in your textbook. By reflecting on the articles you will gain enhanced text information. You can also access this useful form on a product's book support website at www.mhhe.com/cls

NAME:

DATE:

TITLE AND NUMBER OF ARTICLE:

BRIEFLY STATE THE MAIN IDEA OF THIS ARTICLE:

LIST THREE IMPORTANT FACTS THAT THE AUTHOR USES TO SUPPORT THE MAIN IDEA:

WHAT INFORMATION OR IDEAS DISCUSSED IN THIS ARTICLE ARE ALSO DISCUSSED IN YOUR TEXTBOOK OR OTHER READINGS THAT YOU HAVE DONE? LIST THE TEXTBOOK CHAPTERS AND PAGE NUMBERS:

LIST ANY EXAMPLES OF BIAS OR FAULTY REASONING THAT YOU FOUND IN THE ARTICLE:

LIST ANY NEW TERMS/CONCEPTS THAT WERE DISCUSSED IN THE ARTICLE, AND WRITE A SHORT DEFINITION:

We Want Your Advice

ANNUAL EDITIONS revisions depend on two major opinion sources: one is our Advisory Board, listed in the front of this volume, which works with us in scanning the thousands of articles published in the public press each year; the other is you—the person actually using the book. Please help us and the users of the next edition by completing the prepaid article rating form on this page and returning it to us. Thank you for your help!

ANNUAL EDITIONS: Nutrition 11/12

ARTICLE RATING FORM

Here is an opportunity for you to have direct input into the next revision of this volume.
We would like you to rate each of the articles listed below, using the following scale:

1. **Excellent: should definitely be retained**
2. **Above average: should probably be retained**
3. **Below average: should probably be deleted**
4. **Poor: should definitely be deleted**

Your ratings will play a vital part in the next revision.
Please mail this prepaid form to us as soon as possible.
Thanks for your help!

RATING	ARTICLE	RATING	ARTICLE
	1. Can Low-Income Americans Afford a Healthy Diet?		21. Food for Thought: Exploring the Potential of Mindful Eating
	2. Healthy Food Looks Serious: How Children Interpret Packaged Food Products		22. The Best Diabetes Diet for Optimal Outcomes
	3. 10 Urban Food Legends: Things Aren't Always as Simple as They Seem		23. Underage, Overweight
	4. Eat Like a Greek		24. Engaging Families in the Fight against the Overweight Epidemic among Children
	5. Definition of the Mediterranean Diet Based on Bioactive Compounds		25. Birth Weight Strongly Linked to Obesity
	6. Have a Coke and a Tax: The Economic Case against Soda Taxes		26. The Fat Plateau
	7. Pepsi Brings in the Health Police		27. In Your Face: How the Food Industry Drives Us to Eat
	8. Calorie Posting in Chain Restaurants		28. Why We Overeat
	9. A Burger and Fries (Hold the Trans Fats)		29. Influencing Food Choices: Nutrition Labeling, Health Claims, and Front-of-the-Package Labeling
	10. The Potential of Farm-to-College Programs		30. The Benefits of Flax
	11. Color Me Healthy: Eating for a Rainbow of Benefits		31. Brain Food
	12. Keeping a Lid on Salt: Not So Easy		32. "Fountain of Youth" Fact and Fantasy
	13. Fiber Free-for-All		33. Miscommunicating Science
	14. Seafood Showdown: Fatty Acids vs. Heavy Metals		34. H_2 Uh–Oh: Do You Need to Filter Your Water?
	15. The Fairest Fats of Them All (and Those to Avoid)		35. Produce Safety: Back to Basics for Producers and Consumers
	16. Vitamins, Supplements: New Evidence Shows They Can't Compete with Mother Nature		36. Irradiation of Fresh Fruits and Vegetables
	17. Antioxidants: Fruitful Research and Recommendations		37. Is Your Food Contaminated?
	18. We Will Be What We Eat		38. Fixing the Global Nitrogen Problem
	19. Sugar Overload: Curbing America's Sweet Tooth		39. Perennial Grains: Food Security for the Future
	20. Fructose Sweeteners May Hike Blood Pressure		40. Draining Our Future: The Growing Shortage of Freshwater
			41. In Search of Sustainability

ABOUT YOU

Name   Date

_____

Are you a teacher? ☐ A student? ☐
Your school's name

_____

Department

_____

Address   City   State   Zip

_____

School telephone #

_____

YOUR COMMENTS ARE IMPORTANT TO US!

Please fill in the following information:
For which course did you use this book?

_____

Did you use a text with this ANNUAL EDITION? ☐ yes ☐ no
What was the title of the text?

_____

What are your general reactions to the Annual Editions concept?

_____

Have you read any pertinent articles recently that you think should be included in the next edition? Explain.

_____

Are there any articles that you feel should be replaced in the next edition? Why?

_____

Are there any World Wide Websites that you feel should be included in the next edition? Please annotate.

_____

May we contact you for editorial input? ☐ yes ☐ no
May we quote your comments? ☐ yes ☐ no